Occupational Therapy
Student to Clinician
Making the Transition

Occupational Therapy Student to Clinician
Making the Transition

LISA DAVIS, MA, OTR
Executive Director
Therapeutic Resources
Long Island City, New York

MARILYN ROSEE, MS, OTR
Executive Director
Therapeutic Resources
Long Island City, New York

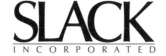

www.Healio.com/books

ISBN: 978-1-61711-025-2

Published by: SLACK Incorporated
                     6900 Grove Road
                     Thorofare, NJ 08086 USA
                     Telephone: 856-848-1000
                     Fax: 856-848-6091
                     www.Healio.com/books

Contact SLACK Incorporated for more information about other books in this field or about the availability of our books from distributors outside the United States.

Library of Congress Cataloging-in-Publication Data

Davis, Lisa, - , author.
  Occupational therapy student to clinician : making the transition / Lisa Davis, Marilyn Rosee.
     p. ; cm.
  Includes bibliographical references and index.
  ISBN 978-1-61711-025-2 (alk. paper)
  I. Rosee, Marilyn, 1954- , author. II. Title.
  [DNLM: 1. Occupational Therapy. 2. Career Mobility. 3. Clinical Competence. 4. Vocational Guidance. WB 555]
  RM735
  615.8'515--dc23
                          2014036635

Printed in the United States of America.

Last digit is print number: 10   9   8   7   6   5   4   3   2

DEDICATION

To my spouse, Sandra Siegal, for inspiring me to be expansive and for showing unending support, patience, and love. You gave me the idea for Therapeutic Resources (TR), encouraged its birth, and have been there cheering us on from day one. To my dad, Irwin, who loved me unconditionally and taught me that anything was possible, and my mom, Roz, who taught me to be optimistic, even on the worst of days. To the entire Rosee clan, a small but growing family who are always there with support and love. (MR)

To my husband, Bill, who wholeheartedly supports me in all of my endeavors. His kindness and love is ever present. To my wonderful childhood friend, Margie, who is always close by in spite of the miles between. (LD)

To my students, who unwittingly gave me the idea for this book, and my mom, who was an exceptional role model for me as a strong professional woman who introduced me to OT and encouraged me to pursue it as a career. To my stepdad, Ralph, who gave me love, laughter, and financial support as I made my way into adulthood. To my dad, who demonstrated the balance of work and play in my early years. (LD)

To the staff of TR and our affiliating therapists, whose dedication to us and the company inspires us to do our best every day. (MR & LD)

Last but not least, to each other. We have worked and laughed together, shared a desk, and been great friends for over 30 years—and we still look forward to each new day and the challenges that await us. We are hoping to continue our journey for many years to come.

CONTENTS

ACKNOWLEDGMENTS

This book represents much of the knowledge we have gleaned in our 30 years of owning a staffing agency that specializes in the placement of occupational therapists, occupational therapy assistants, physical therapists, physical therapy assistants, speech/language pathologists, and special educators. We have loved the opportunity to interact with and place our colleagues in positions in all practice areas and are proud of the great work they have done over the years representing Therapeutic Resources (TR).

We would like to thank all of the staff at TR. Their dedication to the organization is what has made our company stand out and survive for so many years. Our stellar reputation is all due to them. Special thanks to Mary Kelley, our chief operating officer, who keeps the train running and the owners focused; Alan Levenson, whose business expertise and patience transformed us from two occupational therapists with an idea into two entrepreneurial occupational therapists with a successful business; and Caldra Smart, who took the ball and ran with it many years ago to help create the core of TR.

We would also graciously like to thank the occupational therapy programs of Long Island University, Touro College, and LaGuardia Community College, who have given us the opportunity to teach, interact with, and learn from their occupational therapy students. It has been this student interaction that inspired us to write this book. We hope that past and future students find it helpful in making a successful transition from student to clinician.

A big thank you to Tzili Ressler, friend and colleague, who provided us with helpful edits and suggestions.

Lisa Davis, MA, OTR
Marilyn Rosee, MS, OTR

ABOUT THE AUTHORS

Marilyn Rosee and *Lisa Davis*, both occupational therapists, came together in 1985 with an idea. Working together as per diem therapists for a group of nursing homes, they found there were many requests for their services, but only so many hours in the day. Combining their entrepreneurial spirit and skills as occupational therapists, they decided to start their own agency, hiring therapists to work directly for them and placing them in the positions they could not accept themselves. They thought their chances for success were slim, but they decided to try anyway. They named their business Therapeutic Resources.

Before embarking on the new venture, Lisa, a graduate of New York University's graduate program in occupational therapy, was serving as Director of Occupational Therapy at Daughters of Jacob Geriatric Center in New York. Marilyn, a graduate of Columbia University's graduate program in occupational therapy, was a Senior Therapist at Beth Israel Medical Center in New York City. While attending New York University, pursuing a Master of Public Administration in Health Administration, Marilyn was inspired to pursue a nontraditional career path in occupational therapy. Searching for a viable business concept where her talents as an occupational therapist could be utilized, she jumped at the opportunity to work with Lisa to develop their idea to create a rehabilitation staffing agency

After joining together, Lisa and Marilyn continued their full-time consulting positions while spending evenings and weekends interviewing therapists, planning marketing campaigns, and performing bookkeeping tasks. Gradually, their business grew and they were able to afford to rent an office and hire an office manager to help with administrative responsibilities. As each year passed, their staff grew along with their business. Now, almost three decades later, they look at each other across their "partners" desk, enjoy their panoramic view of New York City, and marvel at what they have accomplished as they work together with their office staff to continue their mission. In addition to the hundreds of facilities and municipalities they serve and the respect they enjoy from the therapy community, they are especially proud of their continuing education division, which provides cutting-edge programs for occupational and physical therapists, speech and language pathologists and special educators.

Through it all, Marilyn and Lisa have proudly maintained their identities as "working" occupational therapists through their varied professional positions, including managing a multi-facility rehab department, directing rehabilitation and occupational therapy departments, as well as performing hands-on provision of therapy with pediatric populations. Additionally, they have taught in occupational therapy programs, serving as Adjunct Professors at New York University, Long Island University, Touro College, New York Institute of Technology, and LaGuardia Community College. They have lectured extensively over the years on topics relating to private practice, long-term care management, and most recently, to the skills needed to make a successful transition from student to clinician. They have served as Board Members at the New York State Occupational Therapy District of the New York State Occupational Therapy Association, as well as serving as Co-Chairs of the Geriatric Special Interest Group and the Continuing Education Committee. All of their experiences contributed to the development of this book.

After all these years, Marilyn and Lisa look back with pride at what they have accomplished together and the friendship they have forged.

FOREWORD

It is an imperative need and a great challenge to support the professional development of competent OTs. The complexity of demands in the workforce exceeds the requisite of clinical knowledge and reasoning. Regardless of sophisticated knowledge, use of technology, in-depth understanding of treatment protocols, or even clinical reasoning, our students can only become good clinicians if they understand and demonstrate appropriate professional behaviors.

Productive professional interactions and successful relationships are key elements for a purposeful, effective, and successful career path. Students' discovery that their behaviors, habits, and reactions, at any given moment, can actually impact their effectiveness as professionals and determine their ability to create and access career opportunities is not new in education. What may be new is that professional development and interactions need to become a key element for teaching and learning in OT education.

This book visits the transition from student to clinician, not from a competency-based perspective, but rather from a practical point of view that examines effective and skillful behaviors and habits as well as counterproductive or even distractive actions and communications.

As a more practical approach to professional development, it is easy to read and provides clear learning goals that could serve as benchmarks in the course of students' professional development. It reaffirms the notion that specific learning experiences and practical examples can support students' cultural transformation to a clinician.

The book presents complex concepts in depth and in an understandable manner. It is comprehensive and reflective of the reality in clinical practice. Students can use it to develop a sensor for detecting, in any given interaction, those elements that can hinder success. As such, the book could function as a student manual to create, access, and maintain successful career paths. I appreciated the book for its emphasis on the critical parameters of behaviors, habits, and communications that affect professional interactions. Being an educator for many years, I frequently encounter students' challenges toward their transformation to clinicians—a transformation that requires ample effort and resembles a cultural transition. I have come to believe that it is one of the most challenging learning tasks, as much as this skill set is folded in the nuances of interactions.

I could see this book following students throughout their professional curriculum, and possibly their career, to help them understand the dynamics of their own and others' behaviors and how these dynamics can influence the outcomes of their efforts.

I would like to congratulate the authors for their significant and thoughtful efforts to bring this book to us. It certainly is one of the tools that better our work with students and thus support the growth and prosperity of our profession.

Katherine Dimitropoulou, PhD, OTR/L
Assistant Professor of Regenerative and Rehabilitation Medicine
Columbia University
College of Physicians and Surgeons
Occupational Therapy Program
New York, New York

INTRODUCTION

As you complete your coursework in occupational therapy and begin level II fieldwork experience, your role changes from student to clinician. During this exciting time, you are leaving behind the safety and camaraderie of the classroom to apply your emerging professional skills in a real clinical setting where you will be interacting with fellow professionals.

Most advanced students enter this threshold confident about the foundation they have developed through their professional education. However, the road to a successful career involves more than just mastery of clinical occupational therapy skills. Although schools offering degrees in occupational therapy must focus on providing the prescribed curriculum, new therapists must also master non–occupational therapy skills relating to interpersonal relationships, professionalism, ethics, communication, and emotional intelligence in order to thrive in a collaborative clinical setting. Developing competency in these skills is as important as clinical skills in ensuring professional success.

As owners of an OT staffing agency and as academic educators, we realized the importance of these skills to ensure a smooth and successful transition from student to clinician. This reality inspired us to create a book that would introduce concepts and strategies designed to help students succeed in their fieldwork experience while also addressing the challenges new graduates face in landing their first paid position. *Occupational Therapy Student to Clinician: Making the Transition* is the result of our inspiration. (Note: We have used the terms *occupational therapist, certified occupational therapy assistant*, and *occupational therapy student* throughout the book. At times we have used *occupational therapist* as a general term, meant to include any or all of our colleagues in the spectrum of occupational therapy professionals.)

The book is divided into three sections. In *Section I: Ensuring Success in Your First Job and Beyond*, we cover work-related skills and behaviors that must be honed to succeed in any workplace setting. These skills include learning how to assess and fit into the culture of a new work environment; communicating effectively in a professional setting; dealing with conflict; and understanding team roles and rules, the impact of professional behaviors on reputation, and, importantly, the concepts of social and emotional intelligence and how one's likability will affect career success.

In *Section II: Getting Ready for Your Job Search*, newly graduated clinicians will be presented with strategies to help them organize and implement their job search, conduct themselves on a job interview, negotiate their salary, and understand their benefit package. Another important component that is often not considered by the new graduate is the importance of assessing the culture of a workplace to determine whether a position is the right fit. Armed with these strategies, new graduates will possess a definite advantage over less-prepared job seekers.

In *Section III: Achieving Professional Transitions*, we address issues of continuing competency and the realities of career development. This chapter was designed to help guide decisions that take clinicians beyond their early experiences to ensure a satisfying and long-lasting career in occupational therapy.

Fieldwork educators will find the text helpful as a preparatory introduction and guide to ensure fieldwork placement success for their students. As fieldwork assignments become increasingly difficult to secure, it is crucial to demonstrate that students can be a valuable asset to a placement setting. By addressing important workplace skills, such as teamwork, communication, attitude, initiative, and problem solving, academic programs demonstrate to the clinical community that they understand how important these professional skills are, and are assuming responsibility for ensuring their students possess these skills before they enter the clinic. Realistic examples of workplace situations and role-playing activities help students understand, develop, and refine the work-related skills they need to master.

The book also addresses the needs of academic programs by presenting a variety of Accreditation Council for Occupational Therapy Education standards, along with providing practical strategies for students to reach curriculum objectives.

Although geared toward students and newly graduated occupational therapists and certified occupational therapy assistants, *Occupational Therapy Student to Clinician: Making the Transition* will also serve as an important reference throughout their professional work life, ensuring a satisfying and successful career in occupational therapy.

Note: While the authors would have preferred to use gender-neutral language in the text, as required, they followed current APA guidelines for pronoun use. The authors are hoping that the APA updates their guidelines in the near future to ensure sensitivity toward changing attitudes about gender in our culture.

SECTION I

ENSURING SUCCESS IN YOUR FIRST JOB AND BEYOND

Chapter 1

Organizational Socialization
Learning the Ropes in Your Fieldwork Experience and First Job

LEARNING OBJECTIVES

At the end of this chapter, the reader will be able to:

➤ Define the concept of organizational socialization.

➤ Identify the four behaviors, traits, and skills that indicate the new employee is successfully integrating into the work group.

➤ Name three employee behaviors that foster successful organizational socialization.

➤ Name and define the four stages of organizational socialization.

➤ Describe 10 ways the new employee can make a good first impression.

Entering a new workplace, whether as a fieldwork student or a new graduate, can be a challenging and intimidating time in your professional life. You arrive to a foreign environment as the newcomer and must prove yourself to the rest of the staff and figure out how to fit into the organization. Like a family, every organization has its own unique personality and idiosyncrasies. This is often referred to as the *culture* of an organization. The culture is composed of formal and informal values, ethics, patterns of behavior, rituals, ceremonies, symbols, slogans, and stories. (This will be addressed in detail in Chapter 14.) As a newcomer, it is your job to understand how the organization works and how to work within it. To do that, you must identify the personal and professional adjustments you need to make to get along with your colleagues and supervisors and to fit into the patient-/client-/child-centered model favored by that specific workplace. The process of understanding the culture of this new environment is often referred to as *learning the ropes*, and understanding how to fit into it is sometimes referred to as *organizational socialization*.

This chapter will discuss the importance of organizational socialization, what it involves, and how to facilitate the process to ensure longevity and satisfaction in your first professional position.

Davis L, Rosee M. *Occupational Therapy Student to Clinician:*
Making the Transition (pp 3-14).
© 2015 SLACK Incorporated.

WHAT IS ORGANIZATIONAL SOCIALIZATION?

Entry into a clinical fieldwork experience is just like starting a new job. You are approaching an unfamiliar environment with unknown rules and practices alongside colleagues who have already developed well-established social and professional relationships. No matter what your experience level is, this entry is generally intimidating and stressful. The situation is almost akin to entering a foreign country when you cannot speak the language and do not know the customs. It is helpful to be aware of the difficulties in assuming this newcomer role and to prepare for it by understanding that this is a phenomenon that has a name and is universally recognized in all workplaces.

"Organizational socialization is the process through which a new organizational employee (or fieldwork student) adapts from (being an) outsider to (becoming an) integrated and effective insider" (Cooper-Thomas & Anderson, 2006, p. 492). This is accomplished as the newcomer acquires the knowledge, skills, and behaviors to become an organizational member and insider (Bauer & Erdogan, 2011). The process of acclimating to a new work environment is commonly referred to as *learning the ropes.* The methods to accomplish this transition involve a variety of informal and formal methods initiated by the facility engaging the newcomer as well as through the efforts of the newcomer him- or herself. Employer methods may include orientation sessions, lectures, videos, and printed materials. The newcomer must take the initiative to uncover information about the organization through methods such as observation, listening, and questioning. Successful organizational socialization is a strong predictor of future job satisfaction, commitment, and longevity.

As professionals new to the organization become socialized, their attitudes and beliefs evolve, transforming them from an outsider to an integrated member of the team who is committed to the organization and its goals.

WHAT IS LEARNED DURING THE SOCIALIZATION PROCESS?

Whether you enter a workplace as a seasoned therapist, new graduate, or fieldwork student, every new work environment has different rules and procedures that require an adjustment period in which the newcomer adapts to the organization's unique social norms and expectations. Of course, new graduates have an added burden because their professional experience has been limited to the student role and their clinical skills are still at the novice level. The new graduate must learn the social structure and rules while simultaneously adjusting to the demands to provide patient care at a much higher level of expectation than what he or she experienced as a fieldwork student.

What is learned during the socialization process is sometimes referred to as *socialization content* (Chao, O'Leary-Kelly, Wolf, Klein, & Gardner, 1994). This content is imparted to the newly engaged therapist through a variety of formal and informal processes. These content categories include organizational values, goals, and culture; work group values, norms, and friendships; and skills and knowledge needed to do the job.

During the socialization process, certain traits, skills, and behaviors will evolve and mature, indicating that the process is moving along in a positive direction and the newcomer is successfully integrating him- or herself into the new work environment. These indicators include the following:

- *Task mastery.* The newcomer is exhibiting that he or she is learning key requirements of the job, gaining self-confidence, and attaining a favorable level of job performance. For the new therapist, this might include managing to treat a caseload and perform evaluations within the prescribed time limits, to complete documentation during the work day, or to comfortably communicate within the team setting. For the fieldwork student, this might involve similar types of skill mastery but with lowered expectations and pressure.

◆ *Functioning within the work group.* The newcomer begins to demonstrate an understanding of the way things are done in the workplace by following the lead of team members and coworkers. Indicators of success include adjusting to how the work group performs job responsibilities, gaining the trust of coworkers and superiors, and developing social contacts within the group. Examples might include keeping the therapy area clean by putting things away after every use (if that is the way things are done), keeping one's personal workspace clean and neat, or waiting for the staff at the end of the day to all leave together. Of course, every work group functions differently. This is where observation and questioning can help newcomers identify how the group functions so that they can follow suit.

◆ *Knowledge and acceptance of the organization's culture.* An important step in achieving organizational socialization is to know and understand the organization's culture. With this knowledge comes acceptance and internalization of the culture, resulting in a new identity as an insider. This is accomplished when the newcomer begins to feel a real commitment to the organization. Rather than following the behaviors and actions modeled by seasoned colleagues, the actions are becoming part of the newcomer's repertoire of behaviors and actions in an integrated way. An example of this might include this common scenario: Margaret's fieldwork setting is short-staffed in the morning, and nursing has a difficult time getting her early patients down to the occupational therapy clinic according to their schedule. The result is that she is getting backed up with patients on a daily basis and ends up shortchanging the patients who arrive closest to lunch time. She has tried to resolve the situation to no avail. At first, she does not understand why this problem cannot be solved more easily because it seems like a basic requirement for nursing to get the patients ready for therapy on time. However, with experience in the setting, she decides that rather than complaining about the situation one more time, she will find a way to work within the realities of the facility's staffing dynamics. The next day, Margaret checks in with her supervisor to see whether it would be possible to treat some of her earlier patients on the nursing floor rather than bringing them down to the clinic. She wisely communicates to the nursing staff that she understands they are short-staffed and perhaps this solution would be helpful to both departments. The nursing staff appreciates Margaret's sensitivity toward their difficulties and her supervisor appreciates the initiative she exhibited in identifying a solution that gets patients treated and avoids creating delays or shortchanging sessions for the patients who come later. Margaret looks like a real team player and gets credit for coming up with a solution, solidifying her reputation with the rehabilitation and nursing departments.

◆ *Personal learning.* This is the process whereby newcomer therapists learn about their own motivations, insecurities, anxieties, and strengths in relation to the new work environment. Entry-level occupational therapists can often feel stressed about professional competencies and may fear inadequacy in providing the same level of intervention as more experienced colleagues. Through self-reflection, the novice occupational therapist can adapt and identify proactive strategies that enhance adjustment and integration into the new environment (Anakwe & Greenhaus, 1999).

THE ROLE OF THE EMPLOYER IN THE ORGANIZATIONAL SOCIALIZATION PROCESS

Although the therapist entering a new work environment must take the initiative to successfully integrate into the new workplace, the employer also has a significant obligation to facilitate the socialization process. Neglecting to adequately socialize new employees has been shown to have negative long-term effects on the employment of new hires. Lack of an institutionalized socialization program often results in high levels of unmet employee expectations, which can lead to poor attitudes, negative behaviors, and higher turnover. Because there is a significant cost to the employer to recruit and train new employees, a progressive employer will develop a well-thought-out orientation program designed to make the new hire feel comfortable and prepare him or her to understand the job's expectations, duties, and responsibilities. This initial investment will pay for itself in improved attitude, productivity, and longevity (Cooper-Thomas & Anderson, 2006).

There are many different models employers can use to socialize new hires. The two basic models (as defined by Jones, 1986) include *institutionalized socialization* and *individualized socialization*.

The institutionalized socialization process utilizes a structured step-by-step orientation program, usually performed in a group format with assigned role models or mentors and a specific teaching protocol. Examples of this approach might include the way universities orient incoming college students or the way the military trains and prepares new recruits prior to deployment. As occupational therapists, we may encounter this type of orientation in a very large setting, such as a major medical center or school system, when several newly hired therapists (or fieldwork students) are all starting at the same time. For example, an occupational therapist who accepts a position with a public education department might be scheduled for a group orientation that includes an introduction to benefits, instruction on software and computer systems, and documentation requirements. The new hires are assigned to mentors and given the opportunity to network and bond with their fellow new hires. This structured process helps the new hires understand the working environment while providing support for the transition. This approach will usually result in a positive first impression, which can impact attitude and longevity.

The other approach, which is typically seen in smaller health care and educational settings, is called an *individualized socialization process*. Here, a new employee is placed in the working environment almost immediately, with little or no formal orientation. The newcomer must process and figure out (mostly on his or her own) the norms, values, and expectations of the environment. Within this individualized structure, the new hire is responsible for playing a proactive role in understanding and adapting to the work environment and its culture. He or she must forge bonds and be motivated to seek information and identify how to fit in. Because the fieldwork student is assigned a dedicated supervisor who is responsible for orientation, he or she will ideally experience more support and help in making the adjustment to the organization's way of doing things.

THE ROLE OF THE NEWCOMER IN THE SOCIALIZATION PROCESS

Making the adjustment to a new workplace is influenced by several individual and organizational factors. Researchers have separated these factors into new employee characteristics and new employee behaviors. (Note: For the purposes of this chapter, when the word *employee* is used, it implies a newcomer to an organization, whether a fieldwork student, new graduate, or experienced therapist.)

New Employee Characteristics

Research has shown evidence that workplace newcomers with certain personality traits and prior work experience adjust to organizations more quickly (Saks & Ashforth, 1996, p. 303). Proactive personality refers to a "dispositional tendency for some individuals to behave more confidently, work to control their environment, and seek out information" (Kammeyer-Mueller & Wanberg, 2003, p. 783). These traits can accelerate the socialization process and help the newcomer adapt more efficiently to a new environment.

In addition, other personality traits—including openness, conscientiousness, extraversion, and agreeableness—have been linked to an easier transition to a new work environment. Extroverted newcomers are more likely to seek information, feedback, acceptance, and relationships with coworkers and often tend to be more positive (Kammeyer-Mueller & Wanberg, 2003). Curiosity or the desire to acquire knowledge can also play a role in newcomer adaptation. The curious newcomer will explore an organization's culture and norms and tend to frame challenges in a positive light.

The newcomer's prior work experience will also impact the ease with which he or she adjusts to a new work environment. A newly graduated occupational therapist starting a first job may experience a more difficult adjustment to a new environment than a seasoned therapist who is changing positions. The seasoned therapist has the advantage of prior experiences to draw from, may be more comfortable with the socialization process, and probably has mastered a better understanding of what is expected in a professional work environment.

New Employee Behaviors

The organizational socialization process can be facilitated when newcomers exhibit behaviors that foster the development of relationships, seek information about the new workplace, and seek feedback from peers (Gruman, Saks, & Zweig, 2006).

Newcomers who seek information from coworkers and supervisors will quickly learn about a company's expectations, procedures, and policies. Miller and Jablin (1991) outlined a model of information seeking for new hires that includes concepts such as understanding what is required to function on the job, understanding how to function in relation to job role requirements, and understanding the quality of relationships between current organizational employees. By seeking information, the newcomer can reduce uncertainty about a position, act appropriately based on what is expected, and generally make a smooth transition into a new environment. For example, a newly graduated therapist comes on board 2 days before the Christmas holiday. During that time, there is partying in the department and considerable downtime. The therapist may seek out a more experienced colleague or supervisor to determine whether it is appropriate to participate in the festivities. Without seeking advice and information, the therapist chooses a course of action without the necessary information, potentially behaving in a manner that would be considered inappropriate in that setting. For example, by choosing to participate in the festivities so soon after the start date, an individual could be branded as entitled and arrogant. Lack of participation, however, may brand someone as unfriendly and unsociable. Each interpretation will be based on the culture of the workplace.

Seeking feedback is an important behavior for the new employee. Newcomers might ask peers or supervisors whether a certain performance or behavior is appropriate in the social and political context of the organization. They can then adjust their behavior based upon the feedback received. For example, a fieldwork student treating patients all afternoon opts to put away all used equipment at the end of the day. Later, the student asks peers whether that is an acceptable approach or if it would be more appropriate to put things away between each patient. By seeking feedback, the therapist avoids criticism from peers and demonstrates respect toward the way things are done in that environment.

Networking and relationship building with peers and supervisors can be very important in making the transition to a new work environment. Friendliness and participation in social events on the job can be important building blocks to develop friendships and alliances. When people like newcomers, they tend to protect them, provide them with helpful information, and give them the benefit of the doubt. The importance of being liked cannot be underestimated. For example, Sophie and Ben—two newly graduated certified occupational therapy assistants—start work on the same day. Sophie is very friendly and sociable. She manages to connect with her colleagues fairly quickly and makes a good first impression on her supervisor. During downtime, she is chatting with her peers about their personal lives and sharing about herself. Ben is more shy and studious. During downtime, he is studying up on his patients' conditions and developing treatment plans. Sophie does a good job with her patients in the time allotted but finishes treating all of her patients

20 minutes before the lunch break and spends the extra time chatting with her peers. Ben keeps his patients much longer, finishing up right before the clinic closes for lunch. He does not try to connect to his supervisor and has not had the time to make connections with his peers. After 2 weeks, the new therapists are provided with initial feedback from their supervisor. Ben, the studious hard worker, is criticized for having poor time management skills due to his habit of working right up to the last second with his patients. Sophie gets glowing reviews, even though she is less conscientious. Why? Because everyone likes Sophie better. When you are liked, you are given the benefit of the doubt. Behaviors and work habits that in one light could be considered less professional may be reframed in a more positive light. On the other hand, work habits and behaviors that are generally considered more professional and beneficial for the patient could be perceived as being inefficient. It all depends on how you are viewed. Making yourself liked by your peers and supervisors is an important step in career success. It may not seem fair, but do not underestimate it!

STAGES OF ORGANIZATIONAL SOCIALIZATION

In a famous treatise on organizational socialization, it was proposed that there are four stages through which people assimilate into an organization: organizational anticipatory socialization, organizational encounter, metamorphosis, and disengagement (or exit) (Chaidaroon, 2003). It is helpful to understand these steps to prepare yourself for the realities of a new job or work environment, understand the steps you need to take to succeed, and allay anxieties as you initiate your new job by knowing that "start up" discomfort is universal to all new employees. An explanation of the stages of organizational socialization are as follows:

- *Organizational anticipatory socialization*, the first stage of the newcomer's experience, often occurs during the interview process. At this stage, prospective employees or fieldwork students get their first look at the organizational culture. By doing advance research, the interviewee can uncover information about the workplace's culture and values. Once the position is accepted, the therapist should start exploring the job requirements and considering what it will be like to work for the organization. Information about the facility can be gleaned through many sources, including observations made during the interview process, questions asked of the interviewer and staff (as well as discussions with former employees), outside research about the facility, and review of facility materials.

- *Organizational encounter* occurs when the newly hired therapist or fieldwork student enters the workplace. At this point, he or she is branded as the newcomer and begins the process of becoming acquainted with the organization and his or her role in it. The new therapist has a double challenge in that he or she has to learn about job expectations and how to perform them, as well as having to learn about the organizational culture and how to interact successfully within it. The newcomer has not yet been accepted as a trustworthy or dependable member of the team from the perspective of his or her coworkers. At this time, he or she must obtain information that will help the assimilation process. The information can be culled in a variety of ways, including the following:

  ◊ Observation of coworkers' actions as a model for acceptable behavior within that environment. For example, does the staff eat breakfast at their desks, do they document at the end of the day or during their lunch, or do they stay late to catch up on work?

  ◊ Overt questioning of coworkers and supervisors to uncover the way things are done in that environment. For example, asking the staff what is the appropriate etiquette for personal phone calls, small talk during treatment time, and dismissal procedures (does staff leave promptly at the expected dismissal time or do they stay late to complete their work).

  ◊ Indirect information seeking that employs subtle questioning, hints, and disguises to yield insider information. This may provide answers to questions that you may not be comfortable asking coworkers. People outside of the department (or former employees) can often provide useful information that could fill in the blanks about what is going on inside. For example, is your manager easygoing or a stickler for the rules? You might not want to ask those questions of your coworkers, but a former employee might be happy to provide the information you seek.

The newcomer must be careful during this critical time. The initial stage serves as a proving ground where missteps will be difficult to reverse. For example, Rachel, a newly hired occupational therapist, calls in sick on her second and third day of employment due to food poisoning and is late on the fourth day due to subway delays—all unavoidable occurrences. However, the staff, not knowing her work habits, perceives her to be unreliable. This label sticks with her for a long time.

A Bad Start

Ava was hired as a managing occupational therapist at a long-term care facility. She has expertise in positioning and wheelchair adaptations and was excited about the opportunity to put these skills to work. On her first day, she noticed how poorly the patients were positioned in their chairs. In an attempt to impress her new employer, she got right to work changing wheelchairs and adding adaptive devices and seat cushions. She was very proud of the improvement in the patients' comfort and positioning. A few days later, Ava was called into the administrator's office with the director of nursing present and was admonished for her positioning efforts. While Ava believed that she was showing off her skills and improving quality for the patients, the rest of the staff thought she was disruptive and disrespectful of the staff. Because she did not know procedures yet, she failed to communicate or coordinate with the nursing department about what she was doing and had inadvertently stepped on toes. Although she meant well, Ava got off to a bad start and spent months trying to undo the damage she had done in terms of her relationships with other departments.

During this initial phase, the newcomer must build his or her credibility. This is the time when he or she should go to work, if at all possible (and save calling in sick due to minor illness and family emergencies for when he or she has proven him- or herself in the workplace). Getting to work early, eating breakfast before arriving (even if everyone else is eating at their desks), and taking care of one's appearance to make sure clothes are neat and clean is essential. Coworkers observe little indiscretions, especially when someone is new. As stated earlier, the impression a newcomer leaves in those early days will stay with him or her for a long time. Building up credits early on (through exemplary professional behavior, helpfulness, etc.) will place the newcomer in a positive light and provide him or her with some bargaining chips should they be needed. For example, Phil, a new employee, volunteered to attend a health fair on a Saturday. The staff (who did not want to work on a weekend) appreciated his efforts and gave him the benefit of the doubt when he arrived a little late for work and came back late from lunch.

- *Metamorphosis* is the next stage in the assimilation process. As the newcomer becomes familiar with the organization's culture, he or she begins to make the necessary adjustments and transitions to change from new member to insider. The individual now understands what is expected, has developed some mastery of the job requirements, and has integrated the rules and standards of the workplace into his or her behaviors, which leads to acceptance as a colleague.

- *Disengagement* (or *exit*) is the last step in the organizational socialization continuum. This is when the therapist leaves a job, transfers into another part of the organization, or completes the fieldwork experience. At this point, the assimilation process begins again.

An Occupational Therapist New Grad's Experience Through the Stages of Organizational Socialization

Organizational Anticipatory Socialization

When I was a new graduate, I was quite excited at the prospect of working in my first job as an occupational therapist. I knew I wanted to work in a hospital, and after an extensive search, I landed an interview in a large New York medical center. It was definitely a dream job. On my first interview, I met with the director of occupational therapy, as well as the staff of five therapists. I observed everyone as they treated patients in the clinic and had the chance to chat with the staff and ask questions about the facility. A day or two after the interview, I received a call from the director asking me to come back for a second interview so that she and the staff could decide between me and another more experienced candidate. I was so motivated to get the job that I came back with the goal to sell myself to the staff. A few days later, I landed the job.

In preparation for starting the job, I learned all I could about the facility and the population I would be working with. I would have my work cut out for me to become accepted by the group because they had been working together for a while and seemed very close with one another. There was nothing left to do but try my best to fit in.

Organizational Encounter

The first day at my new job was one of the most uncomfortable days of my life. Although I was an excellent student and had received high marks in all of my affiliations, now it was for real. I was being paid to be an occupational therapist. There was going to be much more expected of me in my performance of evaluations, treating patients, and providing documentation for a large caseload (in a fast-paced acute care environment) than what I was expected to do as a student. There would be no supervisor checking in with me, holding my hand, and advising me.

Upon my arrival that first day, I was sent down to human resources for a half day of orientation. I arrived back in the clinic around noon, where a caseload had already been assigned to me. I did not know the forms, the equipment, or the layout. I was not comfortable asking the staff to help me as they were busy treating their own caseloads. The patients started coming down and I had to move quickly because as soon as one patient was evaluated, another arrived. By the end of the day, I was so stressed and miserable that I did not want to go back the next day.

But, of course, I did go back. The next day was a little less stressful. I arrived early so that I could prepare for my day by exploring the department and gaining an understanding of the equipment and supplies. I was also more emotionally prepared for what lay ahead. During that second day, I was able to keep up with my caseload schedule and felt more comfortable asking questions while trying my hardest to be helpful and friendly in my attempt to break into the group. Actually, all of the therapists, although more seasoned than me, were young and had only been working a year or two. Although they felt light years ahead of me, they actually were not.

Metamorphosis

Within a few weeks, I was feeling much more comfortable at work. I began to understand what was expected of me—how many patients I needed to see, the structure of meetings I needed to attend and participate in, and how to document according to the hospital's requirements to assure reimbursement. I also started to bond with the staff. I was soon

(continued)

An Occupational Therapist New Grad's Experience Through the Stages of Organizational Socialization (continued)

included in lunchtime activities. It was not an easy start, but my workplace soon became my second home and my colleagues become my second family.

Disengagement (or Exit)

I was so comfortable at my job for so long that it felt like I would never leave. Over the years, some of my colleagues had left for other opportunities or moved away. They were replaced by new hires. Suddenly, at the 5-year mark, I decided that it was my time to explore new opportunities. Although it was not easy leaving the comfort of my "home," it was time to start a new adventure. The impetus to finally give notice occurred following a strike by our union. During the month-long strike, I found work as a per diem contractor in a nursing home. The hourly rate was more than I ever imagined earning, and I started to enjoy the freedom and flexibility that being an independent provider afforded me. The day the strike ended, I handed in my letter of resignation and began a new phase in my life. I will always look back on those days with great appreciation for the opportunity I was given to work in such a dynamic and exciting environment.

TIPS FOR THE NEWCOMER TO AN ORGANIZATION

Making a good first impression can involve some very simple and obvious steps. Keep the following in mind when starting at a new workplace:

- *Do not try too hard to show how smart you are.* Often, we start a new job thinking we want to make a good impression by demonstrating how much we know. Although the new employee may know a lot and have useful ideas and suggestions, it is important to sit back and listen. Do not turn off your coworkers by being too aggressive in offering opinions and suggestions. If you are asked for your opinion, feel free to offer it. Otherwise, lay low until you get to know people better.

- *Remember names.* People love the sound of their own name! Remembering names is an important step to making a good impression. Instead of just calling someone to ask a question, say his or her name first. For example, you could say, "Hi, Mohammed. When will Mrs. Rubovitch be ready for occupational therapy?" It sounds so simple, but it can be very effective in developing bonds.

- *Learn who's who and what's where.* Find out who reports to whom and become familiar with the players in the new organization. This will help you determine who to seek out for help, as well as guide you to avoid stepping on toes and making enemies unnecessarily. It is important to ingratiate yourself with supervisors, managers, and directors. They make the hiring and firing decisions. You want them to think well of you.

- *Keep your eyes open.* Watch what is going on. Learn as much as you can through observation.

- *Follow proper organizational channels.* The best way to make an enemy is to go above someone's head to report information or to get an approval. Always go to your immediate supervisor or manager to ask questions. Never go above someone's head, even if you think it will gain you brownie points. Getting the credit is less important (especially initially) than maintaining a good relationship with your superiors.

- *Make friends with aides and administrative staff.* Usually these people have worked in the department for a long time. They know everything about the facility's history, and they can be extraordinarily helpful in orienting you to the department, administration, and facility in general. In addition, when they are your friends, they will watch your back and help you through difficult situations. For example, Sue was on her psychiatric clinical fieldwork experience in a locked unit. One day, she was running a group by herself when one of the members became abusive and violent. Sue became alarmed and was not sure what to do, when suddenly, a male aide swooped in and intervened. Because Sue had made friends with all of the aides upon her arrival, they kept their eyes open to protect her. By working with the aide (and benefitting from his knowledge and experience), Sue was able to diffuse the situation.

♦ *Be friendly and likable.* While this sounds like a simplistic recommendation, it is often difficult to execute. Try some simple steps—say hello to people you know, introduce yourself to people you do not know, smile at people, be positive, and avoid complaining and making negative comments. Just because you think something does not mean you need to say it.

♦ *Arrive early and leave late.* Even though your schedule is from 8 a.m. to 4 p.m., come to work early to prepare for the day and stay a little later—at least initially. It will show that you are not a clock watcher, you take your responsibilities seriously, and are taking all steps to be prepared and complete your work on a timely basis.

♦ *Be helpful.* If you notice someone struggling with something and you are in a position to help, do so. For example, if someone is transferring a patient and you are standing nearby, go over and try to help by stabilizing the chair. If a patient is wheeling into therapy and is struggling, offer to help. This indicates that you are paying attention to your environment and are a team player.

♦ *Volunteer for a project.* If the department is working on something, volunteer to participate. For example, if the department is producing a continuing education event, ask if you can help. It is a good way to show your commitment and make connections.

♦ *Make "to do" lists.* Use lists to make sure you keep up with what is expected of you. At the beginning, when you are trying to prove yourself to the staff, you do not want to forget important promises, obligations, and responsibilities. The best way to ensure that you meet all obligations is to keep a list.

♦ *Do not get discouraged.* Some workplaces are friendlier than others. You may feel like an outsider for longer than you would like. Do not give up. Groups that have been together a long time can be difficult to penetrate, but follow the previous suggestions and eventually you will become one of them (Besette, 2010).

SUMMARY

Fieldwork students and new graduates starting their first jobs are faced with an initial challenge of making the adjustment from student to clinician. This challenge is one that even experienced therapists face when they make changes in their employment status. Starting a new job is almost always a stressful experience. Being unfamiliar with the culture, customs, players, and rules at your new job is uncomfortable, and the tasks required initially to transition into this new environment are challenging. The skills engaged by new hires to make the transition can have important ramifications for future success on that job. In this chapter, we outlined the concept of organizational socialization, what is learned during this process, and what needs to be accomplished. Although we cannot control how our employers handle this important period in our employment, there is a lot we can do to ensure a smooth transition to a new workplace environment. By understanding the process and the universal components that we all experience when starting something new, we can proactively manage our behaviors to pave the way for a positive work experience.

DISCUSSION QUESTIONS/ACTIVITIES

1. Reflect on your fieldwork experiences. Who showed you what to do? How did you learn your role? Describe the specific tactics used to help you get acclimated. Of these tactics, which were the most helpful?
   ◊ If you have had experience running an organization or supervising, what kinds of things did you do to ensure a smooth start for new employees?
   ◊ Share your answers with classmates.
2. Did you notice some students with similar or different responses to the previous questions? Why do you think there are similarities or differences? Do the students who have different answers also have different personalities? Some research indicates that personality traits impact one's ability to fit in. Describe your personality and what aspects might make it easier or harder to adjust as a new employee.
3. Make a list of things you can do as a student to ensure that you will have an easy adjustment to your new work environment.
4. Break into groups of four. Using the example of Ava, the therapist who repositioned patients on her first day and was perceived as disruptive and disrespectful, consider the following:
   a. Describe how she should have responded after being reprimanded.
   b. Identify the steps she should have taken prior to changing the wheelchairs.
   c. What are the best steps to be taken in the first few days of a fieldwork or work experience to ensure your integration into the team?
   Come together as a class; each group should share their responses.

REFERENCES

Anakwe, U.P., & Greenhaus, J.H. (1999). Effective socialization of employees: Socialization content perspective. *Journal of Managerial Issues, 11*(3), 315-329.

Bauer, T. (2004). Organizational socialization. *Encyclopedia of Applied Psychology.* (Vol. 2).

Bauer, T.N. & Erdogan, B. (2011). Organizational socialization: The effective onboarding of new employees. In Sl Zedeck (Ed.), *APA handbook of industrial and organizational psychology, Vol.3: Maintainning expanding and contracting the organization,* APA Handbooks in Psychology, (pp 51-64). Washington, DC, US: American Psychological Association.

Besette, B. (2010, January 10). *5 tips for the brand new employee.* Retrieved from http://workawesome.com/your-job/5-tips-for-the-brand-new-employee/.

Chaidaroon, S.C. (2003). How managers give effective instructions to new employees: Some sample scenarios for teaching supervisory communication. Proceedings of the 2003 Association for Business Communication Annual Convention. Blacksburg, VA: Association for Business Communication.

Chao, G.T., O'Leary-Kelly, A.M., Wolf, S., Klein, H.J., & Gardner, P.D. (1994). Organizational socialization: Its content and consequences. *Journal of Applied Psychology, 79*(5), 730-743.

Cooper-Thomas, H., & Anderson, N. (2006). Organizational socialization: A new theoretical model and recommendations for future research and HRM practices in organizations. *Journal of Managerial Psychology, 21*(5), 392-515.

Gruman, J.A., Saks, A.M., & Zweig, D.I. (2006). Organizational socialization tactics and newcomer proactive behaviors; An integrative study. *Journa. of Vocational Behavior, 69,* 90-104.

Jones, G. (1986). Socialization tactics, self efficacy and newcomers adjustments to organizations. *The Academy of Management Journal, 29*(2), 262-279.

Kammeyer-Mueller, J.D., & Wanberg, C.R. (2003). Unwrapping the organizational entry process: Disentangling multiple antecedents and their pathways to adjustment. *Journal of Applied Psychology, 88*(5), 779-794.

Miller, V.D., & Jablin, R.M. (1991). Information seeking during organizational entry: Influences, tactics and a model of the process. *Academy of Management Review, 16*(1), 92-129.

Saks, A.M. & Ashforth, B.E. (1996). Proactive socialization and behavioral self management. *Journal of Vocational Behavior, 48*, 301-323.

Chapter 2

Polishing Your
Professional Behaviors
Mastering Workplace Skills

LEARNING OBJECTIVES

At the end of this chapter, the reader will be able to:
- ➤ Distinguish the difference between being a professional and acting like a professional.
- ➤ Describe the seven mindsets of trusted professionals.
- ➤ Assess self performance as it relates to professional behaviors, including initiative, empathy, organization, dependability, competence, integrity, and professional appearance.
- ➤ Describe the three components of empathy.
- ➤ Name four important behaviors that indicate dependability.
- ➤ Describe 10 guidelines for professional appearance.

Whether a fieldwork student or experienced therapist, it will always be expected that you present yourself as a professional. That means that your behavior should reflect the commonly held values and beliefs of our profession (Kasar & Clark, 2000). Some of these behaviors are learned as one matures and will prove important in all facets of your life. Many of these behaviors are learned and evolve throughout the academic process and are further refined during fieldwork experiences and employment. Mastery of professional behaviors will have a major impact on your success as an occupational therapist because no matter how technically skilled, knowledgeable, and talented you are, one of the most important factors in determining your success in the workplace is your ability to demonstrate that (among other things) you are reliable, cooperative, organized, and empathic. In Chapter 3, we will focus on the importance of emotional intelligence, self-awareness, and social skills in the development of positive workplace relationships. In this chapter, we will introduce these concepts and address the specific conduct and behaviors expected of you as a professional and how mastery of these skills will enhance your career.

Davis L, Rosee M. *Occupational Therapy Student to Clinician:
Making the Transition (pp 15-30).*
© 2015 SLACK Incorporated.

WHAT IS A PROFESSIONAL?

The word *profession* is derived from "profess," meaning to hold dear a set of beliefs. The beliefs "you hold dear" is what probably guided you toward your choice of a career (Napier, 2011, p. 96). By identifying yourself as a health professional, you carry certain expectations, privileges, and responsibilities (Napier, 2011) and will be held to a certain standard of actions and behaviors.

The field of occupational therapy imposes a number of professional behaviors upon us. In addition to a dedication to others and mastery of a specific base of knowledge, we must "acquire a regard for the dynamics of human relationships and interpersonal skills" (Fidler, 1996, p. 583). To develop these abilities, one needs to integrate the attitudes, beliefs, and values that reflect personal integrity, demonstrate empathy, respect others' points of view, and contribute to the welfare of others. It is these behavioral skills that we will address in this chapter.

THE MINDSETS OF TRUSTED PROFESSIONALS

As occupational therapists and certified occupational therapy assistants, we are considered professionals. We hold a professional license and possess specific skills that make us a unique entity in the workplace. However, being a professional is different from acting like a professional. Professionalism is not just a list of traits, but rather a mindset and a way of approaching the work and its challenges that demonstrate not only technical skills but character traits as well. By embracing the mindset concepts outlined by Wiersma (2011) in his book, *The Power of Professionalism*, occupational therapists can establish themselves as true professionals who stand out in the workplace. These include the following mindsets.

Mindset 1: Professionals Focus on Results

By using your professional skills, along with your passion and values, you aspire to achieve results that are sustainable.

Example: Angie, an occupational therapist, identifies a need to start an activities of daily living training program for nurses' aides on the floor of a long-term unit in a skilled nursing facility. Angie develops the protocol and begins training the aides. The plan is to provide monthly training sessions that will be repeated regularly to reinforce key elements of the program. The hope is that the ongoing training will promote follow-up and buy-in by the aides who will be carrying out the program on the floors. Angie was initially very enthusiastic about the program, but as interest waned on the part of the nurses, Angie's enthusiasm started to wane as well. Her training sessions became inconsistent, and she frequently canceled them at the last minute. In the end, the program failed. Although the initial motivation was strong, the commitment and passion was not there to ensure sustainable results.

In this case, Angie behaved unprofessionally. She lost interest in the project and became complacent, undermining the success of the program. A professional knows that successful implementation of a new program requires perseverance, maturity, and enthusiasm.

Mindset 2: Professionals Act Like They Are Part of Something Bigger Than Themselves

Do not look at what is best for you; commit to the success of your facility. Understand that collaboration and teamwork is what marks you as a professional.

Example: Harrison, a senior occupational therapist, is planning a continuing education event at his hospital. He secures speakers, works to establish the agenda, and begins the marketing process. He is told in the middle of the marketing effort that the physical therapy department will be cosponsoring the event and they are assigning Stu (a physical therapist) to help out. At first, Harrison is resentful that Stu will get as much credit as he does for organizing the event, even though Harrison did all of the preliminary work. By the end of the project, Harrison came to the conclusion that including the physical therapy department in the project was a better idea than going it alone. It expanded the marketing reach of the program, brought in more participants, reduced the amount of work Harrison had to do, and ensured that the entire rehabilitation department would receive the credit for the project by hospital administrators. In the end, the event gave the hospital exposure, generated a small profit, and resulted in a public relations benefit for both the organization and the rehabilitation department. For Harrison, the greater good won out over getting all of the credit himself.

Mindset 3: Professionals Know Things Get "Better" as They Get "Better"

Related to Mindset 2, as you start to perform with the greater good in mind, personal growth and other benefits often appear. In the previous example, Harrison grew professionally during the course of the continuing education project. He learned about producing seminars, made new contacts in the field, and through his collaboration with Stu, he made a new friend. Through that bond, they teamed up on another joint project for the hospital that led to them starting their own continuing education business. Harrison had not thought about how his participation in the event would benefit him personally, but in the end, the benefits materialized organically.

Mindset 4: Professionals Have Personal Standards That Often Transcend Organizational Ones

Professionals have their own personal standards (such as their values and moral beliefs) that are integral to their character and are not dependent on organizational standards. These include the following:

- Having a personalized core set of values
- Doing what is right over what is expedient
- Rising above the fray, staying focused, and avoiding drama

These personal standards keep them focused, even when situations pull them in another direction.

In the previous example, when Harrison was forced to partner with Stu, some of his colleagues suggested that he sabotage the project and point blame at the physical therapist for the failure. Although he initially was caught up in this negative mindset, his need to succeed and be a cooperative team member won out and he refocused himself to participate to the best of his ability. He did not let the negative input sway him.

Mindset 5: Professionals Know the Importance of Integrity

Integrity has everything to do with who you are. When you have integrity, you inspire trust. Doing the right thing just comes naturally. The underpinnings of integrity include the following:

- Authenticity and honesty
- Delivering on commitments
- Refusing to violate the trust others have extended to us

Example: Sandra, an occupational therapist, is providing 1-day coverage at an outpatient facility. While there, the director of the department asks her to cosign the notes of the certified occupational therapy assistant for sessions that were delivered the previous week. Sandra was uncomfortable with this request because she felt it was unethical and violated her integrity. Acting in a professional manner, she told the supervisor that she felt the request was not ethical and she refused to cosign the notes.

Mindset 6: Professionals Aspire to Master Their Emotions, Which Inspires Trust in Others

We often react emotionally to issues and situations based on our history. Emotions can sometimes make smart people stupid. We are responsible for our emotional reactions to experiences and must find a way to control our external response to internal emotional reactions. As professionals, we must master our emotions so that we can remain calm in a crisis or when a situation pushes our buttons. People who know how to master their emotions will do the following:

- Respect clients and colleagues—even when a situation is difficult or challenging
- Maintain their objectivity and keep their wits about them
- Manage their egos and resist the urge for immediate gratification

Example: A child sex offender is brought into the occupational therapy clinic from an incarceration facility so that a splint can be fabricated for a wrist drop. Katy (who has a family history of sexual abuse) reviewed the chart and was shaken by the patient's history. Initially, she did not want to work with the patient. After considering the situation, she chose to fabricate the splint, interacting with the patient in a professional manner. That is what a professional does.

We will cover these concepts in more depth in Chapter 3.

Mindset 7: Professionals Find Pleasure in the Growth and Success of Others

People who have mastered this professional mindset will invest in the growth of others and do not feel threatened by their success. They readily do the following:

- Extend trust to others
- Recognize the value other professionals bring to the table
- Try to lift others up

Example: Eric, an occupational therapist supervisor, learns that one of his mentees, Sumi, is interested in developing an idea she has for a new self-help application. Sumi expresses frustration at not knowing how to start the process. Eric suggests she speak to a friend of his who has developed a successful software business. The friend met with Sumi and provided useful guidance. He reviewed budgets, markets, and legal ramifications and recommended an accountant to help her set up her company, lay out costs, and identify cash needs. Eric wanted Sumi to succeed and helped make it happen.

WHAT ARE PROFESSIONAL BEHAVIORS?

Now that we have covered the mindset principles of professionalism, we will now address specific professional behaviors and skills that are expected of occupational therapists. Professional behaviors are the active manifestations of your beliefs, philosophies, and interpersonal skills. Knowing what it means to be a professional is much different from acting like one. As we have said a number of times already, your success in the world of occupational therapy will be dependent on your understanding and ability to apply these concepts to your practice.

We will review and illustrate all of the components of professional behavior in detail so that you can understand what they mean and how they manifest in the workplace.

Initiative

The *Oxford Dictionaries* define initiative as "the ability to assess and initiate things independently; the power or opportunity to act or take charge before others do; or an act or strategy intended to resolve a difficulty or improve a situation."

In Covey's (2004) book, *The 7 Habits of Highly Effective People,* he discusses the importance of initiative. The person who takes initiative makes things happen. He or she proactively identifies solutions to problems, doing whatever is necessary to be consistent and get the job done. When faced with problems, these individuals do not say, "There is nothing I can do" or, "I cannot change the situation." Rather, they are determined to think of alternatives and will investigate a different approach to find a solution.

In the field of occupational therapy, we have many opportunities to take the initiative to develop strategies, programs, and solutions to address challenges in various settings.

Example: A long-term care facility has many patients who need help to self-feed, but staffing patterns are very low and patients often sit with the food in front of them and do not feed themselves. Because the nurses have so many "feeders," they usually need to rush the patients through their meals. Maria, a certified occupational therapy assistant student at the facility, noticed this problem when on feeding rounds and decided to initiate a new program as her special student project whereby volunteers are trained to cue patients to self-feed. After developing a protocol that was approved by her supervisor and medical director, Maria scheduled training sessions with the volunteers. In these sessions, she reviewed the various conditions that contributed to the resident's decline in self-feeding and demonstrated cueing techniques and assistive interventions that could facilitate the self-feeding process. In the end, residents received more attention during mealtime and were able to participate more in their self-feeding tasks. The volunteers felt satisfied that they were making a contribution and that caretakers could focus on the residents who needed more assistance.

Example: Carlos, an experienced school-based therapist, noticed that a group of new graduates were assigned to his school at the beginning of the year. Because supervision was sporadically provided, he decided to check in with the providers to see how they were managing. They all felt overwhelmed and under-supported. He suggested that they form a peer supervision group to be carried out once per week during their lunch hour. Each therapist would take turns leading the group by either presenting a case or distributing a professional article to be discussed. As a result, the therapists were able to improve their skills while bonding with their colleagues. Even the more experienced therapists were able to learn and improve their skills in the process.

Assessing Your Initiative

1. Do you start projects, evaluations, interventions, and other services without being asked or reminded?
2. Do you plan, organize, and prepare for assessments and interventions to maximize the time scheduled for clients?
3. Do you independently seek information and answers to questions and formulate possible answers before asking for assistance?
4. When a task is completed, do you look for other work or ask whether you can help anyone else?
5. Do you recognize that reading and preparation may need to be done outside of the facility?
6. Do you research clients' diagnoses and needs to gain a better understanding of conditions and how to provide effective interventions?
7. Do you seek feedback from supervisors and use the information to improve your performance (Napier, 2011)?

Empathy

Empathy is a multidimensional concept that has moral, cognitive, emotive, and behavioral components. It involves an ability to understand the other person's situation, perspective, and feelings; communicate in a way that demonstrates understanding; and act on that understanding in a helpful, therapeutic way (Mercer & Reynolds, 2002). A display of empathy on the part of a provider has been shown to increase clients' satisfaction and improve their motivation to participate in their therapy program. Empathy and health care go hand in hand. Rogers describes empathy as

> entering the private world of the other and becoming thoroughly at home in it. It involves being sensitive to the changing meanings which flow in this other person. It means temporarily living in his/her life without making judgments. In some sense, it means that you lay yourself aside. This can only be done by a person who is secure enough in himself that he knows he will not get lost in what may turn out to be the strange and bizarre world of the other. (1975, p. 3)

Morse et al. (1992) have laid out the components of empathy. They see it as a form of professional interaction—a set of skills or competencies rather than a subjective emotional experience or a personality trait that you either do or do not have. The components include the following:

- Emotive: The ability to subjectively experience and share in another's psychological state or intrinsic feelings
- Moral: An internal altruistic force that motivates the practice of empathy
- Cognitive: The intellectual ability to identify and understand another person's feelings and perspective from an objective stance
- Behavioral: The ability to communicate a response to convey understanding of another's perspective (Morse et al., 1992, p. 275)

Kasar and Clark (2000) describe the empathic practitioner as one who is aware of a client's feelings, cares about a client's needs, and creates an open and effective communication.

This requires the ability to actively listen to the client's verbal and nonverbal cues. Townsend (1996) lays out a technique to promote active listening using the acronym SOLER. The steps involve the following:

- S: *Sit* in front of clients, giving the message that you are interested in what they are *saying*.
- O: Sit with an *open posture* with arms and legs uncrossed, implying that you are open to what the client is saying.
- L: *Lean* forward to convey your interest and attentiveness.
- E: Establish *eye contact* to convey a willingness to listen.
- R: *Relax* to demonstrate your comfort with the client.

There are times when even the most empathetic practitioners are not able to muster empathy for a client. This may be due to personal issues and pressures or because of personal values or cultural conflicts with the client (e.g., treating a convicted pedophile who has suffered a stroke while in jail). When this happens, professionals are responsible for identifying their feelings and finding ways to deal with the situation. This may involve removing themselves from the relationship or seeking counsel from a supervisor. No matter what the conflict, it is important to deal with it professionally and respectfully.

Assessing Your Empathy

1. Do you respect the rights, feelings, and opinions of clients and peers?
2. Do you provide assistance, treatment, or services to clients and peers without personal bias or prejudice?
3. Do you listen actively to learn the feelings and needs of clients and peers?

4. Do you avoid demonstrating personal emotions that might interfere with therapy or client service (Napier, 2011)?

Cooperation

Cooperation is the ability and willingness to work together toward a common goal. Cooperation is an essential skill required in any workplace setting. Without cooperation, everyone would do what was good for them, resulting in a chaotic environment where the best interests of the client and the facility would not be served.

Cooperation is demonstrated by "someone who works effectively with other individuals, shows consideration for the needs of the group, and develops group cohesiveness by facilitating the knowledge and awareness of others" (Kasar & Clark, 2000, p. 75). Other professional behaviors and skills, such as dependability, professional presentation, initiative, empathy, clinical reasoning, and verbal communication, are foundational to cooperation.

Cooperation is particularly important when you serve as part of a team process. Much more about this topic is presented in Chapter 5.

Assessing Your Cooperation Skills

1. Do you make positive contributions to the team process?
2. Do you accept group decisions even when your own personal decision differs from the group?
3. Do you focus on common team goals rather than individual goals or needs?
4. Do you give credit to those who deserve it?
5. Do you complete your own share of the work and offer to do more when necessary?
6. Do you return all equipment and supplies to where they belong and in good order so that they are available for the next person who needs them?
7. Do you clearly communicate information needed by peers to carry out their work (Napier, 2011)?

Organization

The *Webster's II College Dictionary* defines *organization* as "the act of arranging or assembling into an orderly structured, functional whole; giving a coherent form to something."

Organizational skills manifest in two types of functions. The first is the ability to initiate the process necessary to create order (Kasar & Clark, 2000). Next comes meaningful action to implement the orderly organization of the task at hand (Kasar & Clark, 2000). Organization represents a key skill in a professional workplace. Organized individuals will determine what is needed and pursue a course of action. They will also have acquired habits that allow them to set aside distractions and obstructions so that they can begin to attack their mission or goal. At this point, the individual may use external aids, such as planners and to-do lists, or may research a solution to guide the completion of the challenge at hand.

Example: Margie was just referred a patient with a C5 spinal injury. She has not had much experience working with this type of patient and has been told that she will need to perform an evaluation the following day. In light of her minimal experience with a spinal cord injury, she decides to spend the night doing research in preparation for the evaluation. She creates a list of the steps she will need to take and the skills required. She takes a number of books home with her to help with her preparation. She reviews textbooks and evaluation tools to determine what needs to be assessed and which tools are most appropriate. She also calls a friend who works in a setting where spinal cord injuries are common. The next day, she comes to work with a plan and has all the needed resources available so that she is ready to perform the evaluation in a professional manner.

- Do you keep information handy, such as in a daily planner or calendar system?
- Do you keep notes and maintain them in an accessible place?
- Are you prepared? Do you carry the supplies you need during the day and restock them as necessary?
- Do you keep things in their place? Do you avoid wasting time and energy in looking for lost items? (Napier, 2011)

Dependability

Dependability is a professional behavior that is essential to all of life's endeavors, but especially as it relates to the workplace. The definition relates to your reliability, trustworthiness, accountability, and sense of responsibility. Behaviors that indicate your dependability include the following:

- Being on time. Whether you show up for work, a meeting, or a treatment session, it is imperative that you are there at the appointed time. This shows respect for your coworkers and clients.
- Showing up. You must be present for events you are scheduled to attend. You should never call in sick unless it is absolutely necessary.
- Take responsibility and fulfill your promises. When you say you will something, do it.
- Communicate appropriately and in advance when you cannot fulfill your obligations or promises so that other arrangements can be made.

The Importance of Timeliness

You must be on time for work and meetings and be able to complete your job responsibilities on a timely basis. Timeliness is impacted by many factors, including culture, upbringing, and a number of interpersonal traits. When working with patients, it is especially important to maintain schedules and keep to time requirements.

Example: Gigi, a certified occupational therapy assistant, is a great therapist, but she is terrible at managing her time. Even though sessions are scheduled and the amount of time mandated to be provided is set, Gigi is consistently off schedule. While Gigi's sessions are scheduled for 30 minutes, she is actually providing 45 minutes. In addition to impacting her other patients, Gigi's time management skills affect the efficient operation of the department and its billing. She believes she is doing the right thing because her patients are improving, but she is actually causing mayhem in her department and on the patient floors. When she keeps a patient longer than scheduled, the patient ends up being late for his or her next appointment, which throws off the schedules of the other departments. As a result, the patient gets back for lunch late, throwing off the medication schedule. Even though Gigi means well, her poor time management has created many problems, both within and outside her department.

- Do you arrive on time at your work site?
- Do you notify your supervisor if you must be absent or late?
- Do you arrive on time for appointments and meetings?
- Do you follow time mandates when providing treatment?
- Do you complete paperwork and documentation on time?
- Do you follow through on assignments, treatment plans, and other services (Napier, 2011)?

Competence

Competence refers to "an individual's capacity to perfom job responsibilities" (McConnell, 2001, p. 14). It is defined in the context of expected knowledge, traits, skills, and abilities. It involves mastery of knowledge related to professional concepts that are specific to our domain of practice. Traits relate to personality, skill, and abilities. Personality characteristics (e.g., self-control, self-confidence, dependability) predispose a person to behave or respond in a certain way. Skills are the capacity to perform specific actions that are a function of one's knowledge and the strategies used to apply that knowledge. Abilities are the attributes that a person has acquired through previous experience and brings to a new task. They are more fundamental and stable than knowledge and skills (Kak, Burkhalter, & Cooper, 2001). Integration of all of these skills, traits, and characteristics results in an individual's competence—his or her ability to perform in a manner that yields desirable outcomes.

Typically, new graduates are at the beginning of their quest for competency (also known as the *novice stage*). With additional training and experience, competency develops. (We cover this issue extensively in Chapter 15.) However, this is not a static concept. Someone may be competent at a given moment in time but that competency improves with additional experience and training. Competence is what you can do, but performance is what you actually do (Kak et al., 2001). Competency is your capacity to perform. Performance can be observed and measured.

Obviously, when you are entrusted with the rehabilitation of clients, it is imperative that you have achieved a level of competency that can assure a performance that will result in the achievement of positive functional outcomes and satisfaction for the client with whom you are working.

How Are Competencies Acquired?

Competency in your profession is an ongoing, lifelong process. It begins with your professional education, nurtured and applied in your clinical fieldwork experiences, and enhanced through on-the-job experiences that may include further independent study, attendance at continuing education courses, and participation in the supervision process, as well as observing and learning from peers.

Competency Assessment Tools

Often, workplace settings will develop competency assessment tools to measure the skill of providers. This is often used in the accreditation process to demonstrate to outside surveyors that providers have the requisite skills to achieve anticipated outcomes. These usually consist of skills checklists, documentation audits, and observation of treatment sessions, along with client satisfaction surveys. These assessments should be used as learning tools by providers to identify strengths and weaknesses and improve performance.

Assessing Your Competence

- Do you review knowledge and skills needed to perform the clinical tasks required of you?
- Do you interview clients appropriately to obtain needed information?
- Do you demonstrate awareness of your limitations and ask for help when needed?
- Do you take appropriate precautions to ensure the safety, comfort, and rights of clients?
- Do you demonstrate flexibility and willingness to accept changing conditions and assignments and adapt to these changes?
- Are you prepared with alternative plans for treatment?
- Do you apply problem-solving skills to complex issues and situations?
- Do you perform all tasks neatly and accurately (Napier, 2011)?

Integrity

Carter (1996), in his book *Integrity*, defines this often-used word by describing the following three simple traits:

1. Discerning what is right and what is wrong
2. Acting on what you have discerned, even at a personal cost
3. Openly affirming that you are acting on your understanding of right from wrong

The term often refers to a refusal to engage in lying, blaming, or other behavior that appears to evade accountability. Integrity is holding true to one's values and doing what you said you would do. We will be covering these issues in great detail in Chapter 9.

As an example of lack of integrity, Selma was an occupational therapy student in an acute care hospital. She was responsible for treating patients on the fourth and fifth floors. One day, Selma came back late from lunch. Not wanting her supervisor to see that she was late, she took off her coat and left it in a patient's room. The next day at morning meeting, the charge nurse for the fifth floor reported that the patient in room 507 was becoming confused as she reported that a girl came in and left her coat, then came back later and took her coat back. Selma never admitted that it was her who put the coat in the room and the nursing staff continued to think that the patient's mental status was compromised.

Assessing Your Integrity

- Do you perform duties ethically at all times?
- Do you respect and maintain confidentiality?
- Do you accept responsibility for your own actions without making excuses or trying to pass blame?
- Do you admit mistakes and are you willing to correct them?
- Do you value and care for the equipment and resources of your agency?
- Do you act with honesty and integrity (Napier, 2011)?

Professional Appearance

First impressions count, and while it may be true that what a person knows is more important than how he or she looks, the reality is that people form opinions about individuals they meet based on appearances. Research has shown that upon an initial consultation with a patient, a first impression is formed based on verbal and nonverbal communication, along with clothing, grooming, and cleanliness (Rehman, Nieteret, Cope, & Kilpatrick, 2005). As you make the transition from a student in a classroom to the fieldwork setting and eventually to an entry-level job as a professional, you may need to make adjustments in the way you attend to your dress and appearance to ensure the trust and respect of clients, peers, and supervisors.

As a clinician, no matter the setting, it is important to portray yourself as well dressed, neat, and clean. This communicates a message to others regarding your self-image, attitude, and competency. A sloppy appearance portrays a message to your clients that they will get sloppy care. In a study published in 2005 in *The American Journal of Medicine*, respondents overwhelmingly favored photographs of physicians dressed in professional attire (shirt, necktie, and white coat for men or skirt or tailored trousers and white coat for women) with photographs of doctors wearing scrubs, a business suit, or informal clothes. The patients also said that they were more likely to divulge their social, sexual, and psychological concerns to the clinicians in the white coats. The conclusion drawn is that how you appear and what you wear impacts how your clients trust and regard you.

Rules for Dress in Professional Settings

Sometimes facilities have a dress code they expect therapists to follow, but more often the mode of dress is left to the individual's discretion. Clearly, therapists working with patients need to dress in comfortable attire that does not impede movement and allows them to perform their responsibilities without worrying about their clothing. However, being comfortable does not mean we cannot look professional.

Costa (2004), in her book *The Essential Guide to Occupational Therapy Fieldwork Education*, lists the following appearance guidelines for clinicians in professional settings:

- Makeup should not be excessive.
- Facial hair on men should be neat and well groomed.
- Fragrances should not be worn because others may have allergies.
- Personal hygiene should include attention to body odor, mouth odor, and cleanliness.
- Body-pierced parts should not be displayed at work (i.e., no nose, tongue, or lip rings).
- Clothing should cover tattoos.
- Revealing clothing or undergarments should not be seen at work.
- Skin should not show as you bend, lift, reach, and twist during patient care.
- Shoes should be supportive, neat, and clean.
- Jewelry needs to be kept tidy and should not interfere with patients during therapy.
- Fingernails must be kept clean and short because long nails can easily tear a patient's skin during treatment.

Some additional recommendations include the following:

- Slogan T-shirts, jackets, and sweatshirts, along with sweatsuits and any sportswear, are not appropriate.
- Tattered, frayed, or wrinkled clothing should not be worn.
- Sunglasses or darkly tinted glasses should not be worn during work hours.
- Identification badges should be worn at all times.

The Impact of the White Coat

In a recent *New York Times* article titled *The Impact of the White Coat,* Blakeslee (2012) illustrates how the clothing a professional wears affects their cognitive processes. In a phenomenon called *enclothed cognition*, it has been shown that when we put on certain clothes we more readily take on a role and improve our basic abilities. In one experiment, undergraduates were randomly assigned to wear a white lab coat or street clothes. They were then given a test for selective attention. Those who wore the white lab coats made half as many errors on trials as those who wore regular street clothes. In another experiment, students wore either a doctor's coat or a painter's coat or were told to look at a picture of a doctor's lab coat. All three groups wrote essays about how they felt about the coats and were then tested for sustained attention. The group that wore the doctor's coat showed the greatest improvement in attention. The conclusion from these trials is that dressing professionally may not only impact how others feel about you, but it may also impact how you feel about yourself, and could actually improve your performance (Blakeslee, 2012, p. D3).

Cultural Considerations Regarding Appearance

Different cultures and religions have different standards as to appropriate dress codes. Be aware of local cultures and the populations you serve when considering what to wear. For example, as a woman working with a Hasidic Jewish or a Muslim population, it is more respectful to wear a skirt and have your arms covered. We will delve deeply into the issues of culture (including dress) in Chapter 7.

Assessing Personal Appearance

- Do you wear clothing that is always clean and appropriate for the work to be performed?
- Do you practice safety and respect for others by avoiding dangling jewelry, long loose hair, strong fragrances, extreme fashion trends, or revealing clothing?
- Do you practice good personal hygiene?
- Do you use appropriate body posture and facial expressions that send reassuring messages to clients (Napier, 2011)?

COMMON ACTS OF UNPROFESSIONALISM SEEN IN THE OCCUPATIONAL THERAPY CLINIC

- Using smartphones for personal calls during work hours (especially during treatment sessions)
- Texting during work hours (especially during treatment sessions)
- Arriving late to work, coming back from lunch late, leaving work early without permission
- Not maintaining a neat and orderly workspace
- Not taking the initiative to complete a task that is expected of you
- Dominating the use of equipment that is to be shared

ARE YOU A DIFFICULT COWORKER?

In a recent survey, it was reported that 93% of employees work with nasty, unreliable, or eccentric people. Only one in four respondents confronted the person (Belkin, 2007). Do you see yourself in any of the types listed below? If so, you might be creating a problem in your department that is impacting morale and negatively impacting your reputation.

- The Forgetful Borrower—borrows things and does not return them.
- The Slacker—lets everyone else do the work and takes the credit.
- The Martyr—thinks he or she is the only one working.
- The Passive-Aggressor—leaves vaguely threatening notes everywhere or constantly complains about his or her insane level of work.
- The Drama Queen—overreacts to seemingly minor incidents.
- The Suck-Up—goes out of his or her way to be recognized.
- The Know-It-All—either points out every little detail or insists on helping you without being asked.
- The Gossiper—always has the dirt on colleagues and cannot resist sharing it.
- The Nose Offender—underdeodorized or overperfumed.
- The Complainer—no matter how good things are, this person complains and is a drag to work with (Warner, 2011).

In a small, unpublished survey we conducted with rehab directors, a number of additional issues were uncovered about unprofessional behaviors in the clinic. Some of these include the following:

- The Messy Clinician—this is the therapist who keeps his or her work area covered with papers and personal items (e.g., extra shoes under the desk, shopping bags with dirty clothes) and leaves therapeutic equipment and supplies where they were last used instead of putting them away. Splinting scraps remain on the counter, towels are left behind, and sheets are not changed. This clinician expects everyone to clean up after him or her. Colleagues do not appreciate the thoughtlessness.

- The Tattletale—nobody likes a colleague who goes to higher-ups to report a problem with another staff member before trying to resolve the issue directly (unless the issue poses immediate harm or danger). For example, Jon, a certified occupational therapy assistant, noticed that his patient now had a hand roll, which he did not provide. He reviewed the chart to determine who had given the device, since occupational therapy was responsible for tracking it, but he found no documentation. In speaking to the patient, he found out that Nikki, the physical therapist, had provided it. Rather than going right to Nikki to find out why she provided a device that the occupational therapist was responsible for, he decided to go directly to the director of rehabilitation to report this infraction. The director did not appreciate the fact that Jon did not deal directly with Nikki, and neither did Nikki. Jon ended up looking bad, and he made a potential enemy in the department.

- The Grandiose Clinician—this is the clinician who has an unrealistic view of his or her abilities and importance, feels superior to others, exaggerates talents and capacities, and is self-centered and often boastful. A rehabilitation director recently shared a story about a new graduate she was thinking about hiring. When the director told the new graduate the salary, the new graduate rolled his eyes and said (with an attitude), "But I have a master's degree!" The director responded, "So does everyone else we are interviewing." The new graduate's attitude was a big turnoff to the director, who decided not to hire him based on that exchange.

- The Entitled Clinician—related to the Grandiose Clinician, this is the therapist who believes that he or she has earned special privileges based on performance. An attitude can border on arrogance. This is the therapist who comes in late every day and does not return from lunch on time. When confronted by his or her supervisor about unprofessional behavior, the clinician responds, "But when I work, I work really hard. I deserve a break." He or she also feels deserving of special accolades for performing expected work duties.

SUMMARY

Being the best at your profession does not guarantee success. Your technical skills must be combined with professional behaviors to ensure that you are respected, admired, and considered worthy for higher-level responsibilities. Often, these skills must be developed as one matures into his or her role as a member of a workplace team. By understanding these issues and focusing or improving on your workplace behaviors, you will enjoy the respect of your coworkers and ensure a career of personal and professional growth.

DISCUSSION QUESTIONS/ACTIVITIES

1. Describe a person you identify as a professional. Explain what attributes he or she exhibits that make you see him or her in this way.

2. Compose a dialogue that reflects an unprofessional interchange between a nurse and an occupational therapist. Role play the scene with two volunteers in class. Discuss what makes the encounter unprofessional. How could it have been handled differently?

3. Describe examples of when you experienced initiative, empathy, cooperation, organization, dependability, competence, and integrity in yourself or observed it in others. Share these examples with one another.

4. Using the Professional Behaviors Competency Checklist on the next page, rate your professional competencies. For any competencies that are below a "Good" level, write a plan to improve. Think about situations where you were disappointed in your professional behaviors. Write up the scenario, how you responded, and how your response could have been better.

5. Using the pictures below, break into groups and answer the following questions:

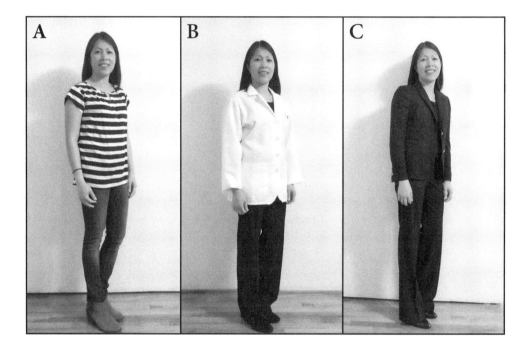

   ◆ Which of these pictures illustrate what you would consider professional attire? Why?
   ◆ What items present an unprofessional look? Be specific.
   ◆ Which of these health care professionals would you trust the most? Why?
   ◆ Which of these individuals would you expect to be the most knowledgeable, competent, caring, and authoritative? Why?
   ◆ What other biases can you identify in yourself, based on these pictures?
   Share your answers with the entire class and compare findings.

Professional Behaviors Competency Checklist

On a scale of 1 to 4, rate your professional competencies in the following areas:
1 = Poor   2 = Fair   3 = Good   4 = Excellent

Positive attitude
_____ Fosters positive communication
_____ Accepts change
_____ Manages stressors in positive and constructive ways

Flexibility
_____ Can adapt and cope with change
_____ Modifies performance after feedback

Professional communication skills
_____ Practices positive verbal and nonverbal communication skills in work interactions
_____ Is concise in verbal and written communication
_____ Handles conflict constructively
_____ Uses assertive communication skills
_____ Written communication demonstrates correct grammar, spelling, and punctuation

A willingness to go the extra mile
_____ Seeks ways to improve
_____ Volunteers for additional responsibilities
_____ Takes on additional responsibilities

Respect of others
_____ Follows the chain of command
_____ Is supportive of others
_____ Can listen to other viewpoints—whether in agreement or disagreement
_____ Respects diversity
_____ Is attentive to others' needs
_____ Is sensitive to others' time frames
_____ Meets deadlines; if unable to meet deadline, informs necessary parties

A team player attitude
_____ Strives to achieve team goals
_____ Is proactive and anticipates needs of others
_____ Pools resources and works efficiently within a group
_____ Assists with resolution development after problem is identified

Personal responsibility
_____ Is aware of strengths and weaknesses
_____ Is punctual
_____ Demonstrates initiative
_____ Follows safety precautions
_____ Respects and maintains confidentiality
_____ Demonstrates an awareness of/follows the code of ethics

Adapted from Sladyk, K. (2002). *The successful occupational therapy fieldwork student.* Thorofare, NJ: SLACK
Incorporated.

REFERENCES

Belkin, L. (2007, February 7). It's not the job I despise, it's you. *New York Times*. Retrieved from http://www.nytimes.com/2008/20/07/fashion/07WORK.html.

Blakeslee, S. (2012, April 2). Mind games: Sometimes a white coat isn't just a white coat. New York, NY: *New York Times*. p. D3.

Carter, S.L. (1996). *Integrity*. New York, NY: Harper Perennial.

Costa, D. (2004). *The essential guide to occupational therapy fieldwork education: Resources for today's educators and practitioners*. Bethesda, MD: AOTA Press.

Covey, S.R. (2004). *The 7 habits of highly effective people*. New York, NY: Free Press.

Fidler, G. (1996). Developing a repertoire of professional behaviors. *American Journal of Occupational Therapy, 50*(7), 583-587.

Initiative [Def. 1]. (n.d.). In *Oxford Dictionaries*. Retrieved from http://www.oxforddictionaries.com/us/definition/american_english/initiative.

Kak, N., Burkhalter, B., & Cooper, M.A. (2001). Measuring the competence of healthcare providers. *Quality Assurance Project. 2*(1), 1-28.

Kasar, J., & Clark, E.N. (2000). *Developing professional behaviors*. Thorofare, NJ: SLACK Incorporated.

Mercer, S., & Reynolds, W. (2002). Empathy and quality of care. *The British Journal of General Practice, 52*(Suppl.), s9-s12.

McConnell, E.A. (2001) Competence vs. competency. *Nursing Management, 32*(5), p. 14.

Morse, J., Anderson, G., Botter, J., et al. (1992). Exploring empathy: A conceptual fit for nursing practice. *Image: the Journal of Nursing Scholarship, 24*, 273-280.

Napier, B. (2011). *Occupational therapy fieldwork survival guide*. Bethesda, MD: AOTA Press.

Organization. (1999). In *Webster's New College Dictionary*. Boston, MA: Houghton Mifflin

Rehman, S.U., Nieteret, P.J., Cope, D.W., & Kilpatrick, A.O. (2005). What to wear today? Effect of doctor's attire on the trust and confidence of patients. *The American Journal of Medicine. 119*(11), 1279-1286.

Rogers, C.R. (1975). Empathic: An unappreciated way of being. *Counseling Psychologist, 5*(2), pp. 2-10.

Sladyk, K. (2002). *The successful occupational therapy fieldwork student*. Thorofare, NJ: SLACK Incorporated

Townsend, M. (1996). *Psychiatric mental health nursing: Concepts of care* (2nd ed). Philadelphia, PA: FA Davis.

Warner, S. (2011). When coworkers go bad. *Advance Magazine*. pp 1-2.

Wiersma, B. (2011). *The power of professionalism*. Los Angeles, CA: Ravel Media.

Chapter 3

Wake Up Your Emotional Intelligence
Developing Competencies for Success

LEARNING OBJECTIVES

At the end of this chapter, the reader will be able to:
- Define the term *emotional intelligence.*
- Describe how emotional intelligence can impact your career.
- Identify the skill sets needed to attain competence in emotional intelligence.
- Name the four aspects of social awareness.
- Discuss the strategies one can use to improve the four core social emotional competencies of self-awareness, self-management, social awareness, and relationship management.
- List 15 emotional intelligence derailers.
- Identify five actions in the workplace that can be counterproductive to relationship building.

After investing so much time and energy in your professional education, you now have the opportunity to demonstrate what you have to succeed in your new profession. It may surprise you to learn that the most important determinant in your success as an occupational therapist and certified occupational therapy assistant (both in your fieldwork assignments and later in your paid work experiences) will not be your clinical skills but your ability to forge effective relationships with colleagues, coworkers, supervisors, patients, and families. No matter what your personal definition of success, whether it is based on financial reward, the mastery of clinical skills, or promotions up the managerial ladder, attainment will be largely determined by how well you have developed your emotional intelligence (EQ) skills.

EQ refers to a set of personal qualities that allow you to understand, control, and manage your own emotions, as well as to recognize the emotions of others in order to see the world through their eyes. EQ facilitates interactions that are sensitive, supportive, empathic, and understanding. People with EQ are usually well liked by peers, supervisors, and patients; make the best managers; and are the most likely to get promoted.

Davis L, Rosee M. *Occupational Therapy Student to Clinician: Making the Transition (pp 31-45).*
© 2015 SLACK Incorporated.

In our professional education curricula, we are taught the art and science of occupational therapy. As we focus academically on all of the required elements of our profession, there is little time spent discussing the acquisition and honing of relationship skills that directly impact upon our ability to work effectively with colleagues, clients, and families. This chapter will introduce the basic concepts underlying social and emotional intelligence, skills that are crucial in helping you manage workplace relationships. By understanding these concepts, you can develop strategies to enhance your own skills and ensure success in the workplace.

Understanding Emotional Intelligence and How it Impacts Your Career and Life

Why is it in life that the most brilliant and well-educated people often struggle with their careers, while other less intelligent people flourish? According to Bradberry and Greaves (2009) in their book *Emotional Intelligence 2.0*, the answer lies in our emotional awareness and understanding and how we apply this knowledge and skill set to manage our behavior and relationships within and outside the workplace. Our ability in these areas is sometimes referred to as *emotional intelligence.*

"Emotional intelligence is your ability to recognize and understand emotions in yourself and others, and to use this awareness to manage your behavior and relationships" (Bradberry & Greaves, 2009). This ability affects "how we handle our behavior, navigate social complexities, and make personal decisions that achieve positive results" (Bradberry & Greaves, 2009, p. 17). EQ is much different from cognitive intelligence (IQ). IQ relates to one's ability to learn. You are born with this ability, and it does not change throughout one's life. EQ is a flexible skill that can be learned and developed (Bradberry & Greaves, 2009, p. 18). In the real world, it has been found that your EQ is more critical to success than your intellectual capabilities. It is the foundation for most work skills and impacts everything you say and do.

From a neurophysiological perspective, in everyday life we must struggle to keep our emotions in control because our brains are wired to react automatically to highly stimulating situations. When an external message travels to the brain, it must go through the frontal lobe before reaching the place where rational, logical thinking takes place. As these signals pass through the limbic system, one experiences raw emotions before they reach the more rational part of the brain. If the brain does not have the time to kick in, an automatic emotional response, or gut reaction, may result. These reactions do not take into account the consequences of the action, and can be counterproductive to fostering positive relationships with others. To avoid unproductive responses to highly charged situations, the emotional and rational brain areas must work together. This coordination results in EQ.

How Does Emotional Intelligence Affect Performance and Success on the Job?

Competency in EQ subskills will play an important part in your career path. Technical and clinical skills play only a part in career success. Most students graduating from an accredited program are skilled and capable at a basic level of expectation. Therefore, it is their emotional competencies rather than clinical ones that separate average new therapists from exceptional ones. In our profession, the exceptional performers are the ones able to deliver their occupational therapy interventions while making strong connections with their patients. They are held in high esteem by coworkers and supervisors, will be most likely to inspire and lead others, and make a positive impact on the work environment. While clinical knowledge and skill is important, clinically strong practitioners can be negatively impacted in their careers by poor interpersonal skills.

Although they may be knowledgeable and talented in the delivery of treatment, without EQ, they will likely experience difficulties in their career path. Based on studies, close to 90% of workplace success is attributable to EQ, proving it to be twice as important as cognitive, technical, and clinical abilities (Bradberry & Greaves, 2009). Furthermore, our EQ is typically the most important factor in determining who gets hired, who gets fired, and who gets promoted (Goleman, 2008).

Examples From the Clinic

Mandy entered her first clerkship experience in a very nervous and agitated state. She had never been in a hospital before (other than to visit her grandmother). She was shadowing her supervisor, who was performing an evaluation. She was surprised when her supervisor handed her a goniometer and asked her to perform measurements on the upper extremity of a young man with Guillain-Barré syndrome. As Mandy entered the room and looked at the patient lying in his bed, she panicked, started to cry, and said, "I can't do it; I don't know how." Her supervisor grabbed the goniometer out of her hands and walked away. Later, the supervisor called the field-work coordinator at the school to schedule a meeting to discuss Mandy's inappropriate emotional outburst. Mandy's lack of awareness led to a panicked response, which was counterproductive to her success at her fieldwork placement. Had she been more aware of her emotions, she could have identified what she was feeling and calmly told her supervisor that she was not ready to perform the evaluation and ask whether she could observe an evaluation, do extra research, and practice before being faced with a real patient. Mandy would have been credited with sharing her needs and could have avoided an unprofessional display of behavior that called into question her suitability as a therapist.

Igor was in his last fieldwork placement as a certified occupational therapy assistant student. The setting was a residence for cognitively and developmentally challenged adults. As a project, Igor designed an Activities of Daily Living group in which three or four patients came together to work on improving their grooming skills. In trying to identify a space for the group, he found that the recreation satellite room was not being used at that time. He gathered the group and began the session. In the middle of the session, the recreation director entered the room in a rage and asked, "Why are you in my space?" He answered that the room was empty, the lights were off, and based on the activity calendar, nothing was planned for that time. She then screamed at Igor in front of his patients and informed him that he must follow proper protocol and send a written memo requesting to use the space. He apologized and took his patients out of the room. Igor was very upset by the exchange. He had never worked in such a formal setting and did not realize that he was not following proper protocol. He felt dejected and embarrassed. In this case, while Igor should have checked further about using the room, the recreation director could have used her EQ skills to calmly and quietly speak to Igor and instruct him on proper protocol and explain why such protocol is important rather than publicly reprimanding in an angry tone and embarrassing him in front of his patients.

Using Emotional Intelligence to Secure a First Job

Kim had been interviewed for a coveted hospital position by the director of an occupational therapy department. The director introduced the candidate to the staff for a group interview after their one-to-one meeting to determine whether there was synergy with the existing staff. The next day, Kim received a call from the director saying that she liked her very much, but the staff did not think she was a good fit. She was asked to come back for a second interview to meet with the staff again over lunch to try and change their minds. Kim was taken aback by the feedback. She wondered why they did not like her and was angry at being put in such a difficult position. How was she going to go back to the facility and face these therapists? Knowing that she really wanted the job, she made a conscious decision not to hold a grudge. She let go of the anger and scheduled a meeting and developed a strategy to try to sell the staff on why she should be hired. Although still

---

Table 3-1

EMOTIONAL INTELLIGENCE

EMOTIONAL INTELLIGENCE SKILLS	YOUR PERCEPTIONS	YOUR ACTIONS
Personal competence	Self-awareness (understanding yourself)	Self-management (managing yourself)
Social competence	Social awareness (understanding others)	Relationship management (managing others)
Adapted from Bradberry, T., & Greaves, J. (2009). *Emotional intelligence 2.0.* San Diego, CA: TalentSmart Inc.		

---

miffed, she was determined to be friendly, enthusiastic, and positive. Lunch with the group went well, and she was eventually hired.

In this case, rather than responding emotionally in anger and coming back with a bad attitude (which would have been counterproductive to her goal), Kim used her EQ to take control of the situation. She tried to identify what in her behavior had triggered the negative vibes, and was determined to show the group who she really was. Months later, the group all laughed about the difficult position they all had been put in.

Understanding the Subskills of Emotional Intelligence

EQ, as defined by Bradberry and Greaves (2009), includes two different skill sets: personal competence and social competence (Table 3-1). By understanding and mastering these skill sets, we can ensure social success at work and in our private lives.

Understanding Personal Competence

Personal competence involves how we manage our own behaviors in response to situations. This combines the mastery of two broad skills: self-awareness and self-regulation (or self-management). Within these two subskills are a number of competencies that must be mastered to maximize EQ.

Self-awareness is the understanding of one's internal state, preferences, resources, and intuitions. While we would like to think that we are aware of our feelings at all times and are in control of our responses, unfortunately that is usually not the case. Self-awareness involves being aware of our mood and our thoughts about our mood (Goleman, 1994, p. 47). It is a nonjudgmental attention to our inner state. Situations that elicit strong emotions in an individual (such as anger, hurt, fear, sadness, or shame) require thoughtful self-reflection to prevent an emotional, out-of-control reaction that could prove counterproductive to important relationships. To control our behavior, we must be aware of what we feel and what we are going to do about these feelings. For example, Jon, a certified occupational therapy assistant, was working with a patient using the standing table. He left the patient momentarily to get an activity for the patient to carry out while using the equipment. Upon his return, Jon found that his patient had been taken off the device and put back in his wheelchair by Chase, the senior occupational therapist, so that he could use the equipment with his patient. Jon was in a rage, as this was the third time that one of his patients was removed from equipment without conferring with him. His inclination was to confront Chase then and there, but he wisely decided to stay quiet until the problem could be addressed at a more appropriate time. In this case, Jon used his self-awareness to determine that he was really angry and needed to do something but wanted to give himself time to choose the most appropriate and helpful reaction at the right time.

Self-regulation or *self-management* involves using your self-awareness to direct your behavior in a positive direction. Rather than responding emotionally to a situation, you take the time to think out and control your responses to pursue larger, more important goals. To do this, you must be able to demonstrate self-control, adaptability, and innovation. In the previous case, Jon decided to approach Chase during one of their breaks to say he had a problem with his behavior and would appreciate it if he checked in with him before removing one of his patients from an activity. Jon and Chase had a productive discussion and resolved their differences. In this case, Jon's self-regulation skills ensured that he got the outcome he sought without undermining his own reputation by responding impulsively with anger.

Understanding Social Competence

Social competence involves how we handle our relationships with others. This requires mastering the following skill sets:

* *Empathy.* Empathy requires personal awareness of self and understanding of others' feelings, needs, and concerns. The inability to register another's feelings is a major deficit in EQ. All relationships are built on rapport, caring, and emotional attunement. The ability to be empathic is an extremely important indicator for success in all of life's arenas, but especially in the health care field. An example of an empathic response might be a situation in which you notice your colleague seems upset. Rather than ignoring the situation, you make contact with him or her in a private space and ask if everything is okay. When the coworker shares a problem with you, you offer to go out to lunch to talk about it. You are recognizing the other person's discomfort and are offering support and an opportunity to let the individual share burdens, if they choose, in a nonintrusive manner.

* *Social awareness.* To be socially aware, one must observe and listen to people and intuit information based on what people are saying, how they are acting, and what they are doing (nonverbally). By observing, listening, and intuiting, you are able to make connections that are appropriate for where the person is at that moment. You must be able to recognize the emotions of others; connect and respond appropriately to their feelings, motives, and concerns; judge their reactions; and respond based on all of the information you are processing about them. In the previous example, you noticed that something was bothering your colleague. You were able to pick up on cues and develop an appropriate response that strengthened the relationship between the two of you. The following are four aspects of social awareness:

  a. *Empathy.*

  b. *Attunement.* Involves listening with full involvement and a sustained presence that facilitates rapport and understanding.

  c. *Empathic accuracy.* Through empathy and attunement, you are able to understand what someone else is feeling and thinking. The most successful people in all fields exhibit strong skills in this area. For example, Linda, an occupational therapist, makes a presentation to a group of colleagues about a patient with whom she is working. During the presentation, she is aggressively challenged by a physical therapist who does not agree with her treatment approach. While Linda was well versed in the case and had thoughtfully considered her treatment plan, she was unhinged by what she perceived as an attack. After the meeting, she was called into her supervisor's office. Her supervisor, intuiting how upset she was, gently spoke to her about the presentation and asked her how she felt about it. The supervisor supported her reality about the inappropriate aggressiveness on the part of the physical therapist and went on to reveal how, in her past, she was similarly embarrassed during a presentation. She offered to help Linda prepare for the next presentation. In this case, the supervisor understood what Linda had gone through and had empathetically supported her and offered assistance for the future.

d. *Social cognition.* This involves exhibiting an understanding of how the social world actually works. People adept at this will know what is expected in most social situations and are able to decode the social signals that are put forth by others. To master this skill, one must be able to gather relevant information and develop the best solutions to social problems and issues. For example, an administrator was fired from a subacute facility for unknown causes. The rehabilitation manager at the facility liked and admired the administrator and contacted him following his firing to commiserate and offer her support and assistance in his finding another position. While she genuinely wanted to help, she intuitively knew that supporting him in his time of distress might be helpful to her career going forward. One month later, he got another job at a larger, more prestigious facility. The first thing he did was call the rehabilitation manager from his old facility to discuss a possible managerial position at the new facility. In this case, although she was not looking for any benefit in the short run, she understood that supporting him at a time when he did not have a position might strengthen their relationship and provide positive benefits in the future (Goleman, 2006).

- *Relationship management.* This involves an awareness of your own emotions and those of others in order to manage interactions successfully, ensure clear communication, and effectively handle conflict. People with strong relationship management skills see the benefit of connecting with different people, even those they do not particularly like in order to build bonds. Solid relationships add to your professional and personal life. Success in this area is the result of how you understand people, how you treat them, and the history you share (Bradberry & Greaves, 2009). The stronger your connection, the easier it is to get your point across. Work relationships can be difficult. Conflicts at work often fester, as people lack the skills needed to initiate constructive conversations. Conflict, anger, and frustration can lead to explosive situations. Relationship management provides you with the skills needed to avoid negative scenarios and make the most of every personal interaction you have.

  ◇ For example, Donna was hoping to be assigned a student to supervise for a fieldwork experience. She was disappointed that she was passed over for a colleague with less experience. Rather than acting out her frustration, she decided to request a meeting with her supervisor to address this perceived slight. She shared her disappointment honestly and directly and asked for feedback or suggestions for how she could improve and prepare so that she might be assigned a student the next time. Although she was upset, she approached the situation with strong initiative, openness, honesty, and maturity.

- *Social skills.* These are used to elicit desirable responses in others. Subskills include influence, communication, conflict management, leadership, change promotion, mindset, bond building, collaboration, and cooperation (Goleman, 2008). People who are able to make good social impressions are able to make connections with others by detecting and responding appropriately to people's feelings, motives, and concerns (which leads to rapport). They can fine tune their social performance in response to other people's reactions to make sure they are having the desired effect and can negotiate solutions and prevent conflicts. These people are usually natural leaders who are able to organize groups in productive ways.

Improving Your Emotional Intelligence

Unlike IQ, the skills needed for EQ can be honed and improved upon. In *Emotional Intelligence 2.0*, Bradberry and Greaves (2009) deliver a comprehensive step-by-step self-help program to increase EQ. By strengthening the four core skills—self-awareness, self-management, social awareness, and relationship management—you can reach your goals and achieve your fullest potential in work and in life. The following is a summary of ways to evaluate yourself and improve upon your skills.

Table 3-2

TWENTY COMPETENCIES FOR EMOTIONAL INTELLIGENCE

COMPETENCY
SELF-AWARENESS
1. **Emotional Self-Awareness:** Recognizes feelings and how feelings affect ourselves, our relationships, and our job performance
2. **Accurate Self-Assessment:** Recognizes strengths and shortcomings and focuses on how to improve
3. **Confidence:** Presents in an assured, forceful, impressive, and unhesitating manner
SELF-MANAGEMENT
4. **Emotional Self-Control:** Stays calm, unflappable, and clear-headed in high-stress situations
5. **Trustworthiness:** Openly admits faults or mistakes and confronts unethical behavior
6. **Adaptability:** Is comfortable with ambiguities and adapts to new challenges
7. **Conscientiousness:** Takes personal responsibility to make sure that tasks are completed
8. **Achievement Orientation:** Works through obstacles and takes risks to continually improve
9. **Initiative:** Seizes or creates opportunities for the future
SOCIAL AWARENESS
10. **Empathy:** Understands others' perspectives; is open to diversity
11. **Organizational Awareness:** Understands the political forces and unspoken rules at work
12. **Service Orientation:** Is proactive about customer satisfaction and addresses underlying needs
RELATIONSHIP MANAGEMENT
13. **Developing Others:** Gives timely and constructive feedback; mentors
14. **Inspirational Leadership:** Communicates a compelling vision; inspires other to follow
15. **Influence:** Finds the right appeal to build buy-in; develops a network of influential parties
16. **Change Catalyst:** Leads change efforts and champions new initiatives
17. **Communication:** Effective give-and-take with others; continually fine tunes his or her delivery
18. **Building Bonds:** Builds strong networks and uses them for answers and support
19. **Conflict Management:** Understands all sides and finds common ideals to endorse
20. **Teamwork and Collaboration:** Is encouraging and draws others into an active commitment for collective effort
Adapted from Bradberry, T., & Greaves, J. (2009). *Emotional intelligence 2.0.* San Diego, CA: TalentSmart Inc.

Self Awareness

Self-awareness strategies involve an understanding of yourself, your motivations, and your emotional triggers and reactions with the assumption that, through understanding, you can control responses and achieve the best social outcomes. Some steps to take (Table 3-2; Bradberry & Greaves, 2009) to improve this subskill include the following:

- Observe how your emotions affect others.
- Lean into your feelings, rather than away from them, to foster understanding.

- Know what pushes your buttons so that you can take control of the situation. Triggers are situations that cause you to get upset, irritated, or impatient. Usually they have involved things other people are doing that irritate you, but sometimes involve the things you notice about yourself. Some examples of possible triggers may include the following:
  - ◇ Getting interrupted
  - ◇ Differing values
  - ◇ Incompetence
  - ◇ Chattiness
  - ◇ Rudeness
  - ◇ Lateness
  - ◇ Sloppiness
  - ◇ Arrogance
  - ◇ Noise (Nadler, 2011)
- Control your triggers. To help you control your triggers to avoid an unpleasant interaction, consider seeking a greater understanding of them. Steps to do this include the following:
  - ◇ Identifying your top triggers.
  - ◇ Determining which triggers create the most intense reactions for you.
  - ◇ Identifying which triggers you have the least patience for.
  - ◇ Identifying which triggers drain you the most (Nadler, 2011).

  By understanding your triggers, you are in a much better position to control them and transfer an emotional response to a more adaptive one.
- Perform an emotional audit. This will help with both self-awareness and self-management. The audit is designed to ask questions that can change your focus when you find yourself in an emotionally charged situation. The goal of the audit is to refocus activity from the "old brain" (amygdala) and provide you with more cognitive control, constructive options, and direction. By asking these questions, you label your thoughts and emotions, bring the issues into your consciousness, evaluate your actions in line with your intentions, and allow yourself to better direct your brain and actions toward a more positive goal (Nadler, 2011). Emotional audit questions include the following:
  - ◇ What am I thinking?
  - ◇ What am I feeling?
  - ◇ What do I want now?
  - ◇ How am I getting in my own way?
  - ◇ What do I need to do differently now (Nadler, 2011, p. 96)?

  For instance, in the example of Kim (the new grad who had to go back for a second interview with the staff who was ambivalent about hiring her), she went through the following process to prepare herself for a difficult situation:
  - ◇ *What was she thinking and feeling?* She was uncomfortable about going back to meet with the staff who she knew were not totally comfortable with hiring her. At first, she considered not going back because she was hurt and angry, but then determined not to let her pride get in the way of a good potential job.
  - ◇ *What did she want?* Kim was very clear that she wanted to work at this facility. It was the dream job for her.
  - ◇ *How was she getting in her own way?* This was a hard one. She had to figure out what she did wrong on the first interview and try to change her behavior. She knew that, when nervous, she sometimes could come off as unfriendly. She also noticed that she was over-dressed for the interview, looking too corporate, which she suspected was off-putting. She

also felt that she talked too much. From her self-analysis, she developed a strategy for the next interview.

◊ *What did she do differently?* First, she changed the way she dressed. While she was not as casual as the staff was, she wore an outfit that would give the appearance that she was ready to work with patients. She came in with a smile and was friendlier with the staff. While waiting for her interview, she noticed one of the therapists struggling with a wheelchair and she offered to help. During the group interview, she made a conscious attempt to listen more, ask questions of the staff, and talk less about herself. At the end of the meeting, she felt that she had done all of the right things and hoped the staff felt the same way.

◆ Check nonverbal communication cues. Your facial expressions, posture, demeanor, clothes, and general appearance say a lot about your internal mechanisms. Try to identify the message you are sending out about yourself. For example, many people do not take criticism well. When feedback is given, an individual may not say anything but may have a smirk or grimace, exhibit poor posture, or turn away from the speaker. This may give the impression that the recipient has an attitude about the feedback. Be aware of your nonverbal responses to ensure that you are not sending the wrong message.

Kim knew that she had a habit of making faces that demonstrated how she was feeling. In the past, when given corrective instruction or constructive criticism, she tended to make a face indicating her annoyance at the feedback. This gave the impression that Kim had a bad attitude and was not open to learning from her mistakes. Going into her fieldwork setting, she was determined that she would make an effort to control her facial responses so she did not give off a negative message. This was not an easy task, but her self-awareness helped her to control her nonverbal behavior to make a good impression on her supervisor.

◆ Seek feedback. There is often a difference between how you see yourself versus how others see you. The most accurate way to see yourself is to ask people who know and work with you to provide feedback. This can be a scary process—finding out what people really think and how they perceive you can be difficult to hear. It is not easy for those providing the feedback either because they are risking their relationship with you. Some questions to ask about yourself include the following:

◊ Are there specific situations where I tend to let my emotions get the best of me?

◊ Is there anything I do too much of? Do I have annoying behaviors? Is there anything I need to tone down?

◊ What do you think is holding me back from managing my emotions effectively?

(Adapted from Bradberry & Greaves, 2009, pp. 127-128.)

Rather than responding defensively, which is normal, try to open up to the feedback and learn from it. Through this willingness, you can reach a new level of self-awareness.

◆ Identify how you handle stress. Are you someone who can handle multiple variables at the same time or do you fly off the handle when asked to do more than one thing? How do you respond to stressful situations? It is helpful to know this so you can control your responses when you find yourself facing such circumstances.

For example, one day, Janet's supervisor assigned her six new admissions and instructed her to schedule and complete the evaluations that same day. She was feeling very stressed about her ability to complete the work and as a result was acting out by screaming at the transporters who were not able to deliver the patients as per her schedule. They in turn responded in anger and lost the motivation to go out of their way to help Janet out of her dilemma. Rather than panic and act out, it would have been more productive for Janet to identify that she sometimes loses it when under stress and develop a plan to get control of the situation. With better self-awareness, she would have been able to speak to her supervisor, acknowledge the importance of completing her work, and share her concern that it might not be possible to complete all evaluations in one day. This way, the supervisor would be informed of the situation and could have helped Janet prioritize, thus reducing her stress. Janet could then attempt to work collaboratively with the transporter, explaining to him what she needed to do, and ask for his suggestions to get the patients down on time. Through self-awareness, she would be able to make changes in her behavior, resulting in a better outcome for herself and the department.

Self Regulation

Self-regulation or self-management strategies involve using your new-found self-awareness to control your responses to situations. Rather than respond impulsively, competency in this area results in an ability to stay composed and calm when involved in stressful situations. This is a crucial skill to master, as the loss of emotional self-control in an impulsive moment can have negative long-term effects on your relationships and career.

For example, Susan, a certified occupational therapy assistant, was very angry at her supervisor for giving her the most difficult patients to work with. However, Susan never confronted her supervisor, continued to accept the caseloads assigned, and felt her anger mount. One day, a new patient was admitted with a particularly difficult diagnosis along with behavioral management issues. Again, the patient was assigned to Susan. Upon reviewing the referral, she stormed into her supervisor's office, who was meeting with a family member, and started yelling that she is sick and tired of being abused and she refuses to accept this referral. The supervisor was surprised and upset at Susan's reaction and took a mental note about the outburst and her lack of self-control. Unbeknownst to Susan, her supervisor was considering her to supervise fieldwork students because of her strong work ethic and clinical skills, but had second thoughts after this incident. Her lack of self-control had a negative effect on her work situation.

To master your self-regulation skills, consider some of the following suggestions:

- Be aware of your own cues indicating that you are being triggered (see previous example) and catch yourself before the buildup of emotions. For example, when getting angry, one might experience certain physical reactions, such as hyperventilating, crying, or developing stomach pains. Knowing what your signals are can help you go into action to get control over your emotions and the situation in that moment.

- Breathe diaphragmatically. When you find yourself in a stressful or emotional situation, try this technique. It brings more oxygen to the brain, reduces stress, and gives perspective on the situation.

- Count to 10. When feeling yourself getting angry, frustrated, and ready to react to a situation, try counting to 10 while breathing. This will cool down your system and give your rational brain time to catch up. It could prevent you from saying something you may regret later.

- Sleep on it. Time brings clarity and perspective and helps you gain control over your emotions.

- Smile and laugh more. A smile can trick your brain into thinking that you are happy. When you are stuck on a frustrating or distressing thought, force yourself to smile. It will help counteract your negative emotional state.

- Set aside time for problem solving. Decisions made during a busy day are never as effective as those made with planning and clarity. Set aside some time in your schedule for problem solving to ensure your decisions are not being impacted by your emotions.

- Take control of your negative self-talk. Negative self-talk can be self-defeating and can send you into a downward emotional spiral, making it difficult to meet your goals. Try the following techniques to turn thoughts around:
  ◊ Turn "I always" or "I never" into "just this time" or "sometimes." For example, change "I always screw up when I make a splint" to "I had a problem fabricating this splint—next time I should be more careful when creating the template so I do not repeat my mistake."

⬦ Replace judgmental statements like, "I'm an idiot" with factual ones like, "I made a mistake."

◆ Learn lessons from all encounters. Be aware of situations and conversations that put you on the defensive. Rather than denying the situation and not taking responsibility for your actions, pay attention to the encounter and see what you can learn about yourself from it. Determine how you could change your response or behavior to achieve a better outcome. For example, when being given negative feedback, rather than making excuses for yourself, ask for specific examples so that you can understand the feedback. Then, go a step further by saying, "Let me get a pad and paper so that I can write this down to avoid the same mistake in the future." (Adapted from Bradberry & Greaves, 2009, p. 97-134.)

Social awareness requires looking outward to recognize and appreciate the emotions of others. This involves putting yourself in the other person's shoes to understand where he or she is coming from and responding in a manner that demonstrates sensitivity and understanding of the person and the situation. In addition to verbal cues, social awareness involves observation of body language, expressions, and tone of voice to uncover important information about the other person.

The following strategies will help to sharpen your skills in the area of social awareness:

◆ Greet people by name. This is one of the most basic and important social awareness strategies. It breaks down barriers, acknowledges who people are, and illustrates your connectedness. For example, Craig, an occupational therapist, enters the dining room of a skilled nursing facility to find out how a patient is eating. He approaches an aide and asks, "How is Mrs. Keene feeding herself?" The aide responds, "Hello to you, too," clearly annoyed. A better approach would have been, "Hi Joey. How are you doing today? I have to do an assessment on Mrs. Keene's feeding skills. Think you can help me?" Guaranteed, you will get much more cooperation while fostering an important ally on the floor.

◆ Stay attuned to body language. Body language is the unspoken way that people show how they are feeling. By assessing body language, we can garner important information about a person and prepare an appropriate response. Body language can show you when it is time to end a conversation or that you are making someone uncomfortable. Be aware and respond accordingly.

◆ Be attuned to timing. The adage goes "timing is everything." When dealing with people, you need to assess whether it is the right time to ask what you are asking. If you know someone just got bad news or is stressed out, it is not in your interest to ask about an unrelated issue. Always consider the timing, the question, and the person's frame of mind.

◆ Plan ahead for social events. Participation in work-oriented social events can help develop workplace connections. Be aware that these events are not just for fun, but also serve as networking opportunities. Prepare for events with a behavioral plan for yourself (e.g., not more than one glass of wine, speaking to at least five new people, connecting with people who seem lost or out of place). Prepare some conversation starters to help you make connections. These can be based on such things as recent news events, issues at your facility, or recent health care legislation. The preparation will allow you to be more comfortable and to demonstrate your social awareness skills.

◆ Practice your listening skills. Listening is about hearing the words, along with the tone, speed, and volume of the voice. When someone is speaking to you, stop and listen. Look the person in the eye and remain fully engaged until he or she is finished speaking. Do not interrupt to answer a call, look at your phone to see who is texting you, or look around at what you may be missing. If you are on the phone speaking to someone, do not multitask by reading or answering e-mails or do anything else that will distract you from the conversation. Always remain focused on the person and what he or she is saying. *The ability to listen intently is probably one of the most important skills that contribute to your success in work and life.*

- Understand the rules and culture of your workplace. As discussed in Chapter 1, this is an important determinant of success at work. Every facility has its own set of rules and expectations. You must learn the rules of the culture by taking time to listen, observe, and understand them. If you are the new kid on the block, think long and hard before you jump in to say or do something controversial. Ask lots of specific questions to be sure that you gain an understanding of what is and is not acceptable in your environment

- Try to understand how others feel. This helps to develop a better understanding of your colleagues and patients, improves your communication skills, guides your interactions, and helps identify problems before they escalate (Bradberry & Greaves, 2009, pp. 135-175).

Relationship management strategies are important in order to achieve success in any work environment. Establishing and maintaining positive relationships with as many of the players at work as possible—from the transporter to the director of the department—can help you in innumerable ways. The following are some relationship management strategies you can use to improve your skills in this area:

- Be open and curious. Share information about yourself and show curiosity about other people. Ask questions to find out more about them and listen to their answers. Use this information in future encounters. People love when you remember something about them—especially when it refers to their family, pets, and vacations.

- Little niceties go a long way. Incorporate "please," "thank you," and "I'm sorry" into your interpersonal relationships. They make people feel appreciated and validated.

- Learn how to take feedback. Feedback can help us improve our performance and our relationships. However, many people are uncomfortable with receiving feedback and become defensive when it is provided. Try to listen to feedback, ask clarifying questions to better understand what is being said, and thank the person for being willing to share his or her observations. After you receive the feedback, reflect upon it, evaluate whether there is some validity to it, and integrate it into your actions. If you have learned something that has changed your behavior or actions, share the information with the person providing the feedback. They will love hearing that you heard them, integrated what they shared with you, and put it into action.

- Build trust with your coworkers. Trust takes time to build and can be lost in a moment. Trust is built with open communication; a willingness to share; consistency in words, actions, and behavior; and reliable follow-through. Trust takes time, and the more you prove yourself trustworthy, the more trustworthy you become.

- Show you care. Do not be afraid to acknowledge people who you admire or who have been particularly helpful or supportive. The simplest gesture can make a big impact and will strengthen your relationship.

- Try to repair a "broken" conversation. When things go wrong and mistakes are made, blame abounds. It is best to try to repair the problem with a "fix it" statement. This may require acknowledging the mistake and identifying solutions. Do not worry about proving yourself right. Think about neutralizing the situation, acknowledging and repairing it. For example, you might want to say, "Maybe I spoke too quickly" or "Maybe my perception is wrong on this." (Adapted from Bradberry & Greaves, 2009, pp. 179-223.)

Read this section a number of times. Think about examples for each of the areas you have encountered in your clinical experiences. Consider your responses and how you could have improved on them.

EMOTIONAL INTELLIGENCE DERAILERS

EQ derailers are attitudes or behaviors that can impact an individual's performance or advancement. These derailers can undermine a whole set of EQ competencies. They must be identified and ameliorated to ensure success in the workplace (Nadler, 2011).

Do you recognize yourself in any of the following descriptions?

- "Smartest person in the room" syndrome: Has to be right all the time, is married to his or her ideas, and is not open to or is distrusting of new ideas
- Lack of impulse control: Emotional reactive, volatile, abrasive, and follows urges to an unhealthy extreme
- Drives others too hard: Micromanages and takes over rather than delegates
- Perfectionism: Sets unrealistic goals; rejects criticism
- Defensive: Blames others; is inflexible and argumentative
- Risk averse: Lacks courage to take risks
- Failure to learn from mistakes: The same kind of mistakes show up over and over again
- Lacks insight into others: Cannot read others' emotions or reactions
- Does not ask for feedback: Misses opportunities to include others for better decisions
- Self-promotion: Is attention seeking; overlooks others' accomplishments for own recognition
- Lack of integrity: Dishonest with self and others
- Failure to adapt to cultural differences: Does not change leadership style appropriately
- Indirect with others: Does not give truthful feedback or initiate difficult, truthful conversations with people
- Approval dependent: Needs too much approval before making decisions
- Eccentricity: Unpredictable and odd in behavior
- Mistreats others: Callous, demeaning, or discounting to others and their needs
- Self-interested: Acts in self-interest instead of in the interest of the whole organization or larger group (Nadler, 2011)

Actions to Avoid in the Workplace

Goldsmith (2007), in his book *What Got You Here Won't Get You There*, outlined a list of typical negative work behaviors that are often counterproductive to building supportive, positive relationships. Check yourself against the list to see if you recognize yourself in any of them.

- Passing judgment or making destructive comments. Cutting or sarcastic remarks are never productive. Before speaking, ask yourself if the comment will help the person you are talking to or about. If the answer is no, keep the comment to yourself.
  - Example: Bettyann, an occupational therapist, and Michael, a physical therapist, are working with the same patient who has increased tone in both upper extremities. Part of the treatment plan is for each discipline to perform passive range of motion to both upper extremities. One day, Michael measures the upper extremity range and finds that a contracture has developed. He approaches Bettyann and says accusingly, "George developed a contracture in his elbow. Obviously, you don't know what you are doing." From that one statement, Michael is exhibiting blaming, judgmental, and negative behaviors. In one act, he destroyed his relationship with Bettyann, which impacted on his relationship with the entire occupational therapy department.
- Speaking when angry. When you are angry, you are usually out of control. It's better to wait for a time when you have cooled off and are more rational. You do not want to gain a reputation in the workplace for being emotionally volatile. In the previous example, Bettyann

was furious at being blamed for the contracture, but rather than reacting immediately, she walked away to assess the patient. She later approached Michael and confronted him about his inappropriate behavior. This was a more productive approach that resulted in a better collaboration in the future.

◆ Being negative. No matter how great a suggestion, there are always people who are ready to say it will not work. If you respond with "no," "but," or "however," you are probably projecting "I heard you, but you are wrong." A better approach is to listen to the idea or suggestion. Hold your negative opinion until you can evaluate it. In the meantime, say, "That is an interesting idea. Let me digest it." That demonstrates an openness and willingness to consider change.

◆ Making excuses. People who tend to make excuses when mistakes are made typically are trying to avoid responsibility for the problem. They will often put the blame on someone else ("The scheduling clerk forgot to remind me that I had this appointment") or blame an inherent fault in themselves that cannot be helped ("Sorry I'm late; my phone didn't alert me to the appointment"). Neither technique is effective in putting a positive light on you as a professional. Take responsibility for mistakes and offer a solution so it will not happen again. For example, "I have a habit of always being late. I'm starting a new system where I review my calendar and write down a daily schedule so I stay on time."

◆ Refusing to express regret. Many people refuse to apologize because they do not want to acknowledge or admit to making a mistake. By not apologizing, you are basically saying to the wronged party that you do not care about him or her. By apologizing, you turn the wronged person into an ally. It encourages everyone to let go of the past and it can positively impact feelings about each other. Again, in the earlier example of the clash between the occupational therapist and physical therapist, following the confrontation, the physical therapist saw how his interaction was inappropriate and offered a sincere apology. This led to the resumption of a civil relationship between the two.

◆ Not listening. When you do not listen, you are sending a negative message to the speaker, demonstrating that they are not important. As a result, you are probably missing out on a lot of important information and turning off a potential ally. It has been said already but bears repeating—learning to listen is one of the most important work and life skills you can develop.

◆ Making a virtue of your flaws. We all have weaknesses. Some people make a virtue of their flaws because the flaws constitute what we think of as "me." If we are chronically late or do not return phone calls, we mentally give ourselves a pass every time we repeat this behavior, saying, "Hey, that's me. Deal with it." But it is not about you. It is about what other people think of you or feel about your actions and how those actions impact them. Consider what other people think about your inconsiderate behaviors and try to "cure" them. It will greatly improve people's perception of you.

SUMMARY

While many people believe that all you need to do to succeed in the workplace is to be good at what you do, in reality this is not the case. While it is true that, as a therapist, you do need to have strong clinical skills, it is also true that there are many technically skilled therapists. What separates the average from the truly exceptional professionals in the workplace is their emotional intelligence. These attributes allow you to navigate the workplace and the world with "integrity, resilience, goodwill, tenacity, agility, openness, and perspective" (Reed & Stoltz, 2011, p 4).

By committing to an understanding of the skills outlined in this chapter, you dramatically improve your chances of getting, keeping, and flourishing as a professional. While the principles outlined in this chapter are meant to be applied to the workplace, their application will enrich all aspects of your life.

DISCUSSION QUESTIONS/ACTIVITIES

1. Describe a time in fieldwork that you had an encounter with either a client or a colleague that caused you to use self-awareness as a strategy.

2. Identify two (out of the four) social competence skill sets that you will need during your fieldwork as you engage in interactions between you and your colleagues. Explain this exchange in detail to a classmate and see if they agree with your description.

3. Choose one of the following scenarios and role play how you would invoke emotional intelligence skills to improve the outcome.

   ◆ Certified occupational therapy assistant: You are instructed to pick up a patient scheduled for therapy. As you arrive on the floor, you see your patient sitting in his wheelchair by the elevator ready to go. As you start to take the patient away, the nurse calls out for you to leave him there because she needs to administer his medication. The patient asks you to please take him to occupational therapy as he has been waiting for a long time and is eager to begin his session. The nurse instructs you to ignore the patient's pleas. You try to negotiate with the nurse by asking her to either bring the medication down to him or give him his medication right away. The nurse complains to your supervisor that she did not appreciate your attitude and demands on her, and you are reprimanded. How would you handle this situation using your EQ skills? Which skill sets would you specifically invoke?

   ◆ Occupational therapist: You are asked to evaluate a child newly admitted to your pre-school. The child arrives clinging to his mother. You introduce yourself to both of them and explain the process. The child begins to cry and the mother requests that the evaluation be canceled. You have been told that the evaluation is already late, the mother has canceled before, and you must complete it today. What skills would you use to try and turn around the situation?

4. Identify a person at one of your clinical settings with whom you would like to develop a better relationship. What are the consequences of this relationship in terms of job effectiveness and satisfaction if you do not improve on it versus if you succeed at improving it? What has stopped you from addressing the relationship in the past?

   Identify three strategies you would use to address the issues within this relationship.

5. Using the six relationship management strategies as a guide, share a situation that has occurred to you either in a clinical or personal situation where some of these strategies were used to develop or improve a relationship.

6. Everyone has situations that trigger emotions for them. Can you identify what your trigger issues are?

REFERENCES

Bradberry, T., & Greaves, J. (2009). *Emotional intelligence 2.0.* San Diego, CA: TalentSmart Inc.

Goldsmith, M. (2007). *What got you here won't get you there.* New York, NY: Hyperion.

Goleman, D. (1994). *Emotional intelligence.* New York, NY: Bantam Books.

Goleman, D. (2006). *Social intelligence: The revolutionary new science of human relationships.* New York, NY: Bantam Books.

Goleman, D. (2008). *Working with emotional intelligence.* New York, NY: Bantam Books.

Nadler, R. (2011). *Leading with emotional intelligence.* New York, NY: McGraw Hill.

Reed, J., & Stoltz P. (2011). *Put your mindset to work.* New York, NY: Portfolio/Penguin.

Chapter 4

Tuning in to Communication Nuances
Connecting With Clients and Colleagues

LEARNING OBJECTIVES

At the end of this chapter, the reader will be able to:

➤ Describe the benefits of good communication with clients.

➤ Describe the impact of poor communication with clients.

➤ State obstacles to good communication with clients.

➤ Outline the five roles that nonverbal language assumes as part of the communication process.

➤ Name four ways to improve delivery of nonverbal communication.

➤ Name five ways to improve listening skills.

➤ Identify six ways to promote effective conversations.

➤ Name seven considerations to improve written conversation.

➤ Define criteria for improving communication with older individuals.

➤ Identify five ways to overcome language barriers.

Effective communication is the foundation of all successful relationships, whether it is with family and friends or colleagues and patients. As occupational therapists, one of our most important goals is to connect and communicate with our patients so that we can establish rapport before embarking on the therapeutic process. Additionally, we must be able to establish positive relationships with our colleagues and supervisor in order to work collaboratively.

In his book, *Words That Work*, Frank Luntz (2007), world-renowned public opinion guru, presents a simple communication premise—"It's not what you say, it's what people hear" (p. xi). No matter the context—whether it is in a work or social setting—and no matter the message, the receiver will interpret it through the "prism of his or her own emotions, preconceptions, prejudices, and preexisting beliefs" (Luntz, 2007, p. xi). According to Luntz (2007), the key to successful

Davis L, Rosee M. *Occupational Therapy Student to Clinician:*
Making the Transition (pp 47-63).
© 2015 SLACK Incorporated.

communication is to put yourself into your listener's shoes and to know what he or she is thinking and feeling. This chapter will present concrete steps to improve your communication skills—written, verbal, and nonverbal—in order to help you succeed in the workplace with clients and colleagues alike.

THE COMMUNICATION PROCESS

Although we all have been communicating with others since infancy, the process of transmitting information from one to another is very complex with many sources of potential error (Wertheim, 2008). Frequently, the meaning of a communication is lost in the transmission and, as a result, the message heard is often different from the one intended. For example, Judy, a therapist working in a subacute facility, says to an elderly patient, "Try to reach your knees." The patient looks up quizzically at the therapist, not knowing what to do. Judy repeats her instruction with the same results. What Judy does not realize was, when she gave her instruction to the patient to reach her knees, the patient heard, "Try to reach the Bolognese."

The therapist can reach many conclusions from this interchange, including that the patient is unable to reach her knees, the patient is resistant, or the patient has dementia and is unable to follow directions. If Judy had just asked the patient, "Did you hear what I asked?" or, "Could you repeat what I just asked you?" she would have gotten much more accurate information.

The Benefits of Good Communication With Clients

* Builds trust between therapist and patient
* Helps the patient disclose important information
* Enhances patient satisfaction
* Involves the patient more fully in his or her therapeutic program
* Leads to more realistic expectations
* Produces more effective carryover

The Impact of Poor Communication With Clients

* Decreases confidence and trust in the care provided
* Deters the client from revealing important information
* Causes patient distress
* Discourages the patient from seeking further care
* Leads to misunderstandings
* Underlies most patient complaints
* Increases the risk of negligence claims

Therapist-Related Obstacles to Good Communication With Clients

* Inadequate training in communication skills
* Lack of sensitivity or empathy
* Unwillingness to recognize patient autonomy
* Unaware of problems arising from differences in language and culture
* Time pressures

◆ Distractions caused by external or personal factors

Patient-Related Obstacles to Good Communication

◆ Interference based on medical condition (confusion, pain, hearing)

◆ Anxiety, embarrassment, or denial about condition

◆ Inexperience in identifying and describing symptoms

◆ Intimidated by health care setting

◆ Impacted by differences in language and culture

◆ Reluctant to ask questions

◆ Concerned about time pressures

(National Health and Medical Research Council, Commonwealth of Australia, 2004)

What Is "Effective Communication?"

The ability to communicate is one of life's basic requirements. Whether in work or leisure environments, one must learn how to communicate effectively to make meaningful connections. Our ability to communicate helps us understand and care for the people in our lives, resolve conflicts, build trust and respect, promote new ideas, and problem solve. However, we often lack the skills to communicate effectively, leading to conflict and misunderstandings. Effective communication is not limited to what you say and hear, but also relates to the emotion and meaning behind what is said. Effective communication requires a set of skills that include the following:

◆ Awareness of nonverbal communication

◆ Ability to listen

◆ Emotional attunement

◆ Verbal communication skills

◆ Written communication skills

Nonverbal Communication Skills

Nonverbal communication is the process of sending and receiving wordless (and mostly visual) messages between people ("Nonverbal communication," 2004). These nonverbal messages can be communicated through gestures and touch, body language or posture, facial expression, and eye contact. An individual's speech can also contain nonverbal elements, known as *paralanguage*. Paralanguage elements include voice quality, rate, pitch, volume, and speaking style ("Nonverbal communication," 2004). Nonverbal communication is significant because it can sway one's impression of what is being communicated through the unconscious information one is exhibiting rather than through what is actually being said. Often, the message presented through nonverbal communication elements can say more than words.

Empirical research indicates that more than 90% of the meaning we derive from communication comes from the nonverbal. People often say one thing but portray the opposite message through their nonverbal behaviors (Wertheim, 2008).

According to Wertheim (2008), nonverbal communication is made up of the following parts:

◆ *Visual*: This refers to body language, facial expressions, eye movements, posture, and gestures.

◆ *Tactile*: The use of touch to impart meaning, such as a handshake, a pat on the back, or a hug.

◆ *Vocal*: How what you say can be altered based on the tone of voice you use and the emphasis you place on particular words. For example, think of a word such as "no." Then, imagine the different ways it might be said based on emotions such as surprise, anger, terror, or amazement.

Table 4-1

EXAMPLES OF NONVERBAL COMMUNICATION AND ITS IMPACT ON INTERPERSONAL INTERACTIONS

EYE CONTACT	Meeting someone's gaze while talking is generally considered a sign of connectedness and an indication that one is truly listening. It can also be a way of judging whether someone is telling the truth or trying to be deceptive. Note: In some cultures, direct eye contact can be construed as disrespectful or threatening.
BODY POSTURE	How you position your body in relation to another can convey a variety of messages. For example, sitting close to someone can convey caring, but in some cultures, close body contact might be construed as threatening. Standing while talking to someone who is sitting can send the message of authority, while arms crossed while speaking may indicate an attempt at keeping one's distance.
GESTURES	The use of one's body can indicate many things to a recipient in an interaction. The shrug of one's shoulders, nod of the head, rolling of the eyes, or finger pointing are all examples of gestures. Such movements can relate messages of doubt, openness, understanding, displeasure, disinterest, etc. Since gestures are interpreted differently by different cultures, an understanding of their cultural implications will help one to communicate appropriately with clients.
FACIAL EXPRESSIONS	Smiles, frowns, and grimaces are all facial expressions that can send messages to the recipient, indicating happiness, warmth, sincerity, displeasure, pain, sadness, etc. Often, we are unaware of our facial expressions, in which case we may send a message we did not intend.
VOICE TONE AND VOLUME	Louder versus softer vocal tones can indicate many things in an interaction. Louder and higher tones when speaking can indicate anger, frustration and assertiveness. Softer and lower tones can indicate poor self-esteem, fear, or calm, or may even be used as a strategy to gain attention.

Adapted from Jacobs, K., & McCormack, G. (2011). *The occupational therapy manager.* 5th ed. Bethesda, MD: AOTA Press.

- *Physical space*: Most people prefer to have a minimum amount of personal space between themselves and others. The need to mark, protect, and control our territory is highly related to cultural preferences.
- *Image*: Our clothing and physical appearance communicates volumes about us in a nonverbal context.

Werthiem (2008) outlines the five roles that nonverbal language can assume as part of the communication process:

1. Nonverbal language can serve as a substitution for words. For example, when expressing condolences, tears in your eyes may communicate how you are feeling better than the words you use.
2. Nonverbal language can repeat the message the person is making verbally. For example, when agreeing with a statement, one can simultaneously shake his or her head, reinforcing the message.

3. Nonverbal language can complement one's spoken words, such as congratulating someone for a job well done while also patting him or her on the back.

4. Nonverbal language can contradict one's spoken words. For example, telling someone you agree with what he or she is saying while simultaneously shaking your head "no."

5. Nonverbal language can provide further support for a verbal message. For example, when someone bangs his or her hand on the table for emphasis to indicate strong disagreement with something (Wertheim, 2008).

We are often unaware of the nonverbal cues that we are portraying. When observing videos of ourselves, we are often surprised at the nonverbal habits, gestures, and facial expressions we are exhibiting. The good news is that, through awareness of our nonverbal behaviors, we can improve our ability to communicate nonverbally. Some suggestions for facilitating communication through nonverbal means include the following:

- *Make eye contact*: Too little eye contact makes one seem evasive, but too much eye contact can appear intimidating. Communication experts recommend intervals of 4 to 5 seconds of fixed eye contact before changing your gaze (Cherry, 2012).
- *Use gestures*: This is your way of making your entire body talk.
- *Avoid mixed messages*: Make sure your words, gestures, facial expressions, and tone matches your message. Smiling when delivering bad news sends a mixed message. Be in tune with the message that is coming from your lips and from your body.
- *Work on improving control of your body language*: Look at yourself in a mirror while you are speaking to someone, or even better, videotape yourself deep in conversation. You will be able to identify how your body gives off nonverbal cues, what they look like, and what they mean. By understanding your body's mechanisms and typical responses, you can begin to work on controlling them.

Listening

The best way to win friends and influence people is to be more interested in listening to them than you are in impressing them (Goulston, 2009). Listening means not just understanding what someone is saying or the information he or she is trying to impart, but also having insight into what he or she is feeling and what underlies its content. Effective listening can do the following:

- Make the speaker feel heard and understood, which helps build a relationship and connection between yourself and the speaker
- Create a safe environment where people are able to express their ideas and opinions and problem solve in effective ways
- Save time by clarifying information and avoiding conflicts and misunderstandings
- Diffuse negative emotions (Robinson, Segal, & Segal, 2012)

Tips for Effective Listening

- Commit to the listening process. Really listen.
- Focus on the speaker and what he or she is saying, as well as his or her body language and other nonverbal cues. By observing the nonverbal cues, you will get a sense of the speaker's emotional state. This gives insight that allows one to read between the lines.
- Create a receptive listening environment. Eliminate all distractions such as cell phones, turn off the television, and put away reading materials. Provide a quiet environment in which to interact.
- Stop talking. Ask the other person clarifying questions; repeat and rephrase answers to make sure you understand what the person is saying.
- Make eye contact.

- ◆ Avoid interrupting. People like to talk about themselves and get their ideas across. Let others get their thoughts out and focus on what they are saying before you respond. Often, we are so busy thinking about what our response will be that we do not pay attention.
- ◆ Avoid being judgmental. Judging the message during delivery interferes with your ability to listen to it.
- ◆ Show interest in what the person is saying. By nodding, smiling, or exhibiting appropriate nonverbal cues and emotional responses to what is being said, you demonstrate that you are listening.
- ◆ Be alert to your own body language. Are you sending listening signals or distraction signals? Are you glancing away, yawning, crossing your arms, or performing acts of distraction? Be attuned to this. Sit with an open position facing the speaker, look into his or her eyes, smile when appropriate, raise eyebrows, or nod in agreement.

Keep in mind that being a good listener can sometimes take practice. Try to apply these recommendations the next time you are in a position that requires active listening and see how the change in your habits impacts the interaction.

Emotional Attunement

We addressed this extensively in Chapter 3, but it bears repeating again and again, as it is so important to many aspects of your personal life and professional career.

Emotions play an important part in our ability to communicate because the way you feel can impact your ability to communicate effectively. Emotions also affect how you understand others and how they understand you. A lack of insight as to why you feel the way you do, and why you react to situations as you do, will impact your ability to communicate with others. Emotional awareness provides you with the tools to understand yourself and others and gain insight into the messages behind your communication. This is easier said than done. Some people spend a lifetime avoiding their feelings. Others spend a lifetime trying to understand themselves. If you only communicate on a very concrete, rational level, you will be less effective in understanding others, resolving conflicts, or getting your needs met (Robinson, Segal, & Segal, 2012).

You may have read Chapter 3, but this is a good time to go back and read it again!

Verbal Communication Skills

As therapists, the ability to communicate effectively on a face-to-face level is crucial to a successful professional career. In your role as an occupational therapist, you will need to find effective ways to communicate with patients, clients, and colleagues.

Braveman (2006) outlined the following strategies to promote effective conversations:

- ◆ Ask open-ended questions to elicit informative answers and to avoid giving the impression that you have already drawn conclusions.
- ◆ Ask for additional details, examples, thoughts, and impressions to show interest and indicate that you are open to what the speaker has to say.
- ◆ Paraphrase or restate what you have heard. This not only gives the speaker the chance to correct misinterpretations, but it also gives you the chance to more effectively process and understand what has been said.
- ◆ Check your perceptions of what the other person is trying to communicate by objectively describing what you are hearing, avoiding expressions of approval or disapproval.
- ◆ Describe behavior without making accusations or generalizations about motives, attitudes, or personality traits.
- ◆ Clarify agreement and summarize discussions by reviewing what has been decided or agreed upon and any course of action that will be taken (Braveman, 2006, p. 314).

As professionals, strong communication skills represent the most important tool in our arsenal to reach and teach. The manner in which one communicates will impact your effectiveness as a therapist, supervisor, supervisee, and colleague. The following basic rules adapted from Luntz's (2007) *Words That Work* can help improve communication skills:

- Keep your message simple. Use small words. Fancy words may make you sound smart, but they often result in misunderstandings. Texting and Twitter have helped us to simplify our messages. The more simply and plainly an idea is presented, the more understandable it will be.
- Keep your message brief. Use short sentences. Never use a sentence when a phrase will do. Look for the right word to make the message clear and keep in mind that one strong visual cue can replace 1,000 words. When it comes to effective communication, "small beats large, short beats long, and plain beats complex. And sometimes a visual beats them all" (Luntz, 2007, p. 8).
- Consistency and repetition reinforce the message. You said it once, but do not be afraid to say it again, and again, and again. Most people are not paying attention to what you say. If you want your message to sink in, keep repeating it. For example, we typically give patients, and their family, instructions on a home program to carry out independently. After the first set of instructions, we assume that the patient knows what to do to carry out the program. Often, that is not the case. It would be more effective to repeat the instructions and ask for feedback to ensure that the message gets through.
- Offer a new way to communicate an old message. People like novelty and they are easily bored, which is why we like to go on different vacations, go to different restaurants, and spend time with different friends. The same goes for the message. Try to provide a different way to communicate the same message. For example, when teaching a home program to your patient, you might explain it the first time, show a video of someone performing it the second time, and ask the patient to teach it to you the third time. By varying the teaching method, you will improve the carryover.
- Visualize the message. Try to create a message that has a visual component. Learning is more effective when you combine verbal and visual messages. For example, when teaching a home program by combining pictures with demonstration and verbal cues, your patient will be much more likely to perform the program effectively.

Some more verbal communication tips are as follows:

- Slow down. When you speak too quickly, you appear nervous and listeners often miss what you are saying. However, do not slow down so much that your listeners feel the need to finish your sentences for you.
- Animate your voice and be dynamic. Your vocal pitch should go up and down. It should not be monotone. Your volume should change as you speak.
- Enunciate your words. Speak clearly. If people do not understand you and ask you to repeat yourself, consider talking into a recorder and analyzing your speech. You may be able to identify some negative speech patterns.
- Pronounce words correctly and use the right words. People will judge your competency and intelligence through your vocabulary, grammar, and the proper use of words.
- Use gestures to indicate your interest and passion. This helps keep the listener engaged.
- Get your emotions in the right place. If you are bored or tired, you may be inadvertently portraying these negative emotions to the listener. Try smiling to improve your vocal tone. It has been proven that smiles can even improve your mood (as well as your message).

The Power of Apologies

In Mark Goulston's (2009) book, *Just Listen: Discover the Secret to Getting Through to Absolutely Anyone,* he shares how effective a simple "thank you" or an apology can be to improve communication and build relationships.

In the course of working with colleagues and patients, you will inevitably make a mistake that impacts someone in your sphere. Simply saying "sorry," while appreciated, may not always patch things up. The hurt, slight, or omission that was experienced from your act needs to be repaired. That is where the "power apology" comes in. A power apology involves the four Rs:

1. *Remorse*: This involves demonstrating to the person that you acknowledge your responsibility for causing him or her hurt or harm and that you are truly sorry. Allow the person to vent to you without responding defensively. That helps the person to get the anger off of his or her chest. By listening patiently, you are acknowledging through your actions that you understand his or her need to unload. This will speed up the forgiveness process.

2. *Restitution*: Find a way to make amends if possible. If the original issue can be repaired, do whatever is in your power to repair it. If not, try to take an action that demonstrates you are trying to make up for the error you made.

3. *Rehabilitation*, or demonstrating that you learned from the mistake you made and are making amends, can be healing to the party who was wronged. It validates that person's position and demonstrates your good faith in not making the same mistake again.

4. *Requesting forgiveness*: To do this, you must sustain your corrective actions until they are integrated into who you are.

By demonstrating remorse, restitution, and rehabilitation, you are on the road to forgiveness.

The Power of Thank You

Saying "thanks" to someone is almost automatic in response to a kindness shown you—whether someone is holding open a door or e-mailing you a telephone number you have been waiting for. How do you respond when someone has done something exceptional for you? How do you communicate your feelings of gratitude, respect, and affinity? Goulston's (2009) book outlines some suggestions for delivering the "power thank you." These include the following:

- Be specific when thanking someone. Rather than just saying, "Thanks," say, "Thank you so much for covering for me when I got the emergency call from my child's school."
- Acknowledge the effort it took for the person to help you, such as, "I know you have such a busy caseload, plus the special project you are working on. I appreciate how hard it was for you to handle the extra work."
- Tell the person the difference his or her act made to you. "I was so scared when I got the call. Your volunteering to take over my patients relieved some of my anxiety."

The power thank you makes the other person feel truly appreciated and it reflects well on you, showing you to be gracious, appreciative, and empathic (Goulston, 2009).

Written Communication Skills

In the electronic age we live in, the development of strong written communication skills has become more important than ever. The quality of our written communications reveals a lot about who we are. Dependence on the written word means that we are increasingly judged on our ability to communicate through this medium. To make a positive impression, you must be able to produce written communications that are clear, concise, and effective.

E-mail and Text Etiquette

Over the past few years, e-mail and text messages have replaced telephone calls, business memos, and letters as the most common form of communication in both business and personal contexts. While there are many benefits to these forms of communication, they are fraught with potential problems as well. The benefit of emails and text messages is the ease and speed with which communication takes place. Problems and issues can be addressed and answered instantaneously. However, the medium can also contribute to miscommunications because it is missing the "nonverbal cues that add meaning to the spoken word" (Jacobs & McCormack, 2011). For example, the sender may be trying to portray humor, but without tonal and facial cues, a message can be misinterpreted as angry or sarcastic. Emoticons are symbols that help provide clues to the message being portrayed. The most common examples are a smiley face (which indicates some kind of good intent) or the laugh out loud (LOL) shortcut, which indicates that a statement is meant to be humorous.

Braveman (2006) presents a list of strategies to avoid when using an e-mail format:

- Never write or send e-mails or text messages when angry.
- Do not make reference to earlier messages without including them as part of the "message thread."
- Proofread messages before sending.
- Be careful using the "reply to all" feature, especially when responding to group e-mails. You may find yourself sending information to unintended individuals.
- Be sure that abbreviations and emoticons are clear and unambiguous.
- Do not copy or forward a message or attachment without permission from the sender.
- Do not use e-mail or text messages to discuss confidential information.
- Do not send or forward e-mails or text messages containing libelous, defamatory, offensive, racist, or obscene remarks.

Formal Business Letters

The formal business letter is becoming obsolete as e-mails take over as the most efficient form of communication. However, there are times when a formal letter is an appropriate choice, especially when communicating to someone outside of your organization.

A formal business letter should follow a professional format. The letter should be on letterhead that identifies the organization or individual the letter is coming from. In addition, a formal letter should include the following:

- The date.
- A salutation that includes the sender's name, title, organization, and address followed by a salutation using a formal designation such as "Dear Mr. (Ms., Dr., etc.) Smith." Try to avoid "To whom it may concern" as it is nonspecific and does not form a bond between you and the recipient.
- The body of the letter will follow the salutation. The letter should conclude with a closing statement such as "Sincerely" followed by your name.
- Sign the letter in between the closing statement and your typewritten name.
- See a sample letter in Chapter 10.

When preparing to write in any format, consider some of the following variables:

- Consider to whom you are writing. Is it an informal e-mail to a colleague, an official report, or a formal letter? The audience determines your tone. Think about who is reading the document and adopt the appropriate level of formality.
- Create a structure. When preparing a written document, think about what your audience knows about the topic. Figure out a logical order that the reader can follow to ensure that he or she understands the basic concepts, followed by the progression of information. An outline breaking down the information into smaller headings and subheadings will help to clarify and keep the reader's attention. Long paragraphs are difficult to read and impossible to skim. Make it easy for your reader to understand your important points.

- Keep it simple. Write in short, concise sentences and paragraphs. See if you can eliminate words and phrases without interfering with the message. Shorter is almost always better.

- Check your clarity. Make sure that the message you are trying to send is evident in your written document. Read it critically to determine if anything might be misunderstood. If you are unsure, have an unrelated party read it to determine if it is understandable.

- Connect to your readers' priorities and needs. If you are trying to convince readers of something, find an angle to make them care. For example, "I know you are concerned about reducing the cost of your expenditure on adaptive devices in our facility. I have developed a new tracking protocol that will help meet that end." You grab readers by focusing on something that is important to them. This "hook" gives them the motivation to keep reading.

- Proofread. A written document with a lot of spelling and typographical mistakes gives the reader the impression that you are sloppy and do not pay attention to detail. By not carefully proofreading, you undermine your reputation and credibility. Read everything over and over. Try reading the document out loud. This makes it easier to identify mistakes. If the document is really important, ask someone else to read it, both to ensure your content is clear and to identify typos or grammatical errors (Manktelow & Carlson, 1999).

Telephone Communication

Speaking on the telephone at work differs significantly from the way you might conduct yourself at home. While we are typically informal and casual in our telephone communications, you are expected to be more formal and professional at work. For example, when answering the phone in your department, you should provide the caller with information about who you are and where you are. For example, "Occupational Therapy, Susan speaking. How can I help you?" When answering the phone at your desk, it is proper to answer with a salutation and your name, "Good morning, Susan speaking." This type of salutation orients the caller to who is on the phone and the department. Your facility may have a preferred way of answering the telephone, so ask your supervisor if there is any formalized approach to telephone etiquette.

Ringing phones can be very annoying as they can interrupt the flow of your activity. The caller is assuming and expecting that you are ready, willing, and able to speak at that moment. By answering the call, you may be forced to break into a live conversation, making someone in your environment wait while you deal with what the caller wants. With today's technology, most phones come with a voicemail feature. By using voicemail, you make the determination of when it is most efficient and practical for you to return the call. When recording your greeting, make sure it is professional. Include your full name and department, and request the caller to leave a message and a telephone number so that you can return the call. Do not forget to call back in a timely manner. The following are some tips for professional phone communication:

- Be prepared to answer the phone by having notepaper and a pen available. This ensures that you get all of the important information, should there be a message, and helps to ensure that the message gets delivered accurately and to the correct party.

- Record your greeting as naturally and professionally as possible, using a friendly tone of voice.

- Do not use words that you are not familiar with in an attempt to sound more intelligent. This could backfire if you pronounce the words incorrectly.

- Do not interrupt the person on the phone. If you must jump in, be sure to say "excuse me" and explain why you are interrupting.

- Listen. Do not text, read, send e-mails, or do anything else when on the phone. The listener can usually tell. Focus on what is being said so that you follow-up or respond appropriately ("How to Sound Professional...," 2012).

PRESENTING TO COLLEAGUES

One of the most frightening events for many therapists is to give a presentation to a group of colleagues. To reduce anxiety and improve communication skills, note the following suggestions.

Preparation

- Find out about your audience. How many will attend and how much does your audience know about the presentation's subject? Make sure that your presentation matches their knowledge level. It should not be too complicated or too simple.
- Determine the expectations of the group.
- Identify where and how you will present. Will the venue affect how you need to prepare?
- Do you have the knowledge to present on the subject? If not, how will you build this knowledge?
- Do you have everything you need for the presentation, such as audiovisual equipment, Internet access, or a projector and screen?
- Does your introduction grab the audience?
- Do you clearly lay out what you intend to get across in the presentation?
- Are the main points in a logical sequence?
- Do the points flow well?
- Do you need to support the main points with visual aids?
- Do you summarize the presentation's conclusion?
- Is the conclusion strong?
- Do you tie the conclusion to the introduction?
- Is your presentation too complex?
- Does it contain jargon that might be confusing?

Practicing

- Have you practiced your presentation? Have you paid close attention to your body language during your practice sessions?
- Have you rehearsed enough to speak smoothly and fluently?
- Have you practiced in front of others? This should be done so that you may receive feedback about your performance.

Presentation Day

- Are your slides, notes, and visual aids in the right order?
- Are you dressed and groomed appropriately?
- Have you left enough time for travel and setup (if applicable)?
- Have you developed a strategy to handle your nervousness?

While Presenting

- Smile and start with a statement that communicates to the audience who you are and what you will be covering.
- Give eye contact to members of the audience.

- Provide handouts (if appropriate) to help the audience follow the presentation and eliminate their need to take notes.
- Use a PowerPoint presentation. By looking at a PowerPoint, the audience takes their eyes off of you and focuses them in another direction.
- Speak clearly at a volume that is appropriate for the room and with an even tone of voice.
- Rely on your notes but do not read the presentation. There is nothing more boring to an audience than a read presentation.

Post-Presentation

- Have you made sure your audience understands your message and have you asked if they have any questions?
- Do you need to follow up with any audience members (Mindtools, 2009)?

COMMUNICATING WITH CLIENTS/PATIENTS

Communication is the key to establishing a therapeutic relationship with the clients with whom you will be working. The therapeutic relationship consists of several components from both your perspective as the practitioner and the client's perspective. One of the most important components is the establishment of a trusting relationship from the outset. The first step in this important goal is establishing communication between the therapist and the client. The relationship with the client is not casual—it is based on the exchange of information that is client focused and time limited (Napier, 2011). Like communication with colleagues, therapeutic communication includes components that are verbal and nonverbal. The development of therapeutic communication with patients will promote motivation and contribute to achieving the best outcomes.

When dealing with patients, the communication process can be further complicated by age and language barriers. When working with an aging population, it is important to consider the physical changes that impact the communication process. The following suggestions, while geared toward the aging client, can actually prove effective in improving communication with any client population with whom you are working.

Tips for Communication With Older Patients

- Allow extra time so your communication is not rushed.
- Avoid distractions. Make sure your time spent with the patient is quality time. Give him or her your undivided attention. Reduce the amount of visual and auditory distractions by conducting your meeting in a quiet environment. Turn off your phone and beeper to avoid interruptions.
- Sit face-to-face. Older patients often have visual and hearing loss. By positioning yourself at their level, you reduce distractions and facilitate communication.
- Maintain eye contact.
- Listen to what the patient is telling you. Do not interrupt the patient when speaking or asking questions.
- Speak slowly, clearly, and loudly. Older people often learn at a slower rate than a younger person. Do not rush through instructions and make sure you are being heard. If you doubt the client comprehends, ask him or her to repeat instructions. Keep in mind that older people are often too embarrassed to ask you to repeat instructions.
- Use short, simple words and sentences.

- Stick to one topic at a time. Information overload can confuse patients. Instead of a long detailed explanation, try to provide the information in an outline form.
- Simplify your instructions and write them down in an easy-to-follow format.
- Use charts, models, and pictures. Visual aids help patients understand your instructions.
- Summarize the most important points.
- Give patients an opportunity to ask questions and express concerns (Robinson, White, & Houchins, 2006).

Tips for Communicating With Children

- Put aside time at the beginning of the consultation to build rapport.
- Listen to and involve the parents.
- Use clear and appropriate language based on the child's age and abilities.
- Let the child take the lead as to where he or she is most comfortable during the assessment (e.g., playing with toys, on a parent's lap).
- Try to maintain yourself at the same level as the child.
- Use an open and collaborative approach incorporating play.
- Take children seriously and do not be patronizing.
- Offer support and praise.
- Be gentle and cue into the child's and parent's pace and needs.

(Adapted from Skillscascade, 2002.)

The Importance of Transcultural Communication

Working with people of differing cultures is a fact of life in health care and an ongoing learning process. No matter the setting, most of us will interact with people from different ethnicities, races, and cultures who may not share our methods of communicating. Many of these people have different culturally influenced patterns of behavior and expectations of the medical system (Luckman, 2000). "To communicate effectively with clients and colleagues from other cultures, it is important to learn about the beliefs and values of different cultural groups, recognize the barriers to transcultural communication, and practice a variety of trans-cultural communication techniques" (Luckman, 2000, p. xi). This topic will be reviewed in detail in Chapter 7.

Overcoming Barriers to Communication

In addition to culture, language, literacy, and physical/cognitive deficits can prove to be a barrier to communication and impact therapy outcomes. As clinicians, it is important that we take the time to get to know our clients and understand their strengths and limitations to ensure that we are able to interact in a manner that leads to the therapeutic outcomes we are seeking (Luedtke, 2012). In addition to accommodating physical and cognitive barriers (for which we receive extensive training as occupational therapists), we will frequently experience barriers relating to language and literacy (Luedtke, 2012).

Language Barriers

It is projected that more than 49 million Americans (18% of United States residents) speak a language other than English at home, with more than 22 million exhibiting limited English proficiency (Flores, 2006). These numbers are even higher in certain parts of the country, such as New York, Florida, and California, where the immigrant population is highest. Language barriers have a definitive deleterious effect on a patient's health care provision. Patients who have limited

English proficiency are more likely to get an incorrect diagnosis and are at greater risk of nonadherence to medication regimens.

Under Title VI of the Civil Rights Act of 1964, discrimination on the basis of national origin is prohibited. The act also guarantees that adequate language assistance must be provided to patients with limited English proficiency. Unfortunately, the availability of translators is limited, especially when dealing with less commonly encountered languages. Often, family members (including children of patients), friends, untrained staff, or strangers are used in clinical encounters to provide interpretation services. These interpreters often have no training in medical terminology or confidentiality, and their presence can inhibit discussions regarding sensitive issues.

To improve communication with clients and patients who have limited English proficiency, review the following tips:

- Identify a client's preferred language at your first encounter.
  - Ask the client for his or her preferred spoken and written language.
  - Display a poster of common languages spoken by clients. Ask your client to point to his or her language of preference.
  - Post translated information relating to the availability of interpreter services and use trained interpreters whenever possible.
- Overcome language barriers.
  - Use simple words; avoid jargon and acronyms.
  - Limit the use of and/or avoid technical language.
  - Articulate words completely.
  - Repeat important information.
  - Provide educational material in the languages your patients read.
  - Use pictures, demonstrations, video, or audiotapes to increase understanding.
  - Give information in small chunks and verify comprehension.
  - Always try to confirm the patient's understanding of the information provided.

(Adapted from Scan Health Plan, 2012.)

Establishing an Environment for Optimal Communication With Patients/Clients

- Approach your patient/client slowly and professionally.
- Make sure that you are sitting at the same level as your patient/client. This communicates that you are with him or her. Do not hover over your patient/client as this sets up an atmosphere of a power inequity that does not demonstrate an empathic approach. It implies that you are in charge and he or she is lesser than you. Your goal is to establish trust and rapport that communicates, "I care about you."
- Introduce yourself, your profession, why you are there, what you are planning to do, and what you expect of your patient/client.
- Be aware of cultural nuances for both parties. Perhaps the patient's religion prevents hand shaking with someone of the opposite sex. If so, respect that and do not attempt to shake hands. Your culture may limit eye contact with an older person, yet the patient may need to see your eyes while talking to you to develop a bond of trust. Read more about this in Chapter 7.

These simple steps will set the stage for a trusting therapeutic relationship.

Literacy Barriers

Health literacy (Luedtke et al., 2012, p. 18) refers to "the degree to which individuals have the capacity to obtain, process, and understand basic health information needed to make appropriate health decisions and (choose) services needed to prevent or treat illness." Some clients may have difficulty understanding information and following directions, which can impede the success of the therapeutic intervention.

As clinicians, we need to assess our client's level of understanding and ensure that our instructions are appropriate for the client's comprehension level. This is especially true when designing home programs that clients will be expected to carry out on their own. When designing educational materials, consider your clients' cognitive abilities, communication skills, and level of education. Cotugna, Vikery, and Carpenter-Haefele (2005) suggest that educational materials provided for clients should be geared to a fifth- or sixth-grade reading level. This improves compliance for all clients by ensuring that instructions are easy to follow (Luedtke, 2012).

SUMMARY

The ability to effectively communicate with your patients and clients will predict how effectively you will be able to motivate and teach them. This will have a direct impact on the achievement of functional outcomes. These same communication skills will impact your standing as a member of your professional team.

Communication is a complicated process that involves more than just what you say. It also involves how you listen, how you portray yourself, how you connect to others, and how you express yourself verbally and in writing. By understanding the components of effective communication, and through practice and discipline, you can improve these skills and become a more effective therapist, coworker, and team member.

DISCUSSION QUESTIONS/ACTIVITIES

1. Write a professional e-mail to the director of rehabilitation, asking him or her whether you can transfer to the subacute unit from the outpatient unit. Explain your reasoning to convince him or her to respond favorably to your request. Send the e-mail to five people you are familiar with to get their feedback on its effectiveness.

2. Partner with a classmate. Prepare an oral report about a fictitious patient's condition and treatment. Present the oral report to your partner for two minutes. Ask for feedback on your performance. Was it easy to follow and understand? Were you presenting any nonverbal cues that enhanced or detracted from the presentation? Did you seem confident and comfortable?

3. Reflect on a time when you felt you were not heard when communicating with someone either face-to-face by phone or via e-mail. What do you think went wrong—the content, choice of words, lack of tone, facial expression? Elaborate on the interaction and what you could have done to communicate differently.

4. Think about a time you interacted with someone you did not know. What did you do to establish the interaction? Describe how you accomplished the connection. How did the person respond to your overture?

5. Review the following scenarios and then answer the questions that follow:

   ◊ *Scenario 1*: You are working with a patient and two others are waiting to start their therapy session with you. The patient you are working with needs to go to the bathroom. Typically, you take the patient and use the experience as activities of daily living (ADL) training. However, today, because of the backup of patients, you are concerned it will take too long. One of your colleagues, who just finished her treatment session, volunteers to take the patient to the bathroom and offers to incorporate your ADL treatment plan into the toileting activity. This frees up your time, ensures the patient gets her therapy minutes, and allows you to work with the next patient.

◇ *Scenario 2*: The recreation therapy department is running a program in which one of your patients is involved. You know that the patient will be going out for an x-ray after lunch and you must provide the patient with a therapy session before that time. You go into the recreation program and tell the patient you must take him to therapy. The patient is upset because he is having a good time at the activity and does not want to leave for therapy. The recreation staff are angry that you assumed that therapy is more important than recreation.

In each instance, how would you handle your thank you or apology? Choose your words carefully to show why you are thanking or apologizing. Are you including the elements outlined in this chapter? Which elements did you include? Now, have your classmate respond with the feelings they think you conveyed.

REFERENCES

Braveman, B. (2006). *Leading and managing occupational therapy services: An evidence based approach.* Philadelphia, PA: F.A. Davis.

Cherry, K. (2012, April 13). *Top 10 nonverbal communication tips: Improve your nonverbal communication skills with these tips.* Retrieved from: http://psychology.about.com/od/nonverbalcommunication/tp/nonverbaltips.htm.

Cotugna, N., Vickery, C., & Carpenter-Haefele, K. (2005). Evaluation of literacy level of patient education pages in health related journals. *Journal of Community Health, 30,* 213-220.

Flores, G. (2006). Language barriers to health care in the United States. *New England Journal of Medicine, 355,* 229-231.

Goulston, M. (2009). *Just listen: Discover the secret to getting through to absolutely anyone.* New York, NY: AMACOM.

How to sound professional on the phone. (2012, April 13). WikiHow. Retrieved from www.wikihow.com/sound-professional-on-the-phone.

Jacobs, K., & McCormack, G. (2011). *The occupational therapy manager.* 5th ed. Bethesda, MD: AOTA Press.

Luckman, J. (2000). *Transcultural communication in health care.* Albany, NY: Delmar Thomson Learning.

Luedtke, T., Goldhammer, K., Fox, L., et al. (2012). Overcoming communication barriers: Navigating client linguistic, literacy and cultural differences. *OT Practice, 17*(4) 15-18.

Luntz, F. (2007). *Words that work: It's not what you say, it's what people hear.* New York, NY: Hyperion.

Manktelow, J., & Carlson, A. (1999). *Writing skills: Getting your written message across clearly.* Retrieved from http://www.mindtools.com/CommSkll/WritingSkills, htm.

MindTools, Inc. (2009). The presentation planning checklist. Retrieved from: http://www.mindtools.com/CommSkll/PresentationPlanningChecklist.htm.

Napier, B. (2011). *Occupational therapy fieldwork survival guide: A student planner.* Bethesda, MD: AOTA Press.

National Health and Medical Research Council. (2004). *Communicating with patients: Advice for medical practitioners.* Canberra, ACT, Australia: Commonwealth of Australia.

Nonverbal communication. (2004). In: *The concise Corsini encyclopedia of psychology and behavior science.* Retrieved from http://www.credoreference.com/entry/wileypsych/nonverbal_c

Robinson, L., Segal, J., & Segal, R. (2012). Effective communication: Improving communication skills in business and relationships. Retrieved from: http://www.helpguide.org/mental/effective_communication_skills.htm

Robinson, T.E. 2nd, White, G.L. Jr, Houchins, J.C. (2006). Improving communication with older patients: Tips from the literature. *Family Practice Management, 8,* 73-78.

Scan Health Plan. (2012). Tips for communicating across language barriers. Retrieved from: https://www. scanhealthplan.com/providers/information-for-office-staff/multi-cultural-resources/language-barriers/.

Skillscascade. (2002). Communicating with children, adolescents and more than one patient at a time. Retrieved from: http://www.skillscascade.com/special.htm#COMMUNICATING.

Wertheim, E. (2008). The importance of effective communication. Northeastern University, College of Business Administrative. Retrieved from web/dba.neu.edu.

Chapter 5

Playing Well With Others
Understanding Your Role as a Team Member

LEARNING OBJECTIVES

At the end of this chapter, the reader will be able to:
- ➢ Define what a team is.
- ➢ Describe four benefits of working in a team.
- ➢ Identify the four steps in the development of a team.
- ➢ Describe six traits that make a team successful.
- ➢ Identify 10 qualities of an effective team member.
- ➢ Identify roles in team dynamics.
- ➢ Predict the characteristics of a group enhancer.
- ➢ Predict the characteristics of a task-oriented group member.
- ➢ Predict the characteristics of a group distracter.

In the previous chapters, we outlined many issues that contribute to your success in the workplace, including interpersonal skills, professional behaviors, and communication skills. Development of these skills will serve you well in all areas of work (and life), but especially as you begin to participate in a team-oriented environment. This chapter will take you a step further to demonstrate the value of the team process in a health care or educational setting, your role in the team, and how to use your skills to become a valued and effective team member.

Teamwork is an important contributor toward enhanced clinical and educational outcomes. No matter what the setting, the division of labor among medical, educational, nursing, and allied health practitioners means that no one profession is primary in the delivery of services—everyone works as a team. However, as important as the team delivery system is, there is little formal training in team skill development in the occupational therapy curriculum. Teamwork skills are generally learned on the job. Because outcomes are dependent on effective interdisciplinary teamwork, there is a need for therapists to prepare for their role as team members (Leggat, 2007).

Davis L, Rosee M. *Occupational Therapy Student to Clinician:*
Making the Transition (pp 65-72).
© 2015 SLACK Incorporated.

WHAT IS A TEAM?

"Teams are groups of people with common goals who work together to achieve those goals. They are an essential component of every health care deliver system" (Napier, 2011, p. 126).

A team is a varied and complex entity. Teams can derive from a single professional group (such as the occupational therapy association planning a local conference), a multidisciplinary group (such as a fall team in a nursing home that tries to identify the reasons for a patient incident), a team with constant membership (such as the board of an occupational therapy association), or a team with constantly changing membership (such as a rotating clinical team). Regardless of the type and nature of the team, they share certain characteristics, such as the following:

- Team members have specific roles and interact together to achieve a common goal.
- Teams make important decisions together.
- Teams possess specialized knowledge and skills.
- Teams differ from small groups as they embody a collective action arising out of task inter-dependency (WHO, 2012).

TEAMS TYPICALLY FOUND IN OCCUPATIONAL THERAPY SETTINGS

There are many different types of teams found in settings where occupational therapists work. The multidisciplinary model involves professionals working independently to accomplish discipline-specific goals. While they are working with the same patients, they may not communicate with one another regarding the care plan and may not be aware of what others are doing. An example of this might be an individual who sustained an injury with multiple upper and lower extremity fractures. The occupational therapist may be working on activities of daily living, such as dressing and toileting, while the physical therapist is working on ambulation and transfers with little or no collaboration.

The interdisciplinary model is a more collaborative approach to care. Under this model, team members work together in setting goals, making treatment decisions, and sharing information related to progress and obstacles encountered to create a holistic approach to the identified issues. Here, communication between all members of the team is crucial. This type of model might be found in a school where the teacher, occupational therapist, social worker, and psychologist work together to identify issues and develop a child's individualized education program. Working with the classroom teacher, the occupational therapist may demonstrate interventions that the teacher can integrate into classroom activities. The teacher can then provide feedback to the occupational therapist so that the approach can be adjusted as changes occur.

In the transdisciplinary model, one team member is appointed the primary provider of the intervention. Team members are cross-trained in different areas that go beyond their own specialty. Roles may be blurred. An example might be when an occupational therapist is called in to evaluate a nursing home resident who is no longer able to mobilize in bed. The occupational therapist may make recommendations for bed mobility training that can be incorporated into the nursing care plan, which would be carried out by the nurse's aide rather than by the therapists themselves. In appropriate circumstances, this can be a cost-effective solution to care.

BENEFITS OF WORKING IN TEAMS

There are many outcomes that can be achieved much more effectively by a team than by an individual. Some of the benefits of team-oriented projects include the following:

- The ability to successfully accomplish projects that an individual cannot easily complete alone. Some workplace tasks are too large and complex for one person to tackle, such as producing a seminar or putting together a health fair.
- The potential for offering more solutions and options—different people looking at the same problem may be able to identify more creative and effective solutions.
- Easier to identify flaws in solutions. A team looking at proposed solutions may be able to identify pitfalls that an individual might miss.
- Development of a workplace community that may be good for morale (Penn State, 2005).

HOW TEAMS DEVELOP AND EVOLVE

Teams are not instantly functional. They grow and develop over time. Tuckman and Jenson (1977) have identified four steps in the development of a team:

1. *Forming*: The time when a group is first forming and getting to know one another (assumptions are being formed about others and alliances are established).
2. *Storming*: As team members negotiate work assignments and express disagreements, conflicts may appear. This is a crucial point in the development of a group. Conflicts can result in improved outcomes, unless the conflicts escalate to a point where the group cannot work effectively together. At that point, conflict resolution must be initiated.
3. *Norming*: After a period of negotiation to resolve conflicts, the team reaches a point where ground rules of conduct are established and members learn to work together. This is when the team starts to become productive.
4. *Performing*: After the group settles down, members can put their energies toward shared goals.

WHAT MAKES A TEAM SUCCESSFUL?

There are certain characteristics that are present in effective health care teams that are able to work together to develop effective solutions to problems. These include the following:

- *Common purpose*: Team members generate a common and clearly defined purpose that includes collective interests and demonstrates shared ownership.
- *Measurable goals*: Teams set goals that are measurable and focused on the team's task.
- *Effective leadership*: Teams require leadership to create and maintain structure, manage conflict, and listen to and support members.
- *Effective communication*: Good teams share ideas and information quickly and regularly, keep written records, and allow time for team reflection.
- *Cohesion*: Cohesive teams have a unique and identifiable team spirit and commitment and have greater longevity as team members are motivated to continue working together.
- *Mutual respect*: Effective teams have members who respect the talents and beliefs of fellow team members. In addition, effective teams accept and encourage a diversity of opinions among members (Mickan & Rodger, 2005).

DEVELOPING TEAM SKILLS

Some teams produce more successful results than others. Brounstein (2002) outlines the qualities that contribute to the success of a team. Many of these skills relate to professionalism and the development of emotional intelligence as outlined in Chapter 3. They include the following:

- *Reliability*: As a team member, you need to attend scheduled meetings, do your share to meet commitments, and follow through on assignments.

- *Consistency*: You need to demonstrate that you will deliver a good performance every time, not just some of the time.

- *Communication*: Team members need to speak up and express their ideas clearly, directly, and honestly. Productive team members are not afraid to make their point but do so in a positive, confident, and respectful manner.

  - ◇ **Example:** Bill was on his second week of fieldwork when he was asked to observe a patient care meeting. Since the patient being discussed was on Bill's caseload, the physician leading the team asked him to provide a report to the team about the patient's progress in occupational therapy. Although nervous, Bill gathered his courage and presented a clear report about the patient's status, goals, and participation level. He expressed concern that the patient was very tired in the afternoon when he was scheduled for occupational therapy and suggested to the team that the morning would be a better time for the patient. While this change would involve some coordination with other departments, the team agreed it was a good suggestion. After the meeting, he was given positive feedback from his supervisor for his professional presentation and initiative in suggesting the change in schedule.

- *Active listening*: This is an essential skill for a team member. Players must absorb, understand, and consider ideas and points of view from others without debate or arguing. One must be prepared to receive criticism without behaving defensively. Team members must learn to listen first and respond second so that a meaningful dialogue can occur.

- *Ability to function as an active participant*: Team players come prepared for meetings, listen, and speak up. They are fully engaged in the work of the team and are proactive. They take initiative and volunteer for assignments. Then, they ask, "What contribution can I make to help the team achieve success?" This indicates that they have enthusiasm and are exuding positive energy, which is contagious and contributes to the success of the group.

- *Willingness to share*: Good team players share information, knowledge, and experience. Often, communication is informal, taking place between meetings, and may include passing along important news and information on a day-to-day basis. This keeps other team members in the loop and ready to work when the official meeting takes place.

- *Cooperation*: Cooperation is the act of working with others to accomplish a job. Good team players identify a way to work with their team members despite differences to get the work done.

- *Paying attention to detail*: The successful attainment of a team goal is the sum of the tasks completed. If members omit details or gloss over task responsibilities, it could impact the success of the activity.

  - ◇ **Example:** Debra's department was putting together a seminar that was being marketed to the public. Each member of the team had an assigned responsibility: one member was responsible for securing the space to hold the seminar, another member was identifying speakers, and so on. Debra's job was to write the brochure. The job had a deadline to ensure that the brochure was mailed out quickly to allow time for registrations to be returned several weeks before the event. While the other members of the team carried out their tasks on a timely basis, Debra procrastinated in completing the brochure, which then went to the printer 1 week late. She also neglected to call the printer and convey that she needed the job done in a rush in order to compensate for the late start. In the end, while the group put together a great program, attendance was very poor because the mailing went out too late. This was all because of Debra's neglect in paying attention to her responsibilities.

♦ *Willingness to use strengths*: Each team member has his or her own interests, skills, and abilities and needs to work with the team to determine who is best equipped to handle particular challenges and issues based on individual strengths.

♦ *Showing commitment to the team*: Strong team players care about their work, the team, and the team's work. They are looking at the outcome beyond their piece of the work. They give a good effort and expect their fellow team members to do the same.

♦ *Strong problem solving skills*: Teams always deal with problems. Solving a common problem is often the impetus for forming the team in the first place. Team members must identify solutions and not dwell on the problems. Blamers and avoiders often do not make good team members. Team players put the problems out in the open; discuss, collaborate, and identify solutions; and form action plans.

♦ *Treating others in a respectful and supportive manner*: Team players always treat fellow team members courteously. They avoid backbiting and complaining about fellow group members. Should a problem develop with a fellow member, team players will try to solve it with that person directly and tactfully. A team player exhibits understanding and support of other team members. Good team players have a sense of humor and know how to have fun, but not at another team member's expense (Brounstein, 2002).

UNDERSTANDING YOUR ROLE IN THE TEAM

The roles that we play in groups are closely related to the roles we play in our social environment. Unfortunately, we are not always aware of our behaviors and how they impact the group process. Our interpersonal styles and defense mechanisms, which develop over many years, can have a profound impact on how productive we are perceived to be in a group setting. It is very helpful for us to begin to self-evaluate so that we understand the roles we are playing in the group. Through understanding, we can make adjustments in behavior and become a productive member of any team we participate in.

According to Napier (2011), in her book *Occupational Therapy Fieldwork Survival Guide*, an individual's role in a group will fall into three general categories. Often, roles change and flow over the course of the process, allowing different members to use their unique skills as needs change.

1. The *group enhancer* assumes roles that enhance the learning process, which are group or team centered with a focus on building group goals. Group enhancers typically exhibit one of more of the following traits:

   ◊ The *encourager* agrees with and accepts the contributions of others. He or she exudes warmth and encouragement, accepting others' points of view.

   ◊ The *harmonizer* mediates between other members to reconcile disagreements.

   ◊ The *compromiser* may yield status by admitting error, disciplining him- or herself to maintain harmony, or offer suggestions to create consensus.

   ◊ The *gatekeeper* facilities participation, proposes regulations, and manages the discussion.

   ◊ The *standard setter* maintains the standards that the group has agreed upon to move the group toward the common goal.

   ◊ The *group observer* maintains records to ensure a history of actions taken so that the group can evaluate its progress.

◇   The *follower* goes along with the group.

2. The *group-centered, task-oriented* member assumes a role that focuses on group tasks and encourages members of the group to produce positive results. Task-oriented group members often assume the following characteristics:

◇   The *information seeker* asks for clarification and seeks the facts pertinent to the group tasks.

◇   The *opinion seeker* asks for clarification of value-oriented issues relating to what the group is trying to accomplish.

◇   The i*nformation giver* offers facts or generalizations that are authoritative, often relating to his or her own experience.

◇   The *opinion giver* states his or her beliefs or opinions with an emphasis on what should become the group's view. This person may ignore relevant information if it does not support his or her theory.

◇   The *elaborator* uses examples to offer a rationale for suggestions and provides ideas related to how an idea might work if actually implemented.

◇   The *coordinator* clarifies the relationship among various ideas or suggestions.

◇   The *orienter* defines the position of the group related to what is happening and raises questions to redirect discussion when the group deviates from its goals.

◇   The *energizer* prods the group into action or decisions and keeps the group stimulated to continue to work toward its goal.

◇   The *procedural technician* performs routine group tasks and helps the process with the "practical" matters, such as distributing materials, cleaning up, and arranging chairs.

◇   The *recorder* keeps the written record and maintains the group memory.

3. The *group distracter* assumes roles that can have a negative effect on group and interpersonal interactions. Group distracters fall into a number of possible roles:

◇   The *aggressor* works through intimidation, deflating the value of other members, taking credit for others' work, or ridiculing the goals of the group.

◇   The *blocker* acts as "the devil's advocate" and dismisses ideas with negative comments or attitudes.

◇   The *recognition seeker* focuses attention on him- or herself through boasting about personal achievements with the goal of enhancing his or her personal status.

◇   The *self-confessor/help seeker* attempts to have the group solve his or her own problems rather than focusing on the task at hand (Napier, 2011).

By understanding the various roles that are assumed by team members and the ways in which these roles enhance or detract from the team process, one can begin to evaluate his or her own roles and behaviors. With self-reflection, participants can begin to change their behaviors if they are not conducive toward making productive contributions to the team process.

SUMMARY

Being a productive team member is a very important skill for occupational therapists and assistants. Working as a team member is a fact of life in most work settings. The team process contributes to better patient outcomes, allows for successful completion of large projects, offers the opportunity for more solutions and options, helps identify flaws in solutions, and helps facilitate a workplace community that is good for morale. To be successful, a team should have a common purpose, measurable goals, effective leadership, effective communication, cohesion, and mutual respect.

In addition to professionalism, the skills required to be a good team member relate to one's emotional intelligence. Like emotional intelligence, these skills can be improved on with insight and motivation. In addition to our team skills, it is important for us to understand the role we assume as part of a team. Some roles contribute to the process in a positive way and some detract from the process. We should all be familiar with the roles we typically assume so that we can determine if we need to make changes in our team dynamic behaviors.

Always seek to assume a positive role within the group, contribute to positive outcomes, and celebrate one another when successes are achieved.

DISCUSSION QUESTIONS/ACTIVITIES

1. Think back to your participation in your fieldwork and academic experiences. Describe team experiences you had and your role within the team. How did your participation affect the team process? Which of your team behaviors are you most proud of? Which team behaviors could you have improved upon?

2. In groups of four, create a sensory kit from objects you find around the classroom. List the objects and describe why they are included in the kit. Next, reflect on the group process. Identify the role each member of the team played in the experience and describe the team-work traits of each of them.

3. Think about an interdisciplinary team process you participated in during your fieldwork experience. Describe the members of the team, their disciplines, their roles, and the team-work traits observed.

4. What are some of the characteristics that contribute to a positive occupational therapist/certified occupational therapy assistant team relationship? Discuss. Describe positive and negative experiences you have had working with certified occupational therapy assistants or occupational therapists.

5. Ask for four volunteers to role play a scenario. Each volunteer will play either the occupational therapist, occupational therapy assistant/student, physical therapist, or nurse.

    ◇ Scenario: The occupational therapist has scheduled a patient for 10 a.m. and has communicated the schedule to the floor nurse. At 10 a.m., the occupational therapy assistant student arrives to work with the patient bedside. The nurse informs him that the physical therapist already picked up the patient. The nurse tells the occupational therapy assistant student that she tried to stop him, but the physical therapist said it is more important that the patient gets her physical therapy as she is going home soon.

    ◇ Play out the scene with the goal of working together with fellow professionals. How would each member respond? What can the occupational therapist and occupational therapy assistant student do to ensure the patient gets her occupational therapy as scheduled?

6. This activity encourages team members to work together toward a common goal. Collaboration, communication, and negotiation are all part of building trust among members of the team.

    ◇ Begin the activity by forming small groups of three to five people. Inform the group that some people are to assume the roles of certified occupational therapy assistants and occupational therapists. Imagine that the occupational therapy department will be moved temporarily to another space during renovations. Each team member can bring one object from the classroom (you are now in) to treat clients in the temporary space. Each team member writes down the article that he or she would like to take and does not share that information with any of the team members until everyone has written the item down. For the next 20 minutes, the team determines its population and practice setting. Then, by using the items chosen by members, strategize a way that the items can be combined together for use in a treatment session. Each group will share with the class how its team chose its population and practice setting and what was combined to use in treatment interventions.

REFERENCES

Brounstein, M. (2012). *Managing teams for dummies.* Hoboken, NJ: John Wiley & Sons.

Leggat, S. (2007). *Effective healthcare teams require effective team members: Defining teamwork competencies.* Retrieved from NIH.gov.pmc/articles/PMC 1800844.

Mickan, S.M., & Rodger, S.A. (2005). Effective healthcare teams: A model of six characteristics developed from shared perceptions. *Journal of Inter-Professional Care, 19*(4), 358-370.

Napier, B. (2011). *Occupational therapy fieldwork survival guide: a student planner.* Bethesda, MD: AOTA Press.

Penn State. (2005). Building blocks for teams: meetings. Retrieved from http://www.archive.tlt.psu.edu/suggestions.teams/student/meetings.html.

Tuckman, B.W. & Jenson, M. (1977). Stages of small group development revisited. In: *Group and Organizational Studies.* 2nd ed. (pp. 419-517).

World Health Organization (WHO). (2012). *Topic 4: Being an effective team player.* Retrieved from http://who.int/patientsafety/education/curriculum/who_mc_topic-4.pdf.

Chapter 6

Turning Conflict Into Opportunity
Rules to Follow to Resolve Rifts in the Workplace

LEARNING OBJECTIVES

At the end of this chapter, the reader will be able to:
- ➤ Define the difference between organizational and personal conflict.
- ➤ Identify five sources of workplace conflict.
- ➤ Describe five different conflict handling styles.
- ➤ Name five healthy responses to conflict.
- ➤ Describe 10 suggestions for resolving conflicts.

A cohesive and effective professional environment requires a team who works cooperatively and collaboratively. Inevitably, when people with differing belief systems, goals, and needs combine, conflict arises. While conflict is usually perceived as a bad thing, it can actually lead to positive outcomes when managed effectively. To successfully participate in any work environment, you must learn to develop your conflict resolution skills so that you can effectively navigate issues that arise with colleagues, clients, and families. This chapter will focus on increasing your understanding of conflicts, how and why they occur, and what skills and techniques you must master to effectively manage them.

UNDERSTANDING CONFLICTS IN THE WORKPLACE

Conflict arises from differences. It occurs when people disagree over their values, motivations, perceptions, ideas, needs, or desires (Segal & Smith, 2011). In the workplace setting, differing needs are often at the heart of disputes. When you can recognize the legitimacy of the conflicting needs and are willing to examine them, pathways are opened to creative problem solving, team building, and improved relationships (Segal & Smith, 2011). Some typical workplace situations that can promote conflict include the following:

Davis L, Rosee M. *Occupational Therapy Student to Clinician:*
Making the Transition (pp 73-85).
© 2015 SLACK Incorporated.

- A coworker who is resentful that a colleague is not performing adequately or carrying his or her load
- A supervisor who is critical during a review of a supervisee's performance
- A coworker who believes another worker is harassing her
- A patient who is making unrealistic demands on a therapist
- A parent who is lacking insight into a child's capabilities, insisting that the therapist deliver an inappropriate intervention

Some important facts to consider are as follows:

- A conflict is more than just a disagreement. It is a situation in which one or both parties perceive a threat (whether the threat is real or not).
- Conflicts continue to fester when ignored. Because conflicts involve perceived threats to our well-being and survival, they stay with us until we face and resolve them.
- We respond to conflicts based on our perceptions of the situation, not necessarily to an objective review of the facts. Our perceptions are influenced by our life experiences, culture, values, and beliefs.
- Conflicts trigger strong emotions. If you are not comfortable with your emotions or are unable to manage them in times of stress, you will experience difficulty in resolving conflicts successfully.
- Conflicts, while often uncomfortable, can present an opportunity for growth. When you are able to resolve conflicts with someone, you build trust with that person. You will feel more secure knowing your relationship can survive challenges and disagreements (Segal & Smith, 2011).

TYPES OF CONFLICT

Conflicts in the workplace generally derive from two root causes: organizational conflicts and personal conflicts.

Organizational Conflict

This involves a conflict that is related to a specific workplace issue. The conflict may be between staff and management, between staff (often as a result of a management decision), or between staff and a patient or family members. It can be caused by an infinite number of factors, including differing goals and priorities, disagreement over implementation of management or policy changes, therapeutic interventions or treatment plans, patient assignments, strategic planning decisions, conflict about supervision styles, or conflict over the best use for (or competition over) scarce resources. The list can go on and on. These types of conflicts can often be resolved internally with skilled conflict management techniques. On the other hand, unresolved disagreements can escalate, leading to more conflict among factions that support differing approaches (Blackard & Gibson, 2002).

Examples of organizational conflicts in the workplace include the following:

- Sarah and Barbara are both vying for an assignment to be placed in the neonatal intensive care unit. Sarah has had extensive advanced training and experience working with fragile infants. Barbara has limited experience with the population but has seniority over her more experienced colleague. Their supervisor decides to give the assignment to Barbara, the provider with less experience, as she is worried about union intervention on behalf of the therapist with seniority. Sarah is so upset that she starts looking for another position where her skills will be better appreciated.

- The occupational therapy department has been awarded a grant of $2,000 to purchase any kind of equipment it would like for the department. The staff is asked to put forth suggestions for what equipment to purchase. The supervisor decides to ignore the input of her staff and purchases equipment that was not on the therapists' wish list (even though the supervisor no longer performs any treatment duties). The staff is angry about the decision.

Personal Conflict

This form of conflict revolves around personal relationships rather than workplace situations. Typical conflicts may stem from differing belief systems, views on social issues, and personal concerns. Personal conflicts usually arise from one of two sources: (1) when functional strife is not resolved or is resolved in a way that one of the parties feels is unfair or (2) from personality or belief conflicts. Since every person is different, differing political beliefs, ethnic background, values, gender issues, religious beliefs, and communication styles can lead to conflict. This conflict can impact the team's ability to collaborate effectively and, if not properly managed or resolved, can even lead to litigation (Blackard & Gibson, 2002).

Examples of personal conflicts in the workplace include the following:

- Paul and Sam, two occupational therapists working in a large metropolitan hospital, have been assigned to share an office. Paul is a conservative Republican. Sam is a liberal Democrat who is very active in local politics. The officemates do not agree on politics, and Sam feels free to express his opinions every chance he gets. This leads to conflicts between the two, which spill over to their relationship in the clinic. This is becoming disruptive to the team and even impacting the patients. Although Paul and Sam will never agree on their political views, they must find a way to behave professionally when at work and resolve the conflict so it does not impact their performance.

- Laurie and Roz, two occupational therapists, share an office in a large metropolitan hospital. Laurie spends a lot of time on the telephone talking to her boyfriend, making weekend plans with friends, and discussing the latest gossip. Roz finds Laurie's constant chatter annoying as it interferes with her note-writing tasks. She also feels resentful that Laurie cuts her treatment sessions short so she can go into the physical therapy office to hang out with her friends in that department. Their supervisor comments that Roz should take a lesson from Laurie, as she seems more efficient than Roz, who often has patients still in the clinic as lunchtime approaches. Roz is now enraged with both her supervisor and Laurie as she feels she works much harder and not only gets no recognition for her efforts, but also gets criticized while Laurie is applauded for her lack of effort. This conflict is having an effect on Roz's morale, as well as that of their other coworkers.

HIDDEN SOURCES OF WORKPLACE CONFLICT

Unresolved conflict can have negative consequences in a workplace environment. Anger, resentment, gossip, rumors, and lack of cooperation can all serve to undermine the operations of an occupational therapy department. Unresolved conflict can be avoided if the source of conflict is addressed. The top five sources of workplace conflict are as follows:

1. *Unarticulated assumptions*: Every conflict has an element of unarticulated assumptions. Each person has a very closely held belief about the way things should work or the way things are. Very few people articulate these assumptions, and when they prove incorrect, frustration and anger can result.

2. *Unmet expectations*: Like unarticulated assumptions, unmet expectations are also at the root of many conflicts. While unarticulated assumptions focus on the way things are done, unmet

expectations are rooted in disappointment about an outcome. When the expected outcome does not happen, people become upset and frustrated and then look for someone to blame.

  ⬦ *What to do:* For such circumstances, one must identify what happened to cause the unarticulated assumption and/or unmet expectation and ask the question, "What about this situation did not meet my expectations?" By talking about it, understanding the process, and clarifying realities, conflict can be avoided or cured.

3. *Perceived lack of respect*: This is a huge driver of conflict. What is considered respectful to one person can be considered disrespectful to another. This is sometimes culturally driven. The bottom line is that you often do not know what others find disrespectful unless you ask. Others do not know that you think they are disrespectful unless you tell them. For example, Elissa, a certified occupational therapy assistant, was eating lunch with her colleagues at the preschool where they worked. She noticed that Joseph, the physical therapist, did not have anything to eat, so she asked him if he would like to share her ham sandwich. Being an observant Jew, he became offended, even though her offer was an innocent act of generosity. Joseph felt disrespected by Elissa and she had no idea why. Later, one of her colleagues explained about Joseph's dietary restrictions. She approached Joseph and apologized, and both learned an important lesson in cultural sensitivity.

  ⬦ *What to do*: Explore whether a perceived lack of respect is *an issue* or *the issue* underlying the conflict. Ask whether perceived lack of respect issues have anything to do with this conflict. Then, you can clarify perceptions.

4. *Playing the blame game*: Fighting to determine fault when something goes wrong does nothing to resolve a conflict. Discussing an issue is productive only if the discussion leads to resolution, which means identifying the problem and moving to solve it.

  ⬦ *What to do*: Move from blame to productive problem solving. The problem is never the person; the problem is the impact of someone's behavior. Make a move toward problem solving by articulating how each person perceives and defines the problem. Then ask, "How can we resolve this?"

5. *Arguing with superiors*: The shortest distance to career suicide is to cross the line that differentiates standing up for yourself from insubordination. Failure to appreciate and respect the power differences in a relationship can be a tactical error. Those who do not feel heard or respected will attempt to be heard through unproductive means, such as talking more, louder, and faster and to more people. This approach can be especially destructive if the dynamic is between a staff member and his or her supervisor or superior.

  ⬦ *What to do:* Respect the position of your superiors. Once decisions are made, you must move from advocating your position to supporting the decision. While you may believe that workplace priorities should be different, unless your job title allows you to make those decisions, sit back and support the decision. It may mean the difference between being employed or being out of work (Browser, 2009).

UNDERSTANDING YOUR CONFLICT HANDLING STYLE

Different people react to conflict situations based on many social/emotional variables. In general, a person's response to conflict will be determined by whether he or she is more concerned with maintaining or improving the relationship with the source of the conflict, or with winning the argument. Behavioral scientists Kenneth Thomas and Ralph Kilman (1999) have identified five styles of response to conflict. These include competition, accommodation, avoidance, compromise, and collaboration. No one conflict style is right or wrong, but some are deemed more appropriate and acceptable when participating in a professional work environment. By understanding conflict styles, professionals can learn how to make choices that are more productive in reducing work conflicts and promoting collaboration.

Competition

People who use this style can come across as aggressive, confrontational, and intimidating. A competitive style is an attempt to gain power and pressure a change at the other person's expense. This style can be appropriate when someone has to implement an unpopular decision or make a quick decision, or if the decision is vital in a crisis situation. The big disadvantage with this style is that relationships can be harmed.

Value of own issue/goal:	High
Value of relationship:	Low
Goal:	I win, you lose

- **Example:** A long-term care facility is planning a renovation of one floor to create a large recreation and therapy wing. Each discipline is determined to secure a bigger space to provide better services to the residents. The recreation therapist feels entitled to the space so residents can enjoy more dynamic programs. The occupational therapists and physical therapists feel the space should be awarded to them so they can improve reimbursement to the facility by providing cutting-edge interventions using sophisticated exercise equipment. Engaging in a competitive approach, the occupational therapist decided to meet with the administrator directly to convince him that the room should be given to the therapy department in order to increase reimbursement. The occupational therapist believes that reimbursement would be a trump card to get the space for her department. While this strategy might work (since reimbursement is an important priority for the administrator), this approach would probably result in conflict with the recreation therapy staff, whom she needs to work with collaboratively.

Accommodation

When you accommodate, you set aside you own personal needs with an attempt to please others. The emphasis here is on preserving the relationship. Smoothing over a situation can result in a false solution to a problem as the accommodator may have feelings about giving in too much. Accommodators are usually unassertive and may play the role of a martyr or complainer. However, this can be a useful style when you want to minimize losses or when you are going to lose anyway, because it preserves relationships.

Value of own issue:	Low
Value relationship:	High
Goal:	I lose, you win

- **Example:** Using the previous situation, an accommodation of this would be if the occupational therapist agreed to give up the space to the recreation department in order to avoid confrontation over the space, especially since the director of recreation has a very strong and difficult personality. By taking this approach, the occupational therapist does not gain any additional therapy space and will probably be resentful down the road, possibly impacting the relationship with the recreation department in unconscious ways.

Avoidance

This is characterized by ignoring or withdrawing from a conflict rather than facing it. The avoider is perceived not to care about the issue at hand. He or she is hoping that the issue goes away or resolves itself without him or her getting involved in the conflict. This approach can be appropriate when you need more time to decide how to respond to a situation or when you know that confrontation will affect a working relationship. This technique can be destructive to your reputation as your apathy might be perceived as a lack of interest.

Value of own issue: Low
Value of relationship: Low
Goal: I lose, you lose

- ◆ **Example**: Using the previous situation, avoidance would occur if the occupational therapist gives up the fight and suggests that the administrator make the decision, without presenting her case for being granted the additional space.

Compromising

This style demonstrates that you are willing to sacrifice some of your goals while persuading others to give up part of theirs. You give a little and get a little. Compromising maintains the relationship and can take less time than collaboration. While it represents an easy way out of a confrontation, it may reduce creative problem solving. By playing to the middle, you may produce a less effective outcome.

Value of own issue: Medium
Value of relationship: Medium
Goal: I win some, you win some

- ◆ **Example:** In the situation described, a compromise would be if the occupational therapist suggests that the extra space be divided between the two departments. While this seems like a fair compromise, it is not an effective solution as neither the recreation nor the rehabilitation department ends up with enough space to make a big difference in their program. The upside is that there is some satisfaction by both members that each gained something.

Collaboration

This style views a conflict as a problem to be solved, with the motivation to identify creative solutions that will satisfy all concerned parties. When collaborating, you do not give up your self-interest; rather, you identify concerns, test your own assumptions, and understand the views of others. It takes time and energy to collaborate, but in the end, results can foster trust, respect, and relationship building.

Value of own issue: High
Value of relationship: High
Goal: I win, you win

- ◆ **Example:** A collaborative solution would result if the occupational therapist and recreation department decide to each use the space at different times of the day. The division of space would meet the needs of both departments and, more importantly, better meets the needs of the patients. The collaborative solution is creative and effective, leaving all parties satisfied with the end result.

RESOLVING CONFLICTS

By understanding why conflicts arise and how conflict handling styles impact conflict outcomes, you can begin to understand your personal preferences and styles and begin to work on improving your own conflict resolution skills. Many people fear conflict and avoid it at all costs. Involvement in a conflict situation is often threatening. Many find it demoralizing, humiliating, and scary. Unfortunately, the aversion to engage in conflicts makes it more difficult to deal with them in a productive manner. However, as we have illustrated in this chapter, conflict is unavoidable and conflict resolution is a skill that will serve you well no matter what the setting.

Healthy and Unhealthy Ways of Managing and Resolving Conflict

Unhealthy Responses to Conflict

♦ An inability to recognize and respond to the things that matter to the other person

♦ Explosive, angry, hurtful, and resentful reactions

♦ The withdrawal of love, resulting in rejection, isolation, shaming, and fear of abandonment

♦ An inability to compromise or see the other person's side

♦ Fear and avoidance of conflict due to the expectation of bad outcomes

Healthy Responses to Conflict

♦ The capacity to recognize and respond to the things that matter to the other person involved in the conflict

♦ Calm, nondefensive, and respectful reactions

♦ Readiness to forgive and forget and to move past the conflict without resentment or anger

♦ Ability to seek compromise and avoid punishing the other

♦ Belief that facing conflict head on is the best thing for both sides (Segal & Smith, 2011)

Other Important Factors in Conflict Resolution

Emotional awareness, as discussed in Chapter 3, is one of the most important factors in resolving conflicts. When you are emotionally aware, you understand your own reactions to difficult situations. The understanding of yourself and your emotional responses helps you to understand the other person in the conflict. It allows you to communicate honestly, negotiate effectively, and influence the outcome.

Your nonverbal communication can have a major impact on the outcome during a conflict. As discussed in Chapter 4, nonverbal cues can often provide more information than the words you use. When in a conflict situation, look for wordless cues such as facial expressions and body language (watch your own as well), and use your best nonverbal skills, such as your tone of voice and facial expressions, to indicate that you want a resolution to the conflict. Your nonverbal communication can reduce the stress for both of the participants, leading to a more effective resolution.

Humor can also be used to reduce tension and anger when in a conflict situation. Playfulness and a sense of humor, when used correctly, can help to reframe the issues and indicate that there is a positive connection between participants. However, you need to be careful with humor to ensure that it will not be misinterpreted to give the impression that you are not taking the situation seriously. Before you make a joke or flippant remark, think about what you are saying to ensure that it will not be construed as passive aggressive, insulting, or demeaning.

Approaching Conflict Resolution

One of the most effective solutions to conflict is to take a rational, problem-centered approach, as outlined in Salmon and Salmon's (2000) book, *The Mid Career Tune Up: Ten Work Habits for Keeping Your Edge*. In it, they present some concrete suggestions for resolving conflicts, as follows:

♦ *Step 1*: Analyze the situation. Start off by describing the conflict and with whom you are having a problem. What triggered the conflict? Is it getting worse?

♦ *Step 2*: Review the impact the conflict is having on your ability to achieve your work goals. Are you being hampered by a lack of cooperation from the other person? Are you wasting valuable time working around the problem?

♦ *Step 3*: Identify any broader impact of the conflict. Is it affecting morale? Is it affecting your ability to do your job?

- *Step 4*: Describe the benefits of resolving the conflict.
- *Step 5*: Brainstorm possible solutions. Be open to new ideas, especially ones you had never considered before.
- *Step 6*: Negotiate a solution.

Earlier in this chapter, we outlined different conflict styles that can be employed to resolve workplace situations. Any one of these approaches might provide appropriate solutions, depending on the situation at hand. You should not decide how you will resolve a conflict until you are faced with it. This determination should be made based on all of the variables of the particular conflict. Some possible approaches include the following:

- *In the assertive approach*, based on your analysis of the conflict, you determine that the problem must be resolved. To do so, you schedule a face-to-face meeting with the person involved. The assertive approach does not mean that you need to be aggressive or confrontational—these stances often are counterproductive for the constructive and productive resolution you are seeking. Instead, prepare for the meeting by doing the following:

  a. Determine what you want to say. What are the key points? Stick to the issue and its impact on the workplace, avoiding personal issues. Provide concrete examples to illustrate your points.

  b. Be prepared to talk from the "I" about how the confrontation is impacting you.

  c. Ask the person a question that invites participation, such as, "What do you think we can do to make things better?" (Problem solving information and tips, n.d.).

- In the *cooperative approach*, you passively accept a solution presented to you. This might be an acceptable solution if the issue is not important enough for you to dedicate time and effort toward a resolution or if it may not be a battle you want to fight at this time.

- In the *collaborative approach*, you can use a combination of the assertive and cooperative approach in that you may be firm about certain issues but willing to compromise with others (Salmon & Salmon, 2000).

11 Tips for Resolving Conflicts

Monarth (2010) described 11 ways to resolve conflicts, restore harmony, and strengthen interpersonal rapport. These skills are very important in maintaining a sense of teamwork and promoting organizational harmony.

1. *Use active listening.* Hearing and understanding the logic and reasoning of both sides is critical to the creation of a mutually satisfying resolution. It is important to listen for what is felt as well as what is said.

2. *Separate the positions from the issues.* Begin with the issue and then view the positions in that context. Using the example of the allocation of space to either the rehabilitation or recreation departments, the occupational therapist's position was that he or she needed the space to expand; however, the real issue was the best use of the space for the residents of the facility. The solution—to use the space in a different way than either party envisioned—successfully addressed the issue. The players needed to change their position for the solution to be accepted.

3. *Understand and validate.* When you serve as an arbitrator of a conflict, it is critical that you not only seek to understand both positions in a conflict, but that you also validate each party's claim to what he or she believes is right. When people feel validated, they let their guard down and stop fighting. This makes it much easier to identify a resolution. Concentrate on resolving the conflict rather than proving you are right.

4. *Empathize.* The power of empathy in conflict resolution cannot be overstated. In the example of the conflict relating to the recreation vs rehabilitation space, by saying, "I understand why

you would want this space for your department. It would add a lot to the resident's experience, but I think my plan would also improve quality of life for the resident," you eliminate a barrier to communication.

5. *Implement boundaries and expectations.* Again, when arbitrating a conflict, be sure to clarify boundaries and expectations for behavior. For example, you might lay out the ground rules that screaming, cursing, and name calling are not acceptable behaviors and represent roadblocks to reaching a resolution.

6. *Be tactful.* Be sensitive to all participants' feelings so that they can remain open to input. Just because something is true does not mean you have to say it. Avoid blaming and direct or back-handed insults. They are all roadblocks to resolution.

7. Explore the issues and alternatives to *devise a mutually agreeable solution.*

8. *Use "I" statements.* When involved in a conflict, it is much more effective to speak from the "I" to express how you feel and how the conflict is impacting you. Do not blame or use "you" statements (e.g., "You never clean up your mess in the clinic when you are finished.") Rather, you should say, "I feel responsible for cleaning up for you so I can treat my patient in a clean environment. I'm starting to feel resentful about this. What can we do to solve this?"

9. *The power of ego stroking.* Giving positive feedback to the person you are embroiled in the conflict with can go a long way to calming down the dynamics.

10. *Attack the issues, not the person.* If the argument gets personal, bring it back to the issue at hand.

11. *End the conflict as quickly as possible.* If you are unable to come to a resolution, agree to disagree, disengage, forgive, and move on (Monarth, 2010).

Try to understand your own conflict resolution style by filling out the Conflict Resolution Styles checklist (Figure 6-1).

STEPHEN COVEY'S THIRD ALTERNATIVE TO CONFLICT RESOLUTION

Another approach to conflict resolution has been put forth by Stephen R. Covey (2004), the well-known author of *The 7 Habits of Highly Effective People.* In his new book, *The 3rd Alternative: Solving Life's Most Difficult Problems* (Covey, 2011), he puts forth the argument that typically a conflict allows for two possible alternatives—my way or your way. While compromise is always an option, many compromises result in a lose-lose solution because each side must give up something important. The 3rd Alternative presents the possibility of a win-win solution in which each side gets everything it wants. The 3rd Alternative is synergistic, meaning that by working in synergy, the result can be better than what could have been achieved alone.

The 3rd Alternative is based on the following four paradigms:

1. Paradigm 1 has to do with self-awareness. "Knowing yourself" requires you to search deep inside to become aware of your motives, uncertainties, and biases. Murray (2012), in his review of Covey's book, reports that in the first paradigm, individuals say, "I have examined my own assumptions. I am ready to be authentic with you." This is where you acknowledge your part in the conflict.

2. Paradigm 2 has to do with accepting and caring for the other person in the conflict. Typically, when there is a conflict, one does not see the person as an individual but as the "other side"— whatever that may be. In this paradigm, there is a switch from combat to collaboration.

3. Paradigm 3 has to do with the engagement of one party by another. Typically, parties in a conflict refuse to listen to one another or focus only on their own side. Covey (2011) contends

CONFLICT RESOLUTIONS STYLES

CHECK OFF THE ITEMS THAT APPLY TO YOU.

- ☐ Do you try to avoid conflict at all costs?
- ☐ Do you easily adapt to other's opinions?
- ☐ Are you aware when others are trying to intimidate you?
- ☐ Do you feel at ease disagreeing with others' point of views?
- ☐ Do you raise your voice when trying to get your point across?
- ☐ Are you tactful and calm when disagreeing with others?
- ☐ Do people think of you as contrary or aggressive?
- ☐ Are you afraid to offer your opinions when others have differing ideas from yours?
- ☐ Are you usually the most vocal or outspoken person in a meeting?
- ☐ Are you able to listen with an open mind to opinions different from yours?

SELF SCORING

BASED ON THE ABOVE, DO YOUR RESPONSES INDICATE THAT YOU ARE:

1. Passive. You tend to back down from conflict and allow others to take over. As a result, your valuable contributions may not be heard.
2. Assertive. You can listen and be diplomatic at times of conflict, but are able to let your opinions be known. People can listen to your arguments without feeling defensive.
3. Aggressive. You are argumentative and intimidating and unable to listen to what others are saying. This can result in turning others off so that they are unable to listen to what you have to say.

Adapted from Dale Carnegie Training. (2008). *Internal Conflict Resolution Guidebook*. Hauppauge, NY: Carnegie & Associates, Inc.

Figure 6-1. Conflict resolution styles checklist.

that "the best response to someone who does not see things your way is to say, 'You disagree? I need to listen to you.'" (Murray, 2012, p. 2) This is when you begin to understand their side.

4. Paradigm 4 is where synergy between the parties occurs. Each party has a more honest perspective of who they are and a realistic appraisal of the other side of the argument. After both parties have sought out and understand each other, the stage is set for a new solution using the strengths of both sides that neither had imagined before.

Using the example of the therapy vs recreation space conflict, if using the 3rd Alternative approach, the parties might ask, "Are you willing to go for a solution that is better than any we have individually come up with yet?" The next step would be to define the criteria—what would better look like? What would be a solution that would keep everyone happy? The next step is to collaboratively create the 3rd Alternative. From here, the parties collaboratively devise solutions, brainstorm new frameworks, think outside the box, suspend judgment, and identify the 3rd Alternative. The collaborative solution to the therapy space dilemma was a good example of this principle. In that situation, both parties came together and devised a solution that was far superior to the original solutions each presented (Covey, 2011).

CONFRONTING CONFLICTS

In his book *Winning with People,* John Maxwell (2004) discusses the benefits of confrontation to resolve conflicts before they lead to a relationship crisis. While it is simple to resolve a conflict from an intellectual point of view, from an emotional perspective ,it can be very difficult. A successful confrontation requires honesty, humility, and dedication to the relationship. He suggests the following steps when confronting someone:

- *Confront someone only if you care about that person.* It is more productive to go into a confrontation keeping the other person's interests in mind.
- *Meet together as soon as possible.* Putting off confrontations only causes the situation to fester.
- *Seek to understand the other's point of view, even if you do not agree.*
- *Outline the issue.* Be positive while describing your perceptions, state how the situation makes you feel, and explain why it is important to you.
- *Encourage the other person to respond to what you said.*
- *Agree on an action plan that identifies the issue and spells out steps to be taken.* The action plan should include a commitment by both parties to put the issue to rest once resolved (Maxwell, 2004).

THE POWER OF AN APOLOGY

With all the energy one needs to invest to deal effectively with a conflict, in the end, an apology can go a long way toward healing old wounds and helping all parties move on. Apologies have helped heal the wounds of atrocities, repaired relationships, resolved interpersonal disputes, and improved customer experiences. However, only some apologies are truly effective.

Research has shown that apologies that include components of compensation, empathy, and acknowledgement of violated norms can be most effective in resolving conflicts (Fehr & Gelfand, 2010, p. 38). Offers of compensation usually refer to the correction of the balance of the relationship through some type of action. It might be as simple as bringing in someone's favorite cupcake with a little sign that says, "I'm sorry," or offering to take that person out for dinner to bury the hatchet. Not only are you saying you are sorry, but you are also doing something thoughtful for the person based on knowing what is important to him or her (Fehr & Gelfand, 2010).

True expressions of empathy demonstrate recognition of and concern for the individual involved in the conflict. The apology can facilitate cooperation going forward. "I'm sorry that I was a selfish officemate. I didn't realize the impact I was having on your work." Statements like this show that you understand the impact you had and are sincere in your commitment to change.

SUMMARY

Our ultimate goal in the workplace is to collaborate with our coworkers to maximize the outcomes for the populations we are serving. Inevitably, conflicts between colleagues, supervisors, clients, and families will occur. These conflicts can serve to reduce productivity and job satisfaction and can result in a negative impact on our client-centered mission. To succeed as professionals, we must enhance our understanding of workplace conflicts and develop our conflict resolution skills. In doing so, we can turn conflicts into opportunities for personal growth and improved clinical outcomes.

DISCUSSION QUESTIONS/ACTIVITIES

1. Review this scenario and then answer the questions that follow.

    You notice that a number of patients are using adaptive feeding devices that you did not provide. You are wondering where they came from since the occupational therapy department is responsible for providing, documenting, and tracking these devices. You ask the dietician about this, and she confronts you saying that the occupational therapy department is not doing its job in providing the devices appropriately, so her department (dietary) has decided to also give out devices as needed.

    ◊ How would you respond to the dietician?

    ◊ How would you resolve this issue?

    ◊ Describe the conflict resolution skills you would use.

    ◊ Role play the discussion with the dietician.

2. Review this scenario in a group format, and develop alternative responses.

    Sophie, an occupational therapist, was standing at the nurse's station reading a patient's chart before performing an initial evaluation. The patient's physician arrived at the nurses station and, seeing that Sophie was reading the chart, he turned to her and said, "Can I have the chart, honey? I need to see the patient." Sophie was initially shocked and then angry about the way the physician spoke to her. She felt that she was not being treated as a professional and interpreted the doctor's words as humiliating and degrading. She shouted back a response to him, saying, "My name is not honey, and this patient is my patient also." The physician smiled and with an amused look said, "Well, what is your name, honey?" Feeling dejected and humiliated, she put the chart down and walked away in anger (Davis, 2011, p. 107). Questions to consider:

    ◊ What was wrong or right with Sophie's response?

    ◊ Identify the conflict within this interaction.

    ◊ Using the five styles of conflict management, state how you would respond to this (using one example for each style).

    ◊ What would be the best way to respond so that the therapist gains self-respect and professionally gets her point across?

    Create groups of four from within the class. Within each group, discuss the questions outlined here. Share findings with the other groups.

3. Think of a time that you experienced a conflict in your life. Write down the behaviors that you think contributed to the conflict. Is there a way you could have changed those behaviors to reduce the conflict? Describe and share your conclusions with a classmate.

4. Think of a time either during your fieldwork experiences or in other aspects of your life that you used the following conflict handling styles: competition, accommodation, avoidance, compromise, and collaboration.

    Describe the situation, the value of the issue, the potential impact on your relationship with the person with whom you are in conflict, your goal in the conflict, and why you chose the style that you did.

REFERENCES

Blackard, K., & Gibson, J. (2002). *Capitalizing on conflict: Strategies and practices for turning conflict to synergy in organizations.* Pasadena, CA: Davies-Black Publishing.

Browser, C. (2009). *Top 10 hidden sources of workplace conflict.* C.W. Bulletin. International Association of Business Communicators.

Covey, S.R. (2004). *The 7 habits of highly effective people.* New York, NY: Free Press.

Covey, S. (2011). *The 3rd alternative: Solving life's most difficult problems.* New York, NY: Free Press.

Dale Carnegie Training. (2008). *Internal conflict resolution guidebook.* Hauppauge, NY: Carnegie & Associates, Inc.

Davis, C. (2011). *Patient practitioner interaction: An experiential manual for developing and art of health care.* Thorofare, NJ: SLACK Incorporated.

Fehr, R., & Gelfand, M. (2010). When apologies work: How matching apology components to victims' self-construals facilitates forgiveness. *Organizational Behavior and Human Decision Processes, 113,* 37-50.

Maxwell, J.C. (2004). *Winning with people.* Nashville, TN: Nelson Books.

Monarth, H. (2010). *Executive presence: The art of commanding respect like a CEO.* New York, NY: McGraw Hill.

Murray, C. (2012). *Steven R. Covey guide you to a win-win,* Soundview featured book review. Soundview Executive Book Summaries. Kennett Square, PA p. 2

Problem solving information and tips. Principles for addressing workplace conflict. (n.d.). Austin, TX: Universtiy of Texas at Austin. Retrieved from http://www.utexas.edu/hr/current/services/dispute/problem.html.

Salmon, W., & Salmon, R. (2000). *The mid career tune-up: Ten work habits for keeping your edge.* New York, NY: AMACOM.

Segal, J., & Smith, M. (2011). Conflict resolution skills: Guiding the skills that can turn conflicts into opportunities., Retrieved from http://www.helpguide.org/articles/relationships/conflict-resolution-skills.htm.

Thomas, K.W., & Kilman, R.H. (1999). *Thomas-Kilman conflict mode instrument (TKI).* Mountain View, CA: CPP Inc.

Chapter 7

Working With Colleagues of All Shapes and Sizes
Diversity in the Workplace

LEARNING OBJECTIVES

At the end of this chapter, the reader will be able to:
- Identify eight specific cultural differences seen in the workplace.
- Describe how these differences impact relationships within the workplace.
- Describe five steps for overcoming cultural differences in the workplace.
- List the different generational groups and their particular traits.
- Identify how the different generational groups are similar and different.
- Describe eight ways to minimize generational conflict.
- Identify ways to promote diversity with the lesbian, gay, bisexual, and transgender (LGBT) community in the workplace.

Every human being is different—that is a pretty obvious statement. However, it is human nature to want people to be just like ourselves—to believe what we believe and to do things the way we do them. Differences can be especially difficult to deal with when they relate to how we perform our work. However, as occupational therapists and occupational therapy students working in diverse environments, we must learn to embrace differences between people resulting from differing cultures, religions, genders, sexual preferences, and upbringing—the list is endless. How do we manage these differences, communicate with one another, and learn to work together collaboratively without rancor and conflict? How can we learn to understand and accept the differences among us and learn from one another to ensure a harmonious and inclusive work environment? That is what this chapter is all about.

UNDERSTANDING DIVERSITY IN THE WORKPLACE

We live in a diverse country that was founded on the freedom of religion and choice, with a rich history of immigration. As a result, it is inevitable that we will be working with people who

Davis L, Rosee M. *Occupational Therapy Student to Clinician: Making the Transition (pp 87-107).*
© 2015 SLACK Incorporated.

are different from us. These differences must be understood and respected to avoid conflict and facilitate our ability to work as a team.

Diversity relates to gender, age, linguistic and cultural backgrounds, disabilities, religious beliefs, and family responsibilities. It also relates to the many other ways we are different, including educational and socioeconomic background, personality, where we live, marital status, sexual preference—the list of possible differences is endless (Workplace Diversity).

When working with people from similar backgrounds, there is a shared understanding of which behaviors, values, beliefs, and lifestyle choices are considered acceptable and appropriate. People who come from different backgrounds and cultures have evolved based on differing social, religious, and political histories; climates and environments; as well as access to resources such as food, water, and housing. Being brought up in different cultures will inevitably result in different ways of communicating as well as different manners and customs.

A progressive workplace will manage diversity issues by recognizing and respecting the value of human differences and actively working to create an environment where all of the abilities and experiences of employees can be shared and applied to their fullest advantage.

Fostering workplace cooperation, acceptance, and teamwork, and accepting differences is not only the productive thing to do, but it is also sanctioned by federal law. Under the Civil Rights Act of 1964, discrimination in hiring for employment is outlawed. This law has evolved over the years to include protections for individuals based on race, religion, marital status, disability, age, pregnancy status, HIV/AIDS status, gender, and nationality. Harassment, segregation, discrimination, and certain pre-employment questions violate Title VII of the Civil Rights Act. According to the law, harassment includes incidents such as racial slurs, derogatory statements, or other offensive behaviors (both physical and verbal). Hostile workplaces that tolerate harassment and discrimination could be found in violation of the law. Practices such as coding or otherwise denoting an employee's race on any document related to employment is deemed as segregation. No individual may be denied employment based on country of origin, birth location, cultural ancestry, or linguistic characteristics. The act also outlaws denial of employment or promotion due to religious affiliation, beliefs or practices, or gender. Religious practices must be reasonably accommodated. It is important for everyone to understand that workplace harassment should not be tolerated and that there are procedures for reporting and remedying them if they occur. Obviously, we should never be part of the problem by initiating behaviors that could be construed or interpreted as harassment or offensive (Illegal Discrimination, 2012).

Cultural Differences

In addition to actual language differences, different cultures communicate and relate to others in different ways. These differences may affect how people greet and address one other, how they communicate feelings, their dietary and dress practices, values, attitudes toward time management, and personal space parameters. Because of these differences, cross cultural miscommunication and misunderstandings can frequently occur when the message from one person's culture is not received in the manner to which it was intended.

Differences that evolve from our diverse culture must be understood in the workplace and include some of the following.

Dress

Some cultures mandate certain dress codes that may be quite different from the typical garb expected within a work environment. These dress codes are usually related to religious requirements. For example, women of the Muslim faith may work in burkas that cover all or most of the body. Orthodox Jewish women may only wear long skirts and long-sleeved garments and must keep their heads covered, whereas men may dress in long coats and hats.

These differing dress requirements must be accommodated in the workplace unless they are in direct conflict with safety precautions. For example, while religion may require a woman's face to be covered, she might be required to show her face for security and identification purposes.

As a newly hired therapist who needs to dress in a manner that differs from his or her colleagues, it is helpful to share information about one's dress code mandates. It is important that you make it clear that your dress will not interfere with work requirements. For example, if you must wear long skirts due to religious requirements that prevent you from wearing pants, make it clear that your clothes will not stop you from getting down on the floor and doing what you need to do with your patients. Being forthright can prevent misconceptions about how your dress might impact your ability to perform job responsibilities.

Religious Practices

Some religions may require that their members pray at certain times during the day, prevent travel and work on the Sabbath, or mandate religious observations involving absences from work or the need to leave early on certain days. Under Title VII, employers are not required to accommodate religious activities when it involves increased financial cost but are encouraged to promote flexibility by allowing employees to make up lost time, flex their schedules, or swap shifts (Steinberger, 2007).

Dietary Practices

Different cultures often exhibit different ways of preparing and seasoning food. For example, some cultures and religions do not allow the consumption of some or all animal products (especially pork and shellfish), while others do not allow the mixture of meat and dairy products. Based on climate differences and gastrointestinal intolerances, certain cultures prefer particular spices and cooking styles. Certain religions may fast during particular holidays or holy periods. Dietary variations are endless and are often observed in the workplace as coworkers share meals together. Many workplaces encourage cross-cultural education relating to dietary differences by promoting holiday parties and celebrations where different ethnic groups share their foods with one another.

Social Values

The social environments in which people grow up and live impact their values. This socialization process affects how one thinks and raises a number of important issues, including social and sexual behaviors; work ethic; attitudes toward pregnancy, child bearing, and child rearing; health and sickness; family roles; and attitudes toward wealth and education. There can be profound differences between cultures based on their ethical beliefs and values. These differences, when shared in the workplace, can result in conflicts that can be counterproductive to working relationships.

Communication Styles

Different cultures communicate in different ways. These differences may impact how people greet one another, how they address each other, what is said, how they express themselves, etc. Some issues to be aware of include the following:

- *Nonverbal communication*: Gestures, tone of voice, eye contact, and facial expressions can vary in meaning across cultures. For example, in India, shaking the head from side to side is an indication of agreement rather than disagreement. Head shaking in agreement can sometimes be used to mask an individual's inability to understand what the other person is saying. Women of Hindu heritage often speak in a soft voice, which makes it difficult to understand and decipher what they are saying. By having an awareness of these nonverbal tendencies, one might avoid confusing messages by verbally clarifying what the person really means.

◆ *Personal space*: In our American culture, there is an unspoken rule about maintaining personal distance in our interactions. Different cultures have differing rules about this, which can create either discomfort (people who come in too close to our personal space) or misinterpretations (people who seem cold and distant). For example, people from the Greek culture tend to be direct and prefer a speaking and sitting distance that is closer than people from other European cultures. Additionally, in some cultures, it is customary to touch during communication, while in other cultures, it is considered taboo (especially between sexes in the Arab and Orthodox Jewish cultures). Traditional Vietnamese people prefer distance during personal and social interchanges. The variations based on culture go on and on.

In the United States, we are typically comfortable with the following space parameters:

◇ The intimate zone extends to 1.5 feet, which allows for perception of breath and odor. This separation is acceptable only in private places.

◇ Personal distance extends from 1.5 to 4 feet. This represents a bubble of space surrounding the body. At this distance, the voice may be moderate and body odor may not be noticed.

◇ Social distance extends from 4 to 12 feet or more. Interaction is impersonal; the volume of the voice must be projected and facial expressions may be lost (Spector, 2004).

It is important that all cultures are aware of what is acceptable space within the culture with whom they are working so they do not make their coworkers uncomfortable.

◆ *Eye contact*: Cultures vary widely on the meaning of eye contact. In many cultures, avoidance of eye contact is a sign of respect, while in other cultures, it is a sign of disinterest and rudeness. While Greeks and Arabs prefer prolonged eye contact, people of Hindu or Japanese descent tend to avoid it.

◆ *Response to emotions*: Different cultures exhibit differing responses to signs of emotion. In the Japanese culture, open communication is discouraged, making it difficult to discern what people think. People of the Turkish culture tend to display emotions openly. Emotions such as happiness, disgust, approval, and sadness are made clear through obvious facial expressions and gestures. In many cultures, agreeing to something (verbally or nonverbally) even if you do not agree is often done to avoid confrontation and disharmony. Some cultures, such as the Vietnamese, often deal with negative emotions by remaining silent. The Navaho culture relies on third parties to relay information between two individuals because a face-to-face disagreement will cause ill feelings. Other cultures value assertiveness as a positive attribute. Self-assurance, confidence, and the ability to articulate ideas and concerns can elevate your professional status, but other cultures may view this assertiveness as rudeness and aggressiveness, especially if that particular culture values passivity as a virtue. It is helpful to know how different cultures deal with workplace communication issues to reduce the chance of a misunderstanding between coworkers due to differing styles.

Language

The content or meaning of language can be interpreted differently based on where it originates. For example, in the United Kingdom, English is the primary language, as it is in the United States. However, the British often use words to connote different meanings than those used in the United States. For example, a "fag" in the United States is a pejorative term for a homosexual man, but the British often use the word "fag" to mean a cigarette. Such cultural differences in the meaning of language can create misunderstandings.

In a clinical setting, it is imperative that you understand how you interact and communicate and how your culture and upbringing impacts on these factors. For example, if your culture favors touching during communication, be aware of that and understand that another culture may view this behavior as aggressive or inappropriate. It can be helpful to notice these differences and communicate the noted differences with colleagues as an educative process. One might say, "I know that I use my hands a lot when I speak and get very emotional. I notice that you tend to handle things in a quieter, gentler manner. I think my way is based on how I learned to communicate from my family. Is your way based on your culture?" Opening up communication to understand differences can go a long way toward fostering harmony.

Family Roles and Obligations

This relates to gender roles, family goals and priorities, roles of the elderly, and acceptance of alternative lifestyles. Some cultures place different values on family, which can sometimes conflict with work obligations. For example, in some cultures, the elderly are highly respected and cared for (and these priorities may take precedent over work responsibilities), while in other cultures, the elderly are shunned and ignored. In some cultures, the father is the absolute ruler, while in other cultures, there is equality between the sexes. In some cultures (such as Vietnamese), the family is the main reference point for the individual throughout his or her life, superseding obligations to country, work, and self (Purnell, 2005).

Differing Attitudes Toward Time

Time management and punctuality are important values in American culture (Purnell, 2005). As a future-oriented culture, we prefer to plan ahead by making schedules, setting appointments, and organizing activities (Spector, 2004) with an awareness that we have responsibilities that must be fulfilled within a particular time frame. As professionals working with patients and clients, we have specific appointments we must keep and deadlines (such as note-writing schedules) that we must adhere to. However, many cultures do not share our orientation to time. Certain cultures are more oriented to the present than the future. The attitude is, "If something interferes with timeliness, so be it." With this orientation, people are likely to be late or miss appointments and deadlines. In a workplace setting, this can be particularly frustrating. While one culture may feel insulted and minimized by people who disregard time requirements, the culture that does not put a priority on time believes this is normal and acceptable behavior. As a professional, this is one area where culture is no excuse for tardiness and failure to complete required tasks. Lack of orientation to time is an issue that must be handled by management to avoid client dissatisfaction, negative reaction from coworkers, and even denial for payment of services. Lack of orientation to time can also become an issue when our patients exhibit the behavior. We are all on schedules, and patients who arrive late for their appointments can have a negative impact on our ability to provide the service as promised. In such cases, the behavior must be addressed directly, with concrete rules for lateness and missed sessions outlined so that the patient understands the consequences.

Biological Variations

Members of different cultural groups often differ biologically (physically and genetically) from one another. Examples of such variations can include body build and structure, skin color, digestive differences, and susceptibility to certain diseases (Spector, 2004). These differences are inherent and can impact many other facets of life, including physical capabilities, diets, and health.

USING STEREOTYPES AS A CULTURAL GUIDE

Stereotyping involves categorization that "organizes our experience and guides our behavior toward ethnic and national groups" (Adler, 1991, p. 5). Stereotypes do not describe individual behavior; rather, they describe the behavioral norm for members of a particular group. Effective stereotyping can be helpful or harmful, depending on how it is used. Used effectively, stereotyping allows people to understand and act appropriately in new situations. A stereotype can be useful when it is the following:

- *Consciously held*: Awareness that one is describing a group norm rather than the characteristics of a specific individual
- *Descriptive rather than evaluative*: Should describe what people from this group will probably be like and not evaluate the traits as good or bad
- *Accurate*: Should accurately describe the norm from the group to which the person belongs
- *Provides a "best guess"* about a group prior to having direct information about the person or persons involved
- *Modified* based on further observation and experience with the actual people and situations (Adler, 1991)

While people are often admonished not to stereotype, it can be a useful initial guide to a situation. Stereotyping has been thought of as a primitive and unnecessary simplification of reality that inaccurately depicts the traits of particular groups. However, there are realities to different cultural norms, especially in relation to communication styles. If these are properly understood, it can be helpful in interacting with people from these cultures until we get to know them as individuals, at which time we can adapt our responses.

For example, certain cultures, such as Japanese or Korean, perceive a lack of eye contact as a sign of respect. While this may be generally true, it would not be true of all members of the particular group. It would be best to respect this general stereotype when first meeting someone from that culture until one can ascertain that the perception does not hold true. Religions also have customs and rituals that should be understood. For example, within the Jewish religion, there are three different denominations that adhere to very different rules and traditions. One cannot assume that all people of Jewish faith are alike. Some members follow strict dress and dietary guidelines, while others do not.

Cultural guidelines (which are widely available in the literature) can be useful in outlining typical behaviors and attitudes exhibited by particular cultures, religions, and races and help us to interact more effectively with that particular group, provided we understand that these guidelines are generalizations that will not always hold true.

STEPS FOR OVERCOMING CULTURAL DIFFERENCES IN THE WORKPLACE

- *Look for commonalities and get to know one another*: We all know that in social and work environments there are certain topics that are best avoided. Religion, money, and politics come to mind right away, but there are also areas where we have much in common with people of different cultures, such as food, family, pets, and sports. Use these safer subjects as a basis for developing a relationship and learning more about the person as an individual.
- *Learn about other cultures*: When we educate ourselves about the culture and history of the people we work with, we automatically understand and know them better. We also gain a better understanding of the world.
- *Listen*: The best way to learn about other people is to listen to them, and not just to what they say—read between the lines. Look at their nonverbal behaviors and what seems to make them comfortable and uncomfortable.
- *Learn to pronounce names correctly*: Everyone wants to be acknowledged and respected. Often, we have a difficult time with names that are different from those with which we are familiar. When that happens, make an effort to pronounce the name correctly. This shows respect for the individual and his or her culture.

- *Do not discuss religion in the workplace*: Work is not the venue for religious discussion, as it could incite arguments, rancor, and rifts that can be difficult to undo.
- *Avoid racially based jokes*: These are offensive and inappropriate at any time, but especially in the workplace. You never know who you are offending when you make a joke. It is better to stay away from sensitive topics.

GENDER ISSUES

Men and women are different, both physically and emotionally. They are socialized differently as children and are given very different messages about how to behave and succeed. As a result, men and women communicate and manage very differently in the workplace. In Deborah Tannen's (1990) book *You Just Don't Understand: Women and Men in Conversation,* she concludes that boys' and girls' early social lives are so different that, even when in the same household, they are actually growing up in different cultures. As a result, conversation between women and men is crosscultural, with the same possibility of misunderstandings that occur between people from different racial, ethnic, and religious backgrounds (Hahn & Litwin, 1995).

Tannen (1990, as cited in Hahn & Litwin, 1995) establishes that men see themselves as engaged in a hierarchical social order in which they are one up or one down in relation to their coworkers. Their communication styles and reactions to others stress the need to "preserve independence and avoid failure" (Hahn & Litwin, 1995, p. 3). Women, on the other hand, tend to see the world as a "network of connections," and their communication and interpretation of others' communication seek to "preserve intimacy and avoid isolation" (Hahn & Litwin, 1995, p. 3). In Carol Gilligan's (1993) landmark book, *In a Different Voice,* she cites research that demonstrates marked differences in the basic operational modes of women and men, starting from when they are young children. In observing girls and boys in play, Piaget and Lever (in separate studies) found that as boys grow they become "increasingly fascinated with the legal elaboration of rules and the development of procedures for adjudicating conflicts," while girls "have a more pragmatic attitude toward rules" (Gilligan, 1993). Girls are "more willing to make exceptions and are easily reconciled to innovations." Boys' play is observed to be more competitive, while girls' play "is more cooperative" (Hahn & Litwin, 1995, p. 3).

As a result of these differences in world view and behavior, it is not surprising that workplace expectations, work style, and characteristics of men and women frequently differ (Hahn & Litwin, 1995).

In Table 7-1, we outline typical feminine vs masculine perceptions about a number of workplace issues. Obviously, these descriptions are guides, as there are many women who exhibit masculine workplace behaviors and men who exhibit feminine workplace behaviors. Because of these differences in values and priorities, workplace misunderstandings are rampant as each gender assumes that the other operates with the same views and behaviors.

Differing Styles in Men and Women

Research has shown that men and women have very different ways of communicating and managing others. When it comes to giving orders, women tend to soften their demands and statements, whereas men tend to be more direct. Since women are conditioned to maintain harmony, softened demands may result in a more tentative communication style. The more direct communication techniques typically favored by men can appear arrogant or bossy to a woman. While both sexes may be equally committed to what they are trying to accomplish, they have been conditioned to communicate it differently. Women also tend to ask more questions than men. The old joke about the man refusing to stop and ask directions when lost, while a stereotype, is based on a communication style often observed. Asking questions means different things to men and women. Men

Table 7-1

GENDER-BASED PERCEPTIONS IN THE WORKPLACE

	FEMININE	MASCULINE
Organizational structure	Participative (see colleagues as complementary)	Hierarchical (see colleagues as potential competition)
Focus on interpersonal attention	Process (care about how people treat each other in carrying out work)	Outcome (care about where they stand in relation to others)
Operating style	Interactional (interact to connect, arrive at understandings)	Transactional (interact to pass information and give directions)
Problem-solving style	Intuitive (trust instincts; will provide proof/explanation as necessary)	Linear (based on methodical thinking; will not trust intuition until proof is presented)
Individual work style	Collaborative (see work as part of a whole; discuss and review with colleagues)	Independent (see work as separate piece; complete work without the help of others)
Management style	Supportive (seek to aid, support, facilitate and provide comfort, meaning, and rewards)	Directive (seek to test, direct, organize, and provide challenges, goals, and incentives)
View of work-related conflict	Disruptive (seek to create harmony; view negative comments as unproductive)	Normal (accept a level of conflict as inevitable; view negative comments as normal part of work)

Adapted from Hahn, S., & Litwin, A. (1995). Women and men. In R.A. Ritvo, A. Litwin, L. Butler, (Eds). *Managing in the age of change: Essential skills to manage today's diverse workforce* (p. 98). Burr Ridge, IL: IRWIN Professional Publishing.

ask questions to gather information. Women ask questions for the same reason, but often ask them when the answer is already known to them in order to show interest in what the other person has to say and to cultivate the relationship (Thiederman, 2008, p. 2).

Men and women also perceive emotions quite differently. In Shaunti Feldhahn's (2009) book, *The Male Factor: The Unwritten Rules, Misperceptions and Secret Beliefs of Men in the Workplace*, she discusses how men believe that if a woman is "excitable or upset at work," she is not able to think clearly. Actually, according to Feldhahn (2009), the female brain is wired to handle a high degree of emotion and still think clearly. Male brains are not wired that way. For men to think clearly, they need to shut down emotions. Men need to understand that women can operate very effectively even when reacting emotionally to a situation. Women need to understand that men have more difficulty handling their emotions while dealing with work challenges. They may choose to ignore their emotions or shut down to operate effectively (Cavey, 2010).

Feldhahn (2009) also postulates that, although men often present a confident exterior, this is sometimes a mask for extreme self-doubt. She found that 75% of the men she studied admitted to feelings of inadequacy with the fear that coworkers will find out that they do not know what they are doing (Feldhahn, 2009). This may be why many men avoid asking questions and are more uncomfortable when questioned about their decisions. Men can perceive these questions as a challenge to their authority or a question about their competency.

How Men and Women Communicate Differently

Research indicates that men and women communicate differently, and these differences impact upon interactions in the workplace (Sherwood, 2012). These tendencies are clearly not absolute as some men exhibit the traits typical of women's communication and visa versa. The observations that follow demonstrate some of what is typically seen:

- *Nonverbal communication*: This involves varying levels of body expression, with women typically functioning at a higher intensity level. Their faces are animated and hands are in motion, with more touching noted. Men tend to be more conservative in facial movement and body contact but are less reserved in their sitting styles, with more of a tendency to spread out and take their space, while women tend to draw in when sitting. Women's nonverbal actions focus on maintaining the relationship by providing attention and encouraging participation. Men's nonverbal communication is focused on preserving calm and preventing emotional escalation.

- *Body orientation*: Men and women are different in the way they align their bodies to others. Women turn toward each other and exhibit continuous eye contact. Men tend to sit at angles, with their eyes roaming. When they interact with each other, these body orientation differences can lead to misunderstandings. The man's lack of eye contact can be interpreted as lack of interest, while his relaxed position, which may help him concentrate, can be construed as standoffish.

  ◊ **Example:** Two therapists, Ralph and Gail, share a work space. Ralph feels comfortable spreading out his work on the desk while conversing with Gail about a recent in-service they both attended. Gail is eager to discuss how they can apply this new knowledge to their patients but feels hurt and minimized because Ralph is not making eye contact with her (even though he is engaged in the conversation). She perceived his spreading out as entitlement and, while annoyed, does not say anything to him as she does not want to make waves. He has no understanding that she is annoyed at him.

- *Arguments*: Women try to get their point across by asking many types of questions: defiant, informational, and rhetorical. The questions are designed to either demonstrate their opposition or to gather data. When engaging in an argument, men tend to be more simplistic and direct. They may be so simple that they often do not recognize that a conflict is ensuing. Once the disagreement is realized, men are more concerned about being right and less concerned about someone's feelings. This perceived lack of compassion upsets women. Because men can be more sensitive to being questioned, they may close down emotionally when this occurs.

  ◊ **Example:** A female supervisor is concerned about the treatment intervention being provided by a newly graduated male therapist. During a supervision session, she asks a number of questions about his goals, approach, and interventions. Rather than engaging in a dialogue with his supervisor, he becomes defensive about his treatment plan and misses out on a learning experience.

- *Apologizing*: After the argument comes the apology. Again, men and women handle apologies differently. Women use apologies to try to create or maintain their connections. Men are wary of apologies as it lowers them to a subordinate position, which may make them uncomfortable. This can lead to a vicious cycle when a man fears losing power and avoids apologizing, which can lead a woman to construe his behavior as insensitive and offensive.

- *Giving compliments*: From a young age, women learn to give compliments. Compliments represent an affirmative and inclusive way of connecting to others. Men are more likely to evaluate a situation rather than handing out compliments. Similarly, they may not seek out compliments because of the possibility that they might get criticized. This complicates communication as a woman may ask questions with the hope of being praised, while the man sees it as an opening to give advice. The advice giver (the man) is automatically shifted to a higher position than the advice seeker (the woman).

◇ **Example:** An occupational therapist (female) and physical therapist (male) are both work-ing with the same patient. The occupational therapist is impressed by the way the physical therapist is progressing the patient's ambulation status and praises the physical therapist on his success. Rather than complimenting the occupational therapist on the great job she has done with the patient's bed mobility and transfer training, he suggests that she follow the protocol he has developed for the patient so that she can also get good results. She comes out of the interaction miffed that he did not recognize her contributions and annoyed that he was instructing her on something she already knew.

◆ *Problem solving*: Men and women approach analytical discussions differently. Men tend to focus on facts, seek immediate resolutions, and go into action. Women desire more interac-tion and discussion to fully understand the problem at hand. As a result of these differences in approaching problem solving, a man may not understand why a woman does not just want to solve the problem. The woman in turn may be hurt by the perceived disregard for her approach to the problem.

◆ *Getting their way*: Men and women have very different ways of trying to get what they want, which can make it more difficult to come to an agreement. Women tend to prefer using a conversational mode, asking questions to get others to acquiesce through agreement. Men often interpret this technique as manipulation. Men are more likely to try to get their way directly and quickly, making statements rather than suggestions to get there. If that does not work they may end the discussion, often in anger.

◇ **Example:** Bruno and Charlotte are working side-by-side in the clinic with two patients. Bruno is working on the mat, and Charlotte is doing tabletop activities. Charlotte says, "It would be great if I could use the mat a bit before Mrs. Gomez's session is over." Bruno interprets this statement as a manipulation, since Charlotte did not directly ask to use the mat but hinted about what she wanted. Bruno becomes annoyed, thinking that now he will be forced to transfer the patient off of the mat and find something else to do with her. He responds with a little annoyance in his voice, "I'll be finished in 15 minutes. Then, you can have the mat for your patient." Charlotte does not understand why he now has an attitude when all she was doing was attempting to gently explore the situation. This demonstrates how each sex tries to get what they want, but misunderstands each other as their styles and strategies are different.

◆ *Chatting*: Most people believe that women are more talkative than men, but research shows this assumption is not true (Sherwood, 2012). Women spend more time talking with friends and family, expressing support, and discussing experiences. Men tend to talk more at work and in formal and social settings with the goal of exchanging information. At home, women generally talk more and can be frustrated with the lack of response from their partners. Women generally prefer to work on their relationships through conversation, while men see less need to speak unless there is a specific purpose, such as a problem to be solved or a deci-sion to be made (Sherwood, 2012).

While communication styles are generally different for men and women, they can avoid mis-understandings; promote effective communication; and avoid distress, anger, and arguments by understanding each other's style and why it has been adopted.

GENERATIONAL ISSUES

When speaking of diversity, we mostly think of issues such as race, ethnicity, and gender. However, a major cause of conflict in the workplace is generational diversity. Within the work-place, there are four distinct generational groups that have very different approaches to work, work-life balance, employee loyalty, authority, and a number of other work-related issues (Notter,

Table 7-2

PERSONAL AND LIFESTYLE CHARACTERISTICS BY GENERATION

	TRADITIONAL-ISTS (1922-1945)	BABY BOOMERS (1946-1964)	GENERATION X (1965-1980)	GENERATION Y (1981-2000)
Core Values	Respect for authority Conformers Discipline	Optimism Involvement	Skepticism Fun Informality	Realism Confidence Extreme fun Social
Family	Traditional nuclear	Disintegrating	Latch-key kids	Merged families
Education	A dream	A birthright	A way to get there	An incredible expense
Communication and Media	Rotary phones One-on-one Write a memo	Touch-tone phone Call me anytime	Cell phones Call me only at work	Internet Picture phones E-mail
Dealing with Money	Put it away Pay cash	Buy now, pay later	Cautious Conservative Save, save, save	Earn to spend

Adapted from Hamill, G. (2005). Mixing and managing four generations of employees. FDU magazine online. Winter/Spring 2005. Teaneck, NJ: Fairleigh Dickinson University. Retrieved from http://www.fdu.edu/newspubs/magazine/05ws/generations.htm.

2002). Generational groups share common experiences that impact their values and attitudes toward life and work. While the cutoff dates for defining generations cannot be exact, there are definite traits exhibited by different generations that generally hold true. These traits are based on how individuals were raised, historical events they experienced, and a huge variety of cultural influences that are specific to the time they were born, as shown in Tables 7-2 and 7-3.

In today's workplace, the generations are as follows:

Traditionalists (Born Between 1922 and 1945)

- ◆ Have worked longer than any other generation
- ◆ Are approaching retirement or are retired and are working part time
- ◆ Have been taught to live within their means
- ◆ Often worked for the same company their entire career
- ◆ Put duty first
- ◆ Sacrificed family and friends for a strong work ethic

The Baby Boomer Generation (Born Between 1945 and 1964)

- ◆ Came of age in the 1960s (Vietnam War, Women's and Civil Rights Movements)
- ◆ Places a priority on higher education
- ◆ Nearing retirement age
- ◆ Believes age is not a barrier when it comes to work

Table 7-3

DIFFERENCES IN GENERATIONS IN THE WORKPLACE

	WORK PLACE BEHAVIORS	STRENGTHS IN THE WORK PLACE	CHALLENGES IN THE WORK PLACE
Traditionalist	• Follows the rules • Respects authority • Hardworking • Values work over family and friends • Sticks with a job throughout their careers	• Loyal • Focused • Not a clock watcher • Will give endless hours to get the job done • Tenacious	• Adverse to conflict • Lacking balance of home and work • Only absent for medical reasons • Not comfortable with technology
Baby Boomers	• Works long hours • Proud of personal achievements • Ambitious • Wants to climb up the ladder of success • Strong work ethics • Optimistic • Expects younger workers to have similar strong work ethics • May have several careers	• Team oriented • Dedicated • Loyal • Will not rock the boat	• Difficulty balancing work and family • Sandwich generation, taking care of parents and children • Adjusting to technology • Adverse to conflict • Fear of being laid off
Generation X	• Prefers changing jobs over the years • Loyal to their peers rather than an organization • Believes work should be fun • Seeks a work / life balance	• Independent • Creative • Strong technical skills • Not afraid to speak up at work	• Does not deal with authority well • Difficulty working with older peers • Comfortable with conflict and office politics • May be unrealistic about job advancement
Generation Y	• Team oriented • Enjoys working on many projects at once • Enthusiastic • Wants to work hard • Enjoys a fun work environment • Risk taker • Not adverse to job hop	• Able to multitask • Tech savvy • Team oriented • Hard working • Desire to grow professionally	• Easily bored • Wants to advance at work and prove themselves later • Needs structure • Can be too direct • Takes shortcuts when writing in a professional way. (Prefers to text and tweet.)

Adapted from Hannam, S., & Yordi, B. (2011). *Engaging the multi-generational workforce: Practical advice for government managers.* Washington, DC: IBM Center for The Business of Government. Retrieved from http://gagmis.org/GA/LinkClick.aspx?fileticket=kcnKy7t0X2k%3D&tabid=70.

Generation X (Born Between 1965 and 1980)

- Often depicted as slackers
- Self-reliant and likes to work alone
- Values flexibility and freedom, especially regarding work
- Likely to have 10 to 12 jobs during their lifetime

Generation Y/Millenials (Born Between 1981 and 2000)

- Fastest growing segment of the workforce
- Values tend to mirror those of their Baby Boomer parents
- Grew up in an age of technology
- Demands flexibility at work but values structure
- Multitasking is second nature
- Works well in team environments
- High expectation of self and employers
- Prefers employers that focus on development and training
- Focus on work-life balance

By growing up in different times with different cultural influences, the generations exhibit very different attitudes and values, which can lead to conflict. Some of the more obvious intergenerational conflicts relate to loyalty to the employer and attitudes regarding work, respect, authority, and training preferences.

Loyalty to the Employer

Traditionalists and Baby Boomers have a history of being extremely loyal toward employers, especially when contrasted with the loyalty exhibited by younger workers. Younger workers view job hopping as a career advancement method (Tolbize, 2008). They have also learned that loyalty to an employer does not guarantee job security (based on observation of what has happened to their parents, many of whom were loyal employees who got laid off). It has been found that about 70% of traditionalists reported that they would want to stay with their current organization for the rest of their working life, compared with 65% of Baby Boomers, 40% of Generation X-ers, and 20% of Generation Y-ers (Deal, 2007).

Younger employees tend to be more "me" oriented, expect to be promoted more quickly than older workers, and are less likely to feel that work should be an important part of their life. A larger percentage reported that they would most likely quit their job if they won a large amount of money (Notter, 2002).

Although loyalty differs across generations, all generations report similar reasons for staying in their organization. Deal (2007) reported that loyalty toward employers improves for all generations when there are opportunities for advancement and promotions to learn new skills and for higher salaries and/or benefits.

Employee loyalty also improves across all generations when an employer's values are perceived as matching the employee's own. Considerations such as a better quality of life, better communication, and more autonomy and control also impact all generations' loyalty. Younger people are more loyal when they feel that their organization respects them for their talent, even if they believe that the organization respects older people more.

Training Styles/Supervision

Generations exhibit different learning styles and training needs. Younger employees often prefer to learn skills on the job, while older employees prefer a combination of on-the-job and classroom instruction. Older employees are less comfortable with feedback as a learning tool and often feel insulted by it, while younger employees seem to desire it. However, younger workers dislike micromanagement and seek strong leadership to provide clear instructions. Baby Boomers seem to value freedom from supervision more than Generation X-ers (Joyner, 2000).

Attitude Toward Work-Life Balance

Younger employees have a definite desire for more balance between their work and life duties and responsibilities. The Generation X-ers saw their parents make sacrifices for their careers that they themselves are less willing to make. Younger people expressed a willingness to work hard but do not want work to interfere with the rest of their lives (Mitchell, 2001).

Attitudes Regarding Respect and Authority

There are definite differences in the way younger workers view managers and management versus the views of older workers. Older workers tend to have great respect for authority, preferring a definite hierarchy. The younger generation of workers is much more comfortable with authority figures and is less intimidated by them. They interact with supervisors, ask questions, and are more comfortable with questioning decisions. They do not view these attitudes as disrespectful. Older workers want their opinions to be given more weight because of their experience and expect younger workers to do as they are told. Younger workers want to be listened to and have attention paid to what they say. Older workers may not agree that equal respect is due and may expect to be treated with more respect based on their years of experience (Tolbize, 2008).

How These Differences Can Lead to Work Conflicts

There are many conflicts that emerge between the generations based on the differing attitudes and values relating to work. Some of these include the following:

- *Work ethic*: Older workers believe you have to pay your dues and that you are rewarded for hard work, time, and effort. Younger workers often expect rewards first and will then generate their efforts and enthusiasm. The older worker learned that work is not the time for socializing on the phone with friends. The younger worker was brought up with technology that allows constant and continuous communication with the outside world.
  - ◇ **Example**: Ann, the senior occupational therapist in a mental health inpatient unit, was supervising Barbara, who was at the site for her fieldwork II placement. During a group therapy session that Ann was leading, she was astounded to observe Barbara texting on the periphery of the group. Following the session, Ann had a discussion with the young therapy student, giving her feedback that her behavior was inappropriate and demonstrated a lack of judgment. Barbara was surprised at Ann's response and did not understand what the big deal was, since she was not the one leading the group. As the placement went on, however, Barbara began to understand why Ann would view her act as a problem and learned to restrict her cell phone use and texting to lunch time.
- *Organization hierarchy*: Older employees tend to accept hierarchies and respect a chain of command. Younger employees often resist formal structures and ignore hierarchies. They prefer more informal relationships with supervisors than previous generations (Lindsay-Lloyd, 2011).
- *Dress codes*: Many organizations have dress codes to ensure that workers look professional. There are generational differences that relate to what is considered proper and appropriate dress. While a Baby Boomer may come to work in Chinos and a neatly pressed top, someone from the millennial generation may believe that designer jeans and expensive sneakers or beach shoes are proper attire. Differing interpretations of what is appropriate can cause conflict between staff.

- *Managing technology and communication*: There are often differing views on the use of communication. Older workers are frequently less tech-savvy, preferring to utilize old methods of communication such as face-to-face conversations and handwritten progress notes versus newer technology such as text messaging and electronic documentation.

- *Breaking out of the student mode*: Younger workers just out of school will often want to continue the culture they experienced as a student. School is about the student and his or her learning and development. Conversely, at work, the focus is on the patients, the team, and the organization. The young workers' personal goals are not the central focus of an organization. At school, you are with peers who are like you. At work, there will usually be a mixture of ages, races, and religions. At school, the focus is on earning grades, whereas work focuses on an identifiable output for which one is responsible. At school, activities are directed, with someone telling you what is expected and what you need to do. Work requires self-direction, problem solving, and critical thinking to successfully fulfill responsibilities. At school, there is a lot of feedback focused on work output. At work, feedback and praise are not always immediate or clear. The evolution from student to paid professional can be a difficult process that can impact relations between generations.

Examples of Generational Differences

Scenario 1

A major project was completed at a hospital where the entire documentation system was dissected and redesigned. The result was a reduction in lost revenue secondary to payment denials. At review time, the entire staff received a bonus for a job well done. The Generation X employee was ungrateful, stating that he should have gotten the bonus when the project was completed, whereas the Baby Boomer was happy to get any bonus at all, reflecting the Generation X employee's preference for instant gratification.

Scenario 2

An intergenerational team in an occupational therapy department is assigned a project to design a new student recruitment and training program. After a few weeks of working together, their manager notes that no progress has been made. Wondering why, upon review, the manager finds that the traditionalists on the team are seeking more specificity about what tasks to complete. The Baby Boomers would like to work more collaboratively, schedule a lot of meetings, and do not mind working after hours. The Generation X-ers do not want to work on the project outside of work and do not want to be called at home. The Generation Y-ers do not want any meetings at all and want to communicate through e-mail and text rather than in person. The manager realized it would be helpful to create a structure for the team and set up rules at the outset to ensure the generations can work together.

Scenario 3

A new graduate is hired in an occupational therapy department. While the starting time is 8:00 a.m., the new hire arrives at work at 8:15 a.m. and then proceeds to eat her breakfast while catching up on documentation. The supervisor is not aware of her tardiness, and the veteran therapists are becoming resentful. When confronted by one of the veterans, the rookie expresses that she works very hard when she is treating her patients, does not see the harm in arriving a little late, and feels she is just as productive whether she is eating or not. The manager needs to address her unprofessional work habits to ensure she adheres to acceptable behaviors and does not undermine department morale.

Minimizing Generational Differences

Working with people of different generations is a reality in the modern work environment. As professionals, we will have to learn to deal with conflicting values and ideas. Differing communication, lifestyle, and work preferences must be addressed, considered, and understood to ensure smooth operations and functional teams. Some suggestions to help facilitate intergenerational harmony include the following:

- Focus on similarities rather than differences. While the generations may have differing priorities and preferences, they have a common goal in the workplace. Remembering the common goal and finding ways to work together, despite differences, can improve outcomes for all.

- Learn from one another and take the best that each generation has to offer. Learning from traditional approaches while remaining open to new innovations is a good solution to work-related problems and can bring the generations together. For example, computer software is the trend in cognitive rehabilitation, but there are times when an old-fashioned memory book or another low-tech intervention might be more effective than a high-tech one.

- Develop a curiosity for things unknown to you. While it is important to learn new technologies, be open to things you do not know and understand. For example, in the past, occupational therapists typically used craft activities as a treatment modality. While this tradition has changed, by learning about how crafts were used, one might identify a useful treatment intervention for a particular patient.

- Ask questions rather than make statements. Often, one's first response is that a new suggestion (whether given by a younger or older person) is useless, old-fashioned, or newfangled. Suggestions by other generations are often met with resistance or ill feelings. Instead of criticizing the idea, ask questions to clarify. With the right questions, your doubts about the idea may become clearer to the person making the suggestion. For example, a colleague suggests that a particular iPad app might be the perfect solution to a patient's inability to perform a task. Rather than reject the idea (because you are unfamiliar with an iPad), ask for a demonstration of how this might work for the patient. Usually, the "techie" is very willing and happy to share the marvels of technology.

- Avoid characterizations based on age. When you have disagreements with someone of a different age, try to focus on the work issue involved rather than thinking that the person holds that view simply because of his or her age. Using age in a discussion can not only be hurtful, but it could also result in legal challenges for your facility.

- Define acronyms. Acronyms can cause confusion, as they can mean different things to different people. Be aware of how you use acronyms when you speak to colleagues and patients. Do not assume that everyone knows what you are talking about. For example, two occupational therapists were overheard speaking in the hall. "I reviewed the IEP for the CPSE case. Since I have an RSA for the child, the DOE wants me to start right away. My BFF is seeing a kid with ASD right in the next classroom. She's doing ABA, but I'm not. We LOLed over the coincidence." Often, these acronyms are understood and help speed up the conversation, but for many people, they are like a foreign language that interferes with communication. In the age of texting, younger people are accustomed to acronyms in their daily life. When using them with other people, explain them at the onset to ensure clear communication.

- Before responding to a sensitive issue, paraphrase the point that you think the other person is trying to make. This can help clarify the issue and ensure that the individuals involved understand each other (Sun, 2011).

SEXUAL ORIENTATION DIFFERENCES

Gay, lesbian, bisexual, and transgender people live in all aspects of society; belong to all economic, racial, and social groups; and are a presence in every work environment. "Sexual orientation refers to the sex of those to whom one is sexually and romantically attracted" (American Psychological Association, 2011). The term *sexual orientation* includes heterosexuality (attraction to the opposite sex), homosexuality (attraction to the same sex), and bisexuality (attraction to either sex). In recent years, the transgender population has been linked to the gay, lesbian, and bisexual communities to form what is commonly known as the lesbian, gay, bisexual, and transgender (LGBT) community. The term *transgender* refers to a range of people who experience and/or express their gender differently from what is expected. This may include expressing to be or living as a gender that does not match the sex listed on one's original birth certificate. This might result in the changing of one's sex through surgery and hormone treatment. Often, the term *transgender* is used to include people who are transsexual, cross-dressers, or otherwise gender nonconforming (Moulton & Seaton, 2005).

Because of pervasive discrimination over the course of centuries, many people within the LGBT community have chosen to hide their identities, especially in the workplace. They may not feel the freedom to share their lives with their coworkers or the safety to bring their full selves into the workplace.

While workplace conflict revolving around LGBT issues are less frequently addressed than other issues such as religion and race, these issues are now in the forefront thanks to greater visibility following successful legal challenges related to marriage equality and military service. It has been found that approximately 4% of the population in the United States is lesbian, gay, or bisexual and 0.3% are transgender, although these figures are assuredly underreported (Catalyst, 2012). The Williams Institute on Sexual Orientation Law and Public Policy has found that 15% to 43% of gay and transgender employees have experienced some form of discrimination or harassment in the workplace (Catalyst, 2012). According to Catalyst (2012), 8% to 17% of gay and transgender employees were not hired or were fired due to their sexual orientation, 10% to 28% were not promoted, and 97% have experienced harassment or mistreatment in the workplace.

Discussions about sexual orientation issues can be difficult in the workplace as they involve different values, beliefs, and opinions. The reality in most workplaces is that heterosexual men and women enjoy membership in the dominant societal group. Their relationships are seen as normal and expected. These perceptions are reinforced by social media and convention. Being part of the subordinated LGBT group can sometimes result in confusion and shame. Assumptions about one's sexual preferences are made based on the dominant group's expectations (i.e., it is assumed that everyone is heterosexual). If a member of the LGBT community chooses to be genuine about his or her lifestyle at work, it will require an action not required of the heterosexual worker—clarification of these assumptions and a requirement to come out (share his or her lifestyle). If one does not come out, he or she is unable to fully share his or her life and is often forced to lie when placed in an uncomfortable or threatening environment (Buccigrosi & Frost, 2003). Since the LGBT community is pervasive throughout our culture with greatly strengthened political and consumer clout, they are becoming more visible and integrated into their communities and are now receiving more widespread protection from discrimination and wider recognition for their relationships.

Working With the Transgender Coworker

Although representing a much smaller percentage of the population than the lesbian, gay, and bisexual community, transgender individuals are becoming much more visible members of our society and workforce. It is believed that 1 in 30,000 males and 1 in 100,000 females seek sex reassignment surgery (Moulton & Seaton, 2005), although this is probably not an accurate statistic, as the population is believed to be undercounted.

Underemployment and unemployment are major issues for transgender individuals, especially during the transition from their biologically assigned sex to their chosen sex. (Transitioning is the process where the individual starts to move toward the opposite gender through a variety of mechanisms, including cross dressing, hormone therapy, and sexual reassignment. The transitioning process is different for each individual.) Transgender people who transition after working somewhere for an extended period of time often encounter discrimination from those who may not understand or accept them. After the transition, the new realities of the person's reassignment can require adaptations, such as determining which restroom he or she uses and how he or she will be addressed. Transgender people usually choose to be referred to by the pronoun that matches their preferred sex (whether they have transitioned or not). It is considered insensitive to refer to someone by the wrong gender once you have established which set of pronouns is preferred.

Often, the transitioning individual will choose to make the change to a new employment situation where he or she is only known in his or her current state of reassignment. While not currently a protected status under federal law, sentiment is changing, with legislation moving toward more extensive protections against employment discrimination. As clinicians and coworkers, we have an obligation to understand and accept differences. Some suggestions for improving relationships with transgender coworkers include the following:

- Learn about transsexualism. There are many publications readily available on the Internet that explain the phenomenon and will help coworkers appreciate the process. Through understanding comes acceptance.

- Maintain an open mind and sense of empathy for what your coworker is going through. Although one may feel uncomfortable around transgender people at first, we must all examine our biases, be respectful, and avoid being judgmental.

- Openly discuss with your transsexual coworker whether he or she is open to answering questions and educating others about his or her status. Often, many misperceptions and misunderstandings can be effectively handled through communication.

Vignette: Joanie was providing coverage in a nursing home during the holiday season. During the staff party, one of the department heads was asked to sing a Christmas carol. He had a wonderful baritone voice, and apparently his performance was a yearly tradition. Joanie noticed that he was wearing a woman's wig and pearls. Later, he came over to Joanie's table to share some pictures of his recent cruise with other staff members. On the cruise, he was dressed in women's clothing, wearing a ball gown and jewelry. He received compliments from the staff about his garb and was asked many questions about the trip. As a member of the LGBT community, Joanie was extremely impressed by the staff's acceptance and inclusiveness. When she was later offered a permanent position at the facility, she grabbed the opportunity. Joanie figured that this was an environment where she would be accepted for her lifestyle choices.

General Suggestions to Promote Diversity With the LGBT Community

In order to foster inclusiveness with the LGBT community, consider the following steps:

- Do not lump all members of the LGBT community into one category. As with any community, all individuals within a group are not the same. Some are single and others are coupled, some have children and some do not, some couples are married and some are not, and some individuals are out and some are closeted. Do not make assumptions—get to know them as individuals.

- Both LGBT and heterosexual communities need to be inclusive of one another. Welcome their spouse equivalents or life partners to group activities and include one another in social activities.

- Expect that some members of the LGBT community may choose to be shy or secretive due in part to negative past experiences and fear relating to their sexual orientation or gender identity. Do not judge someone's unwillingness to come out.
- Refrain from using judgmental language.
- Do not tell, and discourage others from telling, LGBT-related jokes.
- Work to build rapport and trust between the communities. Spend time with each other and get to know about each other's lives.
- Ask individuals (whether heterosexual or LGBT) what terminology they prefer when referring to life partners (e.g., wife, husband, spouse, partner, boyfriend).
- If you want to know something about a person's sexual orientation, gender identity, or personal life, ask him or her directly rather than asking others.
- When someone shares information with you, keep it confidential. Do not out people to others. If someone asks you about someone else, refer him or her back to the person for an answer.
- Avoid making assumptions about a person's sexual orientation or gender based on appearance or behavior.
- Do not assume that a person's spouse or partner is of the opposite sex.

Steps for Members of the LGBT Community to Foster Inclusiveness

- Make the choice to be out to the extent you are comfortable. Be clear with others about what that means, and let them know as changes occur.
- Be honest about whether you want people to ask questions. Be clear whether the information you are communicating is confidential or if it is okay for them to share the information with others.
- Try to be patient, nonsarcastic, and nondefensive when communicating. Some people may want to learn more about you and your community. Help them by sharing information.
- Let supervisors know if you experience discrimination or harassment related to your sexual orientation or gender identity.
- Share equal responsibility with heterosexual coworkers to develop lines of communication, rapport, and trust (Buccigrosi & Frost, 2003).

SUMMARY

   In the workplace setting, there are an infinite number of variables that make us different from our coworkers. Whether it be gender, sexual preference, age, religious beliefs, values, ethnic backgrounds, countries of origin, or primary language, we will find that we are all different from one another. By getting to know people who are different from us, we have the opportunity to expand our knowledge and learn about the world outside of our limited sphere. However, with differences comes conflict. Most people prefer to surround themselves with people who are like them. When differences are experienced, there is sometimes an inclination to want to change the other person or reject his or her lifestyles, habits, values, and traditions. In this chapter, we identified some of the basic differences between people and outlined where these differences derive from and how they evolve. We also identified how these differences can impact our relationships in the workplace setting and how we can improve our relationships through education and understanding. In a heterogeneous country, it is crucial that we address these issues so that we can work together productively for the clients and patients we are there to serve.

Discussion Questions/Activities

1. Think about a time that you interacted with a generational group different from yours. Identify the generation and describe some of the core values observed and how they differ from yours.

2. Role play with a partner a scene in which one plays a Baby Boomer and the other a Millennial. Discuss together how to resolve issues relating to dress attire, timeliness, supervision needs, and communication styles.

3. Based on your culture, how would you describe your communication style? How do you think others perceive it?

4. Give examples of interactions you have had in the clinical setting where there were miscommunications and misunderstandings based on the differing ways of communication between men and women.

5. Form into groups of two students each. Each group will go into a community (different from the one they are accustomed to) and observe daily life in a grocery store. Observe elements such as food choices, dress, communication styles, and gestures, and compare them to what you are accustomed to. Bring back the information to the class and present what was observed and how it is different from what you observe in your own community.

References

Adler, N. (1991). Communicating across cultural barriers. In *International dimension of organizational behavior* (pp. 63-91). Boston, MA: PWS Kent Publishing Company.

American Psychiatric Association. (2011). Practice guidelines for LGB clients: Guidelines for psychological practice with lesbian, gay, and bisexual clients. Retrieved from http://apa.org/pi/lgbt/resources/guidelines.aspx.

Buccigrosi, J., & Frost, D. (2003). *Sexual orientation.* Rochester, NY: wetWare, Inc.

Catalyst. (2012). *Quick take: Lesbian, gay, bisexual & transgender workplace issues.* New York, NY: Catalyst, Retrieved from http://www.catalyst.org/knowledge/lesbian-gay-bisexual-transgender-workplace-issues.

Cavey, J.A. (2010, July 26). Gender differences in the workplace. workforcedevelopment.edublogs.org. Retrieved from http://www.workforcedevelopment.edublogs.org/2010/07/26/gender-differences-in-the-workplace.

Deal, J.J. (2007). *Retiring the generation gap: How employees young and old can find common ground.* San Francisco, CA: Jossey-Bass.

Feldhahn, S. (2009). *The male factor: The unwritten rules, misperceptions and secret beliefs of men in the workplace.* New York, NY: Crown Books.

Gilligan, C. (1993). *In a different voice: Psychological theory and women's development.* Boston, MA: Harvard University Press.

Hahn, S., & Litwin, A. (1995). Women and men. In R.A. Ritvo, A. Litwin, L. Butler, (Eds). *Managing in the Age of Change: Essential Skills to Manage Today's Diverse Workforce* (p. 98). Burr Ridge, IL: IRWIN Professional Publishing.

Hamill, G. (2005). Mixing and managing four generations of employees. FDU magazine online. Winter/Spring 2005. Teaneck, NJ: Fairleigh Dickinson University. Retrieved from http://www.fdu.edu/newspubs/magazine/05ws/generations.htm.

Illegal discrimination in the workplace. (2012). LawFirms.com. Retrieved from: http://www.lawfirms.com/resources/employment/discrimination/illegal-discrimination-workplace.htm.

Joyner, T. (2000). Gen X-ers focus on life outside the job fulfillment. *The Secured Lender,* May/June. Retrieved from http//findarticles.com/p/articles/mi_qa5352/is_200005/ai_n2145543.

Lindsey-Lloyd, K. (2011). *You don't know me: Five generations in the workplace.* Retrieved from slideshare.net. /klinlloyd/you-dont-know-me-generational-conflict-in-the-workplace.

Mitchell, S. (2001). *Generation X: Americans aged 18-34.* Ithaca, NY: New Strategist Publications.

Moulton, B. & Seaton, L. (2005). Transgender Americans: a handbook for understanding. Human Rights Campaign. Retrieved from http://www.hrc.org/documents/Transgender-handbook.pd

Notter, J. (2002). *Generational diversity in the workplace*. Notter Consulting.

Purnell, L. (2005). *Guide to culturally competent health care*. Philadelphia, PA: F.A. Davis & Company.

Sherwood, S. (2012). *Gender and sexuality: 10 ways men and women communicate differently*. Retrieved from http://www.discovery.com/tv-shows/curiosity/topics/10-ways-men-women-communicate-differently. htm.

Spector, R. (2004). *Cultural diversity in health and illness*. Upper Saddle River, NJ: Pearson/Prentice Hall.

Steinberger, J. (2007). *Religion and the workplace*. Retrieved from http://www.entrepreneur.com/article/184334.

Sun, C. (2011). *10+ ways to minimize generational differences in the workplace*. Retrieved from http://www.techrepublic.com/blog/10-things/10-plus-ways-to-minimize-generational-differences-in-the-workplace.

Thiederman, S. (2008). He said, she said. Retrieved from http://www.mexcelle.monster.com/news/articles/1564-he-said-she-said-differences-in-gernder-communication?page=2.

Tolbize, A. (2008). *Generational differences in the workplace*. Minneapolis, MN: University of Minnesota, Research and Training Center of Community Living.

Chapter 8

Doing What Is Legal
Understanding Your Obligations
as a Professional

LEARNING OBJECTIVES

At the end of this chapter, the reader will be able to:

➤ Define and identify the differences between civil law and criminal law.

➤ Name five questions that should be avoided when interviewing a prospective employee.

➤ Identify the three main considerations when determining independent contractor status.

➤ Name the most common causes of lawsuits against occupational therapists.

➤ Identify four ways to reduce the risk of lawsuits as related to occupational therapy practice.

➤ Identify the difference between claims made and occurrence-based professional liability insurance.

➤ Describe examples of fraud and abuse under the Medicare and Medicaid program regulations.

As licensed (or soon-to-be licensed or certified) professionals, occupational therapists and certified occupational therapy assistants operate under the jurisdiction of many regulatory agencies. In addition to the state regulatory board that oversees our licenses, we must be aware of federal, state, and local laws in order to protect ourselves from committing acts that could be interpreted as illegal or lead to professional and personal liability. This chapter outlines how various areas of the law impact occupational therapy practice. Areas covered include employment law, privacy and confidentiality, medical record issues, professional liability, and fraud and abuse.

Davis L, Rosee M. *Occupational Therapy Student to Clinician:*
Making the Transition (pp 109-118).
© 2015 SLACK Incorporated.

UNDERSTANDING THE LAW AND ITS IMPACT ON OCCUPATIONAL THERAPY PRACTICE

What we commonly refer to as *law* consists of a broad set of rules derived from many sources. Congress passes federal laws such as the Social Security Act, Americans With Disabilities Act, and Fair Labor Standards Act. State laws are specific to individual states and include licensure regulations that outline what professionals can and cannot do, along with the sanctions associated with breaches of such regulations, and outlining the continuing education requirements to maintain one's license. Local laws relate to the city or town where the law is passed. They might include anti-smoking legislation, animal control issues, or loitering regulations. Case law is created from judgments made in court rather than those passed by a legislature. For example, the Jimmo vs Sebilus settlement was decided by the U.S. District Court of Vermont and had significant impact on occupational therapy practice. It determined that maintenance therapy must be covered under Medicare, even though it had previously been considered a non-reimbursable expense. The court ruling made it law and overturned decades of practice.

In addition to classifying laws based on which government body passed or decided on it, law can also be classified based on whether it is a civil or criminal action. A civil wrong (often referred to as a *tort*) is based on harm done to a person or a person's property. A civil lawsuit is brought about by an individual or entity against another individual. A criminal wrong is an act that violates criminal statutes (Aiken, 2002, p. 7). Issues that can be classified as civil in nature include contractual issues, negligence, malpractice, labor, and privacy issues. Typically, most cases brought against health care workers are for negligence or malpractice. The allegation typically involves the assertion that the provider failed to provide care that met the standards of the profession, resulting in harm to the patient. Remedies are typically monetary.

Criminal law is concerned with violations against society based on federal, state, or local statute or code. The remedies can include monetary fines, imprisonment, and death. Misdemeanors are lesser crimes punishable by small fines. Felonies are more serious crimes punishable by larger fines and/or imprisonment. A felony conviction may be grounds for revoking a license to practice a health care profession. A health care provider may also be prosecuted criminally for actions such as practicing without a license, falsifying information in obtaining a license, and patient abuse (Aiken, 2002, p. 8).

It is important to understand your state licensing laws and how your personal actions can impact your professional license. For example, some states have strict laws pertaining to driving while intoxicated. Apprehension, charges, and convictions for felonies or serious crimes—such as failure to pay child support—can also have serious professional consequences, including revocation of your professional license.

EMPLOYMENT LAW ISSUES

Discrimination

As discussed in a previous chapter, it is important that we all understand employment law issues and how they impact us in the workplace. Under Title VII of the Civil Rights Act of 1964, employment discrimination is prohibited based on race, color, religion, sex, or national origin. The Age Discrimination in Employment Act protects individuals who are 40 years of age or older and the Americans with Disabilities Act of 1990 prohibits employment discrimination against qualified individuals with disabilities in the private sector and in state and local governments (U.S. Equal Employment Opportunity Commission [U.S. EEOC], 2009). The EEOC enforces these laws in addition to providing oversight and coordination of all employment regulations, practices, and policies. Intentional breach of these laws could result in significant monetary damages for the employer. Even junior members of an occupational therapy department can place an employer in jeopardy if they participate in activities that are construed as discriminatory in nature, even if the breach was unintentional. Staff members are often asked to meet with prospective employees to show them the department, give them a tour of the facility, and get a general sense of who they are. Everyone who meets prospective employees must be mindful of the kinds of questions they can and cannot ask under federal discrimination laws. Questions relating to any of the protected factors must be strictly avoided. Some examples of discriminatory questions include the following:

- What does your husband do? (marital status)
- Where were you born? (national origin)
- When did you graduate from high school? (age)
- Which church do you attend? (religion)
- Do you have any children? (marital status)
- Are you planning on having children? (sex)
- Have you ever been arrested? (civil rights)
- Are you a member of the National Guard? (military status)
- Have you ever filed a claim for workers' compensation? (disability)
- Do you have any physical disabilities that may affect your job performance? (disability)

Anyone in the department who has contact with potential employees must be aware of these laws and understand the implications of their questions to avoid a possible discrimination lawsuit (Jacobs & McCormack, 2011).

Possible Discriminatory Situations

Scenario: An entry-level therapist seeking her first job is being interviewed by three staff members before meeting with the director. One of the staff members observes that the therapist is missing three fingers on the right hand. She asks the interviewee if she is able to splint considering her missing fingers. After hearing that she was not hired, the interviewing therapist is highly insulted and files a discrimination complaint against the facility.

Scenario: A therapist is being interviewed for a position at a local hospital. She had returned to school when her children left for college and was entering the field at middle age. When observing the clinic, she noticed that she was considerably older than the therapists currently working in the department. During the interview, the supervisor (who was 20 years her junior) asked her how she would feel taking orders from someone much younger. After learning she was not hired, the interviewing therapist sent a formal complaint to the facility's executive director and threatened the facility with an age discrimination suit.

Scenario: A rehabilitation director was overheard requesting coverage from a staffing agency. She specified that the agency not send anyone with a foreign accent. A foreign therapist working in the department who also had an accent reported the conversation to the human resources department, which later performed an investigation of the event. The director was written up.

Scenario: A school principal was asked to provide a reference for a therapist who had formerly worked at the school. While the therapist had always received positive yearly reviews and had longevity, the principal proceeded to provide a negative review of the former employee's performance. A friend of the therapist was standing nearby and overheard the conversation and reported it back to her. When the therapist did not get the job, she felt that she was unjustly maligned, so she sued the school for defamation of character.

PRIVACY AND CONFIDENTIALITY ISSUES

Included in the AOTA's *Code of Ethics and Ethics Standards* is the standard that occupational therapists ensure the confidentiality of written communication and documentation and that patient privacy is protected (American Occupational Therapy Association [AOTA], 2010). Privacy refers to the right of patients "to be left alone, free from intrusion, and to choose whether or not to share one's self." Confidentiality refers to a "trust in private communications." When a patient makes a disclosure to an occupational therapy practitioner, the practitioner must not disclose the information to others without consent (Jacobs & McCormack, 2011, p. 503).

This longstanding ethical requirement was strengthened by the passage of the Health Insurance Portability and Accountability Act (HIPAA) of 1996. From this legislation, the U.S. Department of Health and Human Services (HHS) established a set of national standards for the protection of certain health information. These standards are contained in the "Privacy Rule," which addresses the use and disclosure of an individual's health information. A major goal of the Privacy Rule is to assure that health information is protected while allowing for the flow of health information needed to provide and promote high-quality health care and to protect the public's health and well being (HHS, 2013).

The Privacy Rule applies to health plans and to health care providers who transmit health information in electronic forms. All providers of medical or health care services (such as physicians, dentists, and occupational therapists) who electronically transmit health information (bills, progress notes, etc.) in connection with certain transactions are considered a covered entity. These providers are classified as covered whether they electronically transmit these transactions directly or engage a third party, such as a billing service, to do so on their behalf.

What information is protected? The Privacy Rule protects all "individually identifiable health information" held or transmitted by a covered entity or its business associate in any form or media, whether electronic, paper, or oral. Protected health information includes the following:

- The individual's past, present, or future physical or mental health condition
- The documentation of health care provided to the individual
- Anything relating to past, present, or future payment for the provision of health care to the individual

Additionally, it includes any information that identifies the individual or for which there is a reasonable basis to believe it can be used to identify the individual. Individually identifiable health information includes common identifiers such as name, address, birth date, or social security number (HHS, 2003, p. 1).

Disclosure of some information can lead to discrimination in employment and other negative consequences. While individuals cannot sue the provider for violation of HIPAA, the law does provide for civil and criminal penalties for providers who knowingly violate the privacy rules. Health care providers who violate this law could be subject to individual liability for breach of confidentiality or invasion of privacy (a civil lawsuit) or for disciplinary action from their licensure board (Jacobs & McCormack, 2011).

Note: Some exceptions to HIPAA Privacy Rules apply, including the obligation to report child abuse and neglect and the duty to warn potential victims when a credible threat to another individual is made.

MEDICAL RECORDS ISSUES

In addition to the privacy and confidentiality requirements discussed previously, occupational therapists and certified occupational therapy assistants (as well as occupational therapy students) are obligated to adhere to additional medical records regulations. The medical record (chart) is a legal document used to determine if health care providers have carried out their obligations to the patient and followed policies, procedures, guidelines, and standards. Medical records cannot be thrown out, altered, or destroyed. Legally, the pieces of paper within the medical record belong to the health care facility, but the patient owns the information that is recorded in the chart (Aiken, 2002, p. 79).

In the past, patients did not have access to their medical records, but today, they may request to see their chart. Most facilities have a policy regarding access to a patient's medical information. As a provider of health care within a facility, you should be aware of the policies to ensure that you are following proper procedures when patients request access to their medical records. Once patients have been discharged, they may obtain a copy of the medical record by requesting it (Aiken, 2002, p. 79).

Charting documentation requirements may vary based on facility policies and reimbursement requirements. However, the following are charting essentials that all professional should follow:

- Chart the care that you provide and any unusual events. If there are contraindications (such as nonweightbearing status), indicate acknowledgment in your documentation to demonstrate you are following proper precautions. If you notice anything unusual in the patient's status or the patient complains of pain that is not typical, be sure to report the occurrence through the proper channels and document your actions in relation to the occurrence. This protects you in the event of a legal action and ensures communication with other disciplines.

- Do not falsify records. Once a notation is written, it cannot be changed. Changing or falsifying records after the fact can be considered fraud and can have serious consequences for the provider. Occasionally, an employer may request that a provider change the documentation in response to a retrospective audit or lawsuit. From a legal and ethical standpoint, this should never be agreed to.

- Making corrections. If entering the wrong information in a chart, never use correction fluid or cross out the errors with markers. Proper correction entails drawing a line through the incorrect information, dating and initialing it, and then writing the correct information.

- Record information carefully. Since one of the functions of the medical record is to protect the provider when a negative outcome occurs, be sure to document any information that might protect you in a possible lawsuit. For example, if a patient is not cooperating with his or her treatment program, is missing sessions, or is not performing the required home exercises, these observations should be noted in the chart. In the case of a lawsuit, this documentation may be helpful in mounting a defense for the provider.

- Document incidents. When documenting a negative incident such as a fall, it is best to objectively state the course of events without placing blame. For example, "when transferring Mrs. Frankel from bed to chair, her legs buckled during the turn toward the wheelchair. Therapist was able to support patient's weight and was able to get her into the chair, without patient actually falling to the ground." It would be helpful to state that the patient is typically able to perform transfers with minimal assistance. This type of reporting is factual and does not place blame vs a statement such as "patient was transferring from bed to wheelchair. Aide had neglected to remove leg rests, causing patient's legs to get caught." Or, "Aide did not place wheelchair at a right angle to the bed, forcing patient to pivot over a much larger space than what she is accustomed to. In all probability this led to the subsequent fall." This information could be used in a negative way should a lawsuit ensue (Aiken, 2002, pp. 85-89).

- Medical charts can never leave the premises and must be kept locked and secured when not in use. If performing home care services where files are kept at home, they must be maintained in a lock box.

- Electronic records must be password protected. Computer screens must be positioned so that others cannot see any patient identifiable information. A screensaver should be used after a short down time to avoid having patients' names visible (Aiken, 2002, pp. 85-94).

PROFESSIONAL LIABILITY ISSUES

As professionals living in a litigious environment, it is important to develop an awareness of professional malpractice risks. By understanding and developing risk management strategies during practice, we protect ourselves from unnecessary lawsuits.

Understanding Negligence

As discussed previously, in the United States, we have two sets of laws that govern our behavior toward one another—civil and criminal. According to civil law, everyone in society is responsible for exercising their duty to care for their own safety and the safety of others. Failure to do this is called *negligence*. When harm comes to another person from one's negligence, it can give rise to a cause of action or lawsuit. Health care professionals are responsible for complying with the standards of care of their profession, meaning that they must exercise the ordinary care that a prudent person in the same profession would exercise under similar conditions. Each profession has its own rules of conduct and practice. Falling below these reasonable practitioner standards is referred to as *medical negligence*, *professional negligence*, or *malpractice* (Ranke & Moriarty, 1997, p. 672).

For occupational therapists, negligence "is doing or not doing, something that an occupational therapist of ordinary skill, care, and knowledge should or should not do under similar circumstances" (Ranke & Moriarty, 1997, p. 672). To prove negligence, the injured party must show that the therapist deviated from accepted standards of care. In a trial, the standard of care is determined by expert testimony. To determine whether a therapist has deviated from the standard of care, several factors are considered, including the following:

- How does an occupational therapist of ordinary care, skill, and knowledge perform the function in question?
- What rules or regulations does the hospital, employer, or rehabilitation department set forth, and have these been followed in the situation at hand?
- Is there occupational therapy literature or texts that provide the standards of treatment?
- Does the AOTA set forth guidelines or standards of practice relating to the situation at hand?
- Is there a state licensure board that determines practice guidelines (Ranke & Moriarty, 1997, p. 672)?

Once liability is established, the next consideration is determining who is responsible for the liability. When determining who is liable for the damages suffered in a negligence suit, the law looks to the relationship that the occupational therapist had with his or her employer. Is the relationship one of an employee and employer or it is an independent contractor relationship? When a therapist is an employee of a facility, the relationship is defined by the law of agency. When the employer engages an employee to perform services and controls the physical conduct of the employee in the performance of the services, an employer-employee agency relationship exists. In this case, the employer can be held liable for the negligence of its employee if the negligence occurred during the course and within the scope of the employer's business. The injured party may file a lawsuit against the employer without naming the therapist as a defendant (Ranke & Moriarty, 1997, p. 672). In this case, the facility can theoretically seek indemnification from the therapist. This rarely happens as the facility will usually have malpractice insurance to cover the negligence of its employees.

In the case of the independent contractor, although the employer theoretically has no control over the methods utilized by the independent contractor, negligence can still be extended to the employer. Two issues are in play here. The important issue is whether the independent contractor is truly independent or whether he or she is controlled in some ways by the employer. For example, the employer may be furnishing equipment and space, engaging the provider over a long period of time, paying him or her on a regular basis, and paying him or her for work performed as part of the facility's regular form of business. For example, an occupational therapist is engaged by an outpatient clinic to provide evaluation and treatment services. The therapist chooses to hold herself out as an independent contractor. However, the clinic provides the space, equipment, referrals, and documentation tools and performs the billing function. Additionally, the facility employs staff members who perform the same tasks as the independent contractors. In the case of a negligence suit, the facility could most likely be considered the de facto employer and would be responsible for the liability from the independent contractor.

Even though independent contractors can be classified as employees of the facility in cases of negligence, it is vital that they carry their own liability insurance as the facility is not responsible for defending the independent contractor should they also be personally named in a lawsuit.

Although lawsuits against occupational therapists and certified occupational therapy assistants occur infrequently, the most common causes leading to them include lack of knowledge, failure to communicate, misuse, or carelessness. Examples include the following:

- Burns from modalities such as hot packs
- Falls during therapy
- Improper treatment or reinjury of a preexisting condition
- Injuries secondary to equipment malfunction
- Sexual misconduct allegations (Ranke & Moriarty, 1997, p. 674)

When considering these sources of lawsuits, therapists can reduce risk by adhering to some of the following suggestions:

- When using physical agent modalities, especially hot and cold packs and electrical stimulation, appropriate protocols must be followed and the patient should be adequately supervised during the treatment. Be sure that standards of care are followed.
- Regarding equipment failures causing injuries and falls, equipment should be inspected and maintained and records of such maintenance be retained. Therapists should be aware of the proper use of equipment and have proof of training.
- When training others about equipment use, be sure to provide specific documentation regarding what was taught and who was trained. Make sure you are aware about which equipment requires physician orders and be sure to secure them. Also, be sure that faulty equipment such as broken wheelchair brakes and leg rests, are taken out of service.
- All plans of care must consider the medical condition of the patient and preexisting conditions. Complaints of pain or discomfort must be taken seriously, and uncomfortable interventions should be discontinued.
  - ◇ For example, a lawsuit was filed when a physical therapy assistant was treating a patient with metastatic breast cancer. During a transfer, the patient complained of pain in her upper leg. The therapist continued to work with the patient and failed to inform the nursing staff or physician of the reported pain. It was later found that the patient suffered a pathological fracture, and the facility was sued along with the therapist.
- Therapists must be aware of the ethical and legal ramifications of sexual conduct with clients (Ranke & Moriarty, 1997, p. 677).

Understanding Insurance Options for Professional Liability

Whether an occupational therapist or certified occupational therapy assistant is an independent contractor or an employee of a facility, it is always wise to secure professional liability. As a general rule, the greater the independent judgment a professional exercises in the performance of duties, the greater the need for insurance. However, it is also true that professionals who are employees can be named individually in a lawsuit. Whether independent contractors or employees, by purchasing their own liability insurance, providers ensure that they have legal representation (the cost of which can easily exceed the value of the lawsuit) which is covered in most policies. It also ensures that the provider's interests are being protected, since the facility's insurance will focus on protecting their interests, not necessarily those of the therapist. Another reason for purchasing your own insurance is that it protects you no matter what happens to the facility. For instance, if you leave the employment of a facility before a lawsuit is filed or the facility no longer exists when the lawsuit is filed, the covered provider ensures that he or she is protected from possible financial consequences.

Insurance for occupational therapists and certified occupational therapy assistants is relatively inexpensive. It is recommended to opt for the maximum amount offered on the professional policy when purchasing coverage, which is usually $1 million per incident with a $3 million per year cap. It is also a good idea to purchase umbrella liability, as it is not unusual for even minor lawsuits to amount to more than what the basic policy offers even when the maximum coverage is taken. Insurance programs are readily available through a variety of sources, including professional associations.

It is important to remember that all liability insurance policies are not the same. Before purchasing a policy, it is recommended that you identify whether the policy you are considering offers the coverage you need. Some issues to consider include the following:

- Whether the insurance purchased is a claims-made or occurrence policy. A claims-made policy provides coverage for claims made in the period the policy is in force. Once premiums stop (if insurance is cancelled for any reason), the company is no longer responsible for acts that occurred when the policy was in force. In other words, if a provider had coverage in 2011 that was cancelled in 2012 and the suit occurred in 2013 (although the act in question occurred in 2011), the policyholder will not be covered as the actual lawsuit occurred after the coverage was cancelled. You must maintain your policy to assure coverage for past events.

- Occurrence coverage provides coverage based on when the act occurred, regardless of when it is reported. For example, an incident occurred in 2012, when you had coverage. The coverage was cancelled in 2013 and a suit was filed in 2014. The policy holder will still be covered for the event, even though the policy is no longer in force.

- The distinction between a claims-made and occurrence policy is a very important factor when choosing the insurance to purchase. Although the claims-made policy may be less expensive, it might not be in your best interest to take the risk.

- Investigate the financial strength of the insurer. You want to be sure that it will be there to defend and pay possible claims when they are needed.

Fraud and Abuse

As the cost of health care skyrockets, the largest payers of health care—the federal and state government under the Medicare and Medicaid programs—have stepped up initiatives to uncover fraud and abuse in health care. Due to the increasing regulations and laws relating to fraud and abuse, occupational therapists and certified occupational therapy assistants, as well as durable medical equipment vendors and all other health care providers and facilities, face increasing scrutiny in their billing and documentation practices.

Under Medicare law, fraud is defined as "making false statements or representations of material facts to obtain some benefit or payment for which no entitlement would otherwise exist. These acts may be committed either for the person's own benefit or for the benefit of some other party" (HHS, 2012, p. 1). In other words, fraud includes obtaining something of value through the misrepresentation or concealment of material facts. Examples include billing for services that were not furnished and/or supplies that were not provided and knowingly altering claims forms to receive higher payment amounts. In occupational therapy practice, the most common examples of fraud include billing for occupational therapy services not provided, misrepresenting the patient's diagnosis to justify the occupational therapist's services, and "up coding" (submitting billing using incorrect codes in order to benefit from higher reimbursement rates) (Jacobs & McCormack, 2011).

Abuse is described as a practice that "either directly or indirectly results in unnecessary costs to the Medicare Program" (HHS, 2012, p. 511). Abuse includes any practice that is not consistent with the goals of providing patients with services that are medically necessary and meeting professionally recognized standards at fair prices. Examples include misusing codes on claims, charging excessively for services or supplies, and billing for services that were not medically necessary. In occupational therapy practice, typical examples include performing occupational therapy assessments more often than necessary (i.e., every 2 weeks), charging Medicare patients higher rates than non-Medicare patients, and performing unnecessary interventions, such as activities of daily living training on comatose patients (Jacobs & McCormack, 2011).

Both fraud and abuse can expose providers to criminal and civil liability. Various laws have been implemented to address Medicare fraud and abuse. These include the False Claims Act, Anti-Kickback Statute, Physician Self-Referral Law (Stark Law), Social Security Act, and the U.S. Criminal Code. Violations can result in nonpayment of claims, civil monetary penalties, and criminal and civil liability.

In addition to these civil and criminal penalties, the HHS Office of Inspector General can permanently exclude individuals who engage in inappropriate or illegal conduct from participating in federal health care programs. Providers are required to be screened by employers to determine if they are on the exclusion list. Any therapists on this list will be unemployable by any entity that accepts Medicare or Medicaid funds.

Summary

This chapter was designed to assist occupational therapists and certified occupational therapy assistants in understanding the legal issues that face them as professionally licensed individuals. Through this understanding, we are able to take proper steps to ensure our compliance with a number of federal and state mandates, identify our own risk within our professional practices, develop our own risk management strategies, and develop procedures to proactively protect ourselves and our licenses from possible charges of ethics violations, fraud and abuse, lawsuits, and discrimination in employment.

With staff shortages, increased productivity requirements, and an environment fraught with potential for error, the health care setting presents many opportunities for unintentional negligence that can lead to injuries, as well as financial and professional liabilities. It is important that we are aware of our professional standards of care, workplace policies and procedures, job descriptions, and our role within the environment in which we work. If we practice in a responsible, defensive, and professional manner, we will ensure the well-being of our patients and avoid professional and personal liabilities.

Discussion Questions/Activities

1. Write a paragraph describing a situation you observed in your fieldwork experience that presented a potential liability. Share with classmates.
2. Choose a role-play partner. One will play the director of a department and the other will play an interview candidate. Conduct a mock interview in front of the class. The class should identify potential questions asked that breach federal discrimination laws.
3. Cite two examples of civil suits and two examples of criminal suits that can impact occupational therapists.

4. Scenario: Helene, an occupational therapist, was providing home care services to Mr. Marc, an elderly gentleman who had recently sustained a double below-knee amputation. She wanted to work on transfers using a sliding board the patient had received from the hospital. The sliding board was a different model than the one she had worked with before, but she was confident that she could master the different device. When assisting with the transfer, Mr. Marc slid to the floor and fractured his pelvis. Do you think this is a case of negligence? Why or why not?

REFERENCES

Aiken, T.D. (2002). *Legal and ethical issues in health occupations.* New Orleans, LA: Saunders.

American Occupational Therapy Association [AOTA]. (2010). Guidelines to the occupational therapy code of ethics. *American Journal of Occupational Therapy, 60,* 652-658.

Equal Opportunity Commission. (2009). Federal laws prohibiting job discrimination questions and answers. Retrieved from http://www.eeoc.gov/facts/qanda.html.

Jacobs, K., & McCormack, G. (2011). *The occupational therapy manager.* Bethesda, MD: AOTA Press.

Ranke, B., & Moriarty, M. (1997). An overview of professional liability in occupational therapy. *American Journal of Occupational Therapy, 51*(8), 671-680.

U.S. Department of Health and Human Services (HHS). (2013). *OCR privacy brief: Summary of the HIPAA privacy rule.* Washington, DC: US Department of Health and Human Services. Retrieved from http://www.hhs.gov/ocr/privacy/hipaa/understanding/summary/index.html.

U.S. Department of Health and Human Services (HHS). (2012). *Medicare fraud & abuse: Prevention, detection and reporting.* Washington, DC: U.S. Department of Health and Human Services., Centers for Medicare and Medicaid Services, Medicare Learning Network.

Chapter 9

Doing What Is Right
Identifying and Resolving
Ethical Issues

LEARNING OBJECTIVES

At the end of the chapter, the reader will be able to:

> ➢ Define morality and ethics.
> ➢ Name the seven professional behaviors expected of occupational therapists as part of the Occupational Therapy Code of Ethics.
> ➢ Define organizational ethics.
> ➢ Identify three ways that organizational ethics can impact occupational therapy practice.
> ➢ Describe ways to avoid conflict of interest when selling equipment to patients.
> ➢ Outline steps to take to resolve ethical dilemmas.

As occupational therapy students and later as occupational therapists and certified occupational therapy assistants working in a variety of settings, we will be faced with many situations that challenge our personal and professional ethical standards. As the availability of health and educational care dollars shrink, our ethics are challenged even more by the need to generate revenue and perform our practice efficiently. This chapter outlines our ethical responsibilities as occupational therapists, the typical ethical challenges we may face in the course of our practice, and mechanisms used to identify and resolve the ethical dilemmas we encounter.

OVERVIEW OF ETHICS AND MORALITY

Morality is defined as the "differentiation of intentions, decisions, and actions between those that are good (or right) and those that are bad (or wrong)" (Johnstone, 2008, p. 102). Furthermore, morality is "concerned with relationships between people and how, ultimately, they can best live in peace and harmony" (Purtilo, 2005, p. 8). Guidelines of morality are designed "to preserve the fabric of society" (Purtilo, 2005, p. 8). Personal morality consists of the "virtues, values, and duties"

Davis L, Rosee M. *Occupational Therapy Student to Clinician:*
Making the Transition (pp 119-129).
© 2015 SLACK Incorporated.

that one has adopted based on culture, customs, laws, rules, and beliefs, or more simply put, is based on the "way things were done" in their family (Purtilo, 2005, pp. 9-10).

Ethics is the study of and reflection on morality that "provides rules or guidance for how one should act in consideration of others but not necessarily how one feels like acting" (Jacobs & McCormack, 2011, p. 470). In other words, an individual may want to act in a way that is not considered ethical, but he or she instead chooses to take the ethical path for a variety of reasons, including societal or peer pressure, concern about his or her reputation, or guilt about possibly doing the wrong thing.

Occupational therapists and certified occupational therapy assistants are often faced with ethical issues that challenge their morality and ethical standards. An ethical dilemma involves knowing the right action to take but feeling conflicted by the knowledge that the most ethical course of action may not be in one's own best interest or that of the organization for which he or she works.

OCCUPATIONAL THERAPY CODE OF ETHICS

As health professionals, we are members of a trusted group that comes with a specified set of moral and ethical expectations. These expectations are outlined in the AOTA's (2010) *Occupational Therapy Code of Ethics and Ethics Standards*. The code "is an aspirational document to guide therapists and occupational therapy students toward appropriate professional conduct in all aspects of their diverse roles. It applies to any conduct that may affect the performance of occupational therapy as well as to behavior that an individual may do in another capacity that reflects negatively on the reputation of occupational therapy" (AOTA. 2010, p. 1). The specific purpose of the document is to do the following:

- Identify and describe the principles supported by our profession
- Educate the general public and members regarding established principles to which occupational therapy personnel are accountable
- Socialize occupational therapy personnel to expected standards of conduct
- Assist occupational therapy personnel in recognition and resolution of ethical dilemmas (AOTA, 2010)

Specific to the *Occupational Therapy Code of Ethics and Ethics Standards*, the following professional behaviors are expected:

- *Beneficence*: Occupational therapy personnel shall demonstrate a concern for the well-being and safety of the recipients of their services. This section covers actions that promote good and prevent or eliminate harm. Specific items in this section include (among other things) providing appropriate assessments on a timely basis, providing services within one's level of competence and scope of practice, using evidence-based evaluation and intervention techniques, and reporting any unethical or illegal practices to appropriate authorities.

- *Nonmaleficence*: This relates to an obligation to refrain from harming others. Unlike beneficence, which requires action to incur benefit, nonmaleficence requires no action to avoid harm. Specific items include avoiding the infliction of harm to recipients of occupational therapy services; ensuring continuity of services; avoiding relationships that exploit others physically, emotionally, psychologically, financially, or socially; avoiding engagement in any inappropriate sexual relationship (with patients or coworkers); not allowing personal problems and limitations to interfere with professional duties; avoiding undue compromising influences such as drugs or alcohol; avoiding situations where one is unable to maintain professional boundaries with patients, students, and colleagues; and avoiding exploitation of relationships for one's own gain.

- *Autonomy and confidentiality*: This relates to the concept that providers must treat clients according to their wishes, within accepted standards of care while protecting client confidential information. This involves forming a collaborative relationship with recipients and their caregivers in setting goals and priorities; providing full disclosure of the benefits, risks, and outcomes of any intervention; obtaining consent for administering services; respecting the recipient's right to refuse services; providing students with access to accurate information regarding educational requirements; obtaining informed consent from participants in research activities and respecting their right to withdraw; ensuring that confidentiality and the right to privacy are respected and maintained; and maintaining the confidentiality of all communications.

- *Social justice*: Also called *distributive justice*, this area refers to the fair, equitable, and appropriate distribution of resources. This principle infers that individuals are provided services in a fair and equitable manner. This would involve ensuring the common good; taking responsibility for educating the public about the value of occupational therapy services; promoting activities that benefit the health status of the community; advocating for just and fair treatment for all patients, clients, employees, and colleagues; advocating for recipients of occupational therapy to obtain needed services; and providing pro bono services when possible.

- *Procedural justice*: This outlines our responsibility to comply with institutional rules; local, state, federal, and international laws; and AOTA documents applicable to the profession. Procedural justice is based on the concept that procedures and processes are organized in a fair manner and that policies, regulations, and laws are followed. Although not implicitly stating that law and ethics are synonymous, occupational therapists have an ethical responsibility to uphold reimbursement regulations and all laws governing the profession. Under this section, we must be familiar with and apply the code and ethics standards to our work settings; be familiar with and abide by institutional rules relating to ethical practice; be familiar with policies and procedures for handling concerns about code of ethics standards, as well as procedures for handling ethics complaints; hold appropriate credentials; take responsibility for maintaining continuing competence; provide appropriate supervision for individuals for whom we have supervisory responsibility; work with employers to prevent discrimination and unfair labor practices; maintain ethical principles and standards of the profession when participating in business arrangements; and refrain from working for or doing business with organizations that engage in illegal or unethical business practices.

- *Veracity*: This relates to the virtues of truthfulness, candor, and honesty. Occupational therapists are responsible for providing comprehensive, accurate, and objective information when representing the profession. Under the code, occupational therapists must accurately represent their credentials in all forms of communication; refrain from participating in the use of false, deceptive, or misleading forms of communication; record and report all information relating to professional activities in a timely manner; ensure that documentation for reimbursement is in accordance with laws, guidelines, and regulations; ensure that marketing and advertising are truthful and accurate; describe the type and duration of occupational therapy services accurately in professional contracts; be honest, fair, and accurate when gathering and reporting fact-based information; give credit and recognition when using the work of others in written, oral, and electronic media; and not plagiarize the work of others.

- *Fidelity*: This deems that occupational therapy personnel shall treat colleagues and other professionals with respect, fairness, discretion, and integrity. This includes respecting the traditions, practices, and responsibilities of their own and other professions; preserving, respecting, and safeguarding private information; discouraging, preventing, exposing, and correcting any breaches of the code of ethics standards and report such to appropriate authorities; avoiding conflicts of interest; avoiding using one's position or knowledge gained from that position in a way that gives rise to real or perceived conflict of interest; using conflict resolution or other dispute resolution resources to resolve organizational and interpersonal conflicts; being a diligent steward of human, financial, and material resources of employers; and refraining from exploiting these resources for personal gain (AOTA, 2010).

LICENSURE AND STATE ISSUES RELATING TO ETHICS

As professionals, we are responsible for following the code of ethics of our professional organization. However, for all of us living in a state where occupational therapy is a licensed, certified, or registered profession, we are responsible for abiding by the practice acts and ethics requirements of the states where we practice. Every occupational therapist and certified occupational therapy assistant must be aware of the professional conduct and disciplinary provisions of his or her state's practice act, which may differ from the AOTA's *Code of Ethics*. A breach of one's state licensure laws or practice act could result in revocation of one's license in that state (Mongello, 2007, p. 1).

For example, in Arizona, "failing to document or maintain patient treatment records or failing to prepare patient or client reports within 30 days of services or treatment" can be grounds for license revocation (Mongello, 2007). Many states have standards for failing to keep written records that justify the course of treatment for the patient. In Pennsylvania, certain violations of unprofessional conduct can result in a fine, jail time, or both, along with license suspension or revocation (Mongello, 2007, p. 1). In Iowa, occupational therapists are responsible for informing the physician making the referral if a requested treatment is believed to be inadvisable or contraindicated. In such cases, the occupational therapist is empowered to refuse to carry out orders that he or she believes to not be in the best interests of the patient. In Ohio, a provider who practices in an area where he or she is incompetent or untrained may be subject to disciplinary actions. Additionally, sexual misconduct with patients is covered by many states' code of misconduct for therapists (Fowler, 2007).

Additionally, occupational therapists and certified occupational therapy assistants must be aware of and comply with state laws relating to the supervision of certified occupational therapy assistants. Supervision and documentation (cosignature) requirements differ on a state-by-state basis. Although the AOTA and regulatory agencies such as Centers for Medicare and Medicaid Services have their own regulations for the use of certified occupational therapy assistants, keep in mind that the minimum standard therapists need to follow is based on their state regulations (Fowler, 2007).

Important points to remember are as follows:

- All therapists must be aware of their state's regulatory and disciplinary standards to protect their license and ability to practice in their state. (Note: The statues and regulations on disciplinary provisions for each state are available on AOTA's website under State Policy [Mongello, 2007].)
- Remember that you carry your professional obligations 24/7, even when you are not providing therapy. In many states, individuals who are found guilty of criminal offenses, such as driving while under the influence of alcohol, disorderly conduct, or child abuse, may be jeopardizing their professional license. As a professional, you are held to a higher standard than nonlicensed individuals, even in your private life.

ORGANIZATIONAL ETHICS

Organizational ethics involves the ideals and values that create the ethical climate of an organization and that impact its business practices. These ethics can affect billing practices, marketing, managed care decisions, and institutional policies (Jacobs & McCormack, 2011). As health care professionals, our most important priority has always been the recipient of care. This focus on the patient or client assumes priority over all other concerns, including the interests of the facility that employs us. However, this patient-centered ethic can sometimes conflict with the goals of the facilities where we work, especially if they are for-profit organizations. Milton Friedman, a famous economist, stated that, "there is one and only one social responsibility of business—to use its resources and engage in activities designed to increase profits" (Ozar, Berg, Werhane, & Emanuel, 2000, p. 5). However, this philosophy may create a conflict in a health care or educational environment where the culture has historically been oriented toward serving the needs of the clients/patients rather than the profitability targets of the organization. Generally accepted business management strategies often do not work in a health care or educational culture and can result in demoralization and strained relations between professionals and the executives who manage the facility. In a changing health care environment, facilities are under pressure to control costs and maximize reimbursement. As payers (Medicare, Medicaid, and managed care organizations) reduce reimbursement to health care facilities, managers must identify strategies to maintain solvency. These strategies can sometimes result in questionable policies, which conflict with professional ethical standards.

Common issues that relate to organizational ethics and impact occupational therapy practice may involve the following:

♦ Unrealistic productivity expectations that may be counterproductive to the patient's needs or may challenge billing and documentation veracity

♦ Pressure to provide treatment that exceeds a therapist's competency or scope of practice

♦ Inadequate supervision or the use of unqualified personnel to provide skilled services (Jacobs & McCormack, 2011, p. 474)

For example, in a recent report by the Office of the Inspector General, the investigative arm of the U.S. Department of Health and Human Services, it was alleged that $1.5 billion was inappropriately paid to nursing facilities in 2009 under the Part A Medicare benefit; furthermore, the investigation targeted therapy reporting and use as key problem areas (Levinson, 2012, pp. 11-13). In the report, it was found that patients received inappropriately high levels of rehabilitation intervention. Not so coincidentally, these intense therapy levels correlated with the highest reimbursement rates under Medicare during a Part A skilled nursing facility stay. Furthermore, the report contended that therapy was provided to patients not in need of such services and that, in some cases, claims did not meet Medicare coverage criteria (HHS, 2012). Deborah Slater, MS, OT/L FAOTA, liaison to AOTA's Ethics Commission, states that, "Therapists must reinforce that their clinical judgment will determine decisions on therapy needed by skilled nursing facility patients and (they) should not be pressured to provide more or less than what can benefit a patient. Occupational therapy intervention, documentation, coding, and billing should accurately reflect the patient's clinical status, (and must be able to) withstand scrutiny by payers, and align with our professional, ethical standards" (Slater, 2006, p. 2). However, the pressure placed on therapists to deliver the levels of therapy needed to ensure the highest reimbursement potential is a very powerful force in our industry. Therapists are often deemed uncooperative when they express an unwillingness to participate in a facility's strategy to maximize reimbursement.

Some typical scenarios that might challenge ethical standards include the following:

♦ A therapist is working in a long-term care facility where reimbursement is based on the intensity of therapy provided. The supervisor has instructed the therapist to place a newly evaluated patient on an ultra–high-intensity (720 minutes per week) therapy program. The therapist does not feel that the patient has the potential to improve and that the high-intensity program will be too rigorous considering the patient's current medical condition. However, the therapist is aware that if she ignores the advice of her supervisor, she will be branded uncooperative.

♦ A managed care patient is admitted to a facility. His insurance only covers him for a 30-minute session daily. The evaluating therapist believes the patient needs 1 hour per day but knows that the facility will not be reimbursed for the additional time. If the therapist documents the need for more therapy minutes than the facility will be reimbursed for, they may be blamed for making a poor case management decision.

♦ A therapy program in a subacute facility engages an occupational therapy aide to assist with treatment. A newly hired occupational therapist notices that the aide is now running the daily feeding group without any occupational therapists present, yet the time provided is being captured as a restorative treatment for reimbursement.

- A newly graduated certified occupational therapy assistant is providing treatment in a pediatric setting. She has been told that she would get supervision on a weekly basis and that all of her notes would be reviewed and cosigned. After a month on the job, she is told that she does not need supervision and observes that her notes are being cosigned by a therapist who has not observed her treatment.

- A therapist is working in an outpatient setting with orthopedic patients. She has been told that she has to treat at least three patients at a time, setting two up on an activity while working hands-on with another patient. She then fills out billing time sheets, which imply that she has provided one-on-one sessions to all the patients.

- A therapist is working with a 2-year-old child providing early intervention. Based on a standardized assessment, it is found that the child is functioning within normal limits in all areas. The therapist decides that it is time to discharge the child from program. The parent becomes very upset about the discharge, and the supervisor instructs the therapist to keep the child on for another 6 months even though all goals have been met.

- A therapist is evaluating a child for early intervention. Using standardized tools, the initial evaluation determines the child to be functioning within normal limits. The agency would like to put the child on a program and asks the therapist to reevaluate the child, implying that the therapist find a way to qualify the child for services.

- A covering therapist was engaged by a facility when one of the staff members had a prolonged absence. The covering therapist resigned without completing his documentation. The supervisor asks another therapist who was working at the facility to write the notes on patients he did not treat.

- A therapist notes that her colleague is documenting more time than he is providing to patients to qualify for higher reimbursement.

These and many other ethical challenges will be faced by occupational therapists, certified occupational therapy assistants and students as they encounter the financial realities of today's health care environment. It is important to understand that there are many outside variables that impact our decision-making process, and they may interfere with the moral priorities and professional standards embedded in us as health care professionals. Even more impactful to us personally is the risk that some of these ethical dilemmas may actually represent a breach of federal and states laws, jeopardizing our reputation, licenses, and ability to practice our profession, as well as exposing us to possible civil and criminal penalties. Even when the financial survival of the organization is at stake, monetary gains and the financial well-being of our facility should not outweigh patients' health and outcome priorities (Ozar & Berg, 2000) or our professional futures. We must relate back to our professional code of ethics and our state practice acts when making care delivery decisions and balance these with the priorities and needs of the facilities that employ us.

ETHICAL ISSUES IN PRIVATE PRACTICE

Ethical Considerations When Engaging in Business Transactions With Clients

Today, many occupational therapists in private practice will sell recommended products to their patients. When selling goods directly to patients, it is important to consider whether there are any potential conflicts of interest. A conflict of interest occurs when an individual or organization is involved in multiple interests, one of which could possibly corrupt the motivation for an act in another. Although the conflict may not necessarily lead to corruption, there is a risk that professional judgment or actions will be unduly influenced by the secondary interest (Lo & Field, 2009). With proper action, a conflict of interest can be diffused before any corruption occurs. It is not inherently corrupt for a therapist to sell equipment to a patient, especially if the item is related to the treatment being provided. However, to diffuse the perception of conflict of interest, occupational therapists selling equipment or devices from which they profit as a part of their private practice should disclose to their patients what their relationship is with the equipment company and whether they stand to profit from sales of equipment. They should be sure that the prices charged are in line with competitors and that a list of other sources offering the same product line is provided, giving the patient a chance to compare prices and benefits. If those standards are met, conflict of interest is avoided (Austin, 2006).

Fee Splitting

Fee splitting occurs when a professional pays a second party for providing a referral. Fee splitting is considered unethical and in many states is illegal as it is perceived to adversely affect patient care and well-being since there is financial incentive to refer to someone who may not be the most appropriate care provider for their particular issue. Additionally, a professional should not receive free care (from a professional) in return for providing referrals. This is also considered fee splitting.

Some examples of fee splitting include the following:

- An occupational therapist is working independently in a hand surgeon's office. The therapist rents space in the office and, when referrals are received from the physician, she pays him 10% of her therapy fee as a referral reward.
- An occupational therapist who only performs evaluations refers all of her cases needing therapy to a friend who owns a pediatric practice. The pediatric therapist sends the referring therapist a $100 gift certificate every time she gets a referral.
- An occupational therapist has developed a successful practice treating temporomandibular-related issues. She refers many of her patients to a local dentist, who in turn provides free dental services to her and her family.

RESOLVING ETHICAL DILEMMAS

Within the course of our occupational therapy practice, we will surely be faced with ethical dilemmas we will need to resolve, whether they involve making a decision about our own action in relation to self-interests, an institutional issue that involves us, or an unethical act that we witness. Frameworks have been developed to help us analyze ethical dilemmas we face and provide the structure to identify an action plan to be implemented. Kornblau and Starling (2000), in their book *Ethics in Rehabilitation*, layout a format that specifically relates to rehabilitation professionals. Their suggested steps are as follows:

1. Identify the problem. The first step is to ask yourself the question, "Am I facing an ethical dilemma?" Does the problem violate your personal integrity and conscience? Sometimes what may seem an ethical issue may turn out to be a legal or personal issue (Morris, 2007).

2. What are the facts of the situation? The next step is to clearly state the dilemma to clarify it and analyze the facts. Often, when the facts come out, the clarification is enough to resolve the question.

3. Identify the values being challenged—both your own and those of the people around you. Values reflect personal beliefs based on one's culture. One set of values may violate another person's value system, but it may not necessarily represent an ethical breach (Morris, 2007).

4. Who are the interested parties and what are the consequences and/or benefits of the possible breach? Who are the players in the ethical dilemma—the patient, your supervisor,

administration, colleagues, family members, the payer of services, or yourself? How does this possible ethical breach impact the various players?

5. Is there a legal issue?
   ◇ Does this possible breach in ethics also represent a legal issue? Does the issue in question violate a practice act or state licensure laws?

6. Do I need more information? Are there policies and procedures, laws, regulations, or documents that would help me clarify the issue? How can I find the information? Do I need to question other people involved in the situation? Do I need to do more research? Do I need to consult with a mentor, lawyer, or expert on this issue?

7. Brainstorm possible action and develop your action plan. After gathering all of the facts and pertinent information, you may determine whether an action is appropriate and what that action should be. Keep in mind that if you are challenging current policy within your facility or the actions of someone else, you may be placing yourself in a difficult position. Consider the consequences of each action before implementing it. The goal is to develop a course of action that will resolve the dilemma (Morris, 2007).

8. Analyze the action steps before implementing them.
   ◇ Have you eliminated obviously wrong or impossible choices?
   ◇ How will each alternative action impact your patients, workplace relationships, and personal and professional reputation?
   ◇ Do your choices abide by your code of ethics, state practice act, and any pertinent regulations?
   ◇ Are your choices consistent with your moral, religious, and social beliefs?

9. Choose a course of action and implement it (Kornblau & Starling, 2000).

   In addition to performing your own analysis, it is crucial that you share your perceptions with sources such as your supervisor, peers, or even the ethics committee at your facility. Trusted colleagues can help you maintain objectivity, make suggestions for alternative solutions, and guide you to choose a path of action based on facts and logic rather than emotions.

   Use one of the many tools that have been developed to help you identify and clarify the situation being faced, provide a structured approach to analyze the principles that may have been breached, analyze the alternatives, determine an action, and assess the outcome. Using a form such as this can be helpful to ensure that all issues have been considered prior to taking an action. We have included an example of such a form, the Ethical Dilemma Worksheet, at the end of this chapter (see pp. 128-129).

ENFORCEMENT PROCEDURES FOR THE OCCUPATIONAL THERAPY CODE OF ETHICS

As discussed, the *Occupational Therapy Code of Ethics and Ethics Standards* were designed to "protect the public and reinforce its confidence in the profession, rather than to resolve private business, legal, or other disputes" (AOTA, 2010). The code also guides occupational therapists and students toward appropriate professional conduct. The enforcement process was created to ensure objectivity and fairness to all individuals who may be a party to an ethics complaint. These procedures are established and maintained by the ethics commission of the AOTA. All occupational therapists should be fully familiar with both the code of ethics and the enforcement process. Ethics complaints can be submitted using the AOTA form entitled "Formal Complaint of Alleged Violation of the Occupational Therapy Code of Ethics and Ethics Standards." If deemed credible, the AOTA will conduct an investigation and plan an action as per its document entitled "Enforcement Procedures for the Occupational Therapy Code of Ethics and Ethics Standards."

Reporting Unethical Conduct

In addition to the enforcement procedures outlined by the AOTA, there are other avenues for reporting unethical conduct. If the person you are reporting on is an occupational therapist or certified occupational therapy assistant, a formal complaint can be submitted to the state licensure board where the therapist is licensed. This can be in addition to a formal complaint submitted to the AOTA.

All professions have ethical standards to uphold. If the provider is from another discipline, the alleged event can be reported to the state licensure board, state professional association, and/or credentialing body of the specific profession. Medicare fraud can be reported to the Office of the Inspector General that handles Medicare and Medicaid fraud and abuse prevention, detection, and reporting. If you wish to file a complaint about a facility, it is best to contact the state agency that licenses the facility, such as the State Education Department or the Department of Health.

Summary

As licensed professionals, we are held to ethical standards that go beyond what is expected of the average person. It is crucial that we understand our ethical obligations, are able to identify ethical dilemmas, and know how to resolve them in a manner that protects not only ourselves, but our colleagues and the facilities where we work as well. These standards should provide a framework for guiding one's practice.

Discussion Questions/Activities

1. Using the scenarios presented on pp. 123-124, please consider the following questions:
   a. If faced with these ethical dilemmas, what would you do?
   b. What would you do if your facility did not support your stand?
   c. Which principles of the code of ethics are involved in each example?
2. Research your state's practice act. What specific requirements and limitations are established for occupational therapists and certified occupational therapy assistants?
3. Go to the U.S. Department of Health and Human Services, Office of the Inspector General website and download one of the most recent reports relating to rehabilitation services. Review the report and identify the issues being investigated. Were there any findings related to ethical issues? Which ethical issues (using AOTA's Code of Ethics) are involved? Have you ever observed any of the examples outlined in the report?
4. Identify an ethical challenge you have experienced in your life. Using the Ethical Dilemma Worksheet on the next page, as a model for resolving ethical issues, consider the following:
   a. What was the dilemma? State the facts and identify the values that were challenged.
   b. Who were the players in the dilemma? What were the consequences of the dilemma?

ETHICAL DILEMMA WORKSHEET

1. **What is the problem?**
2. **What are the facts of the situation?**
3. **Who are the interested parties?**
    Facility?
    Patient?
    Other therapists?
    Observers?
    Payers?
    Other:
4. **What is the nature of their interest? Why is this a problem?**
    Personal
    Business
    Economic
    Intellectual
    Social

Interested Parties	Their Interests

5. **Ethical?**
    Does it violate a professional code of ethics? Which section(s)?
    Does it violate moral, social, or religious values?
6. **Is there a legal issue?**
    What is the practice act/licensure law and regulations? Section(s)?
7. **Do I need more information?**
    What information do I need?
    Is there a treatment, policy, procedure, law, regulation, or document that I do not know about?
    Can I obtain a copy of the treatment, policy, procedure, law, regulation, or document in writing?
    Do I need to research the issue further?
    Do I need to consult with a mentor, an expert in this area, and/or a lawyer?
8. **Brainstorm possible action steps.**
9. **Analyze action steps:**
    Eliminate the obvious wrong choices.
    How will each alternative affect my patients, other interested parties, and me?
    Do your choices abide by the code of ethics?
    Do your choices abide by the practice act and regulations?
    Are my choices consistent with my moral, religious, and social beliefs?
    Eliminate obviously wrong or impossible choices.

(continued)

ETHICAL DILEMMA WORKSHEET (CONTINUED)

10. **Choose your course of action:**

    The Rotary four-way test:

    >   Is it the *truth*?

    >   Is it *fair* to all concerned?

    >   Will it build *goodwill* and better *friendship*?

    >   Will it be *beneficial* to all concerned?

    Is it win-win?

    How do you feel about your course of action?

Adapted from Kornblau, B., & Starling, S. (2000). *Ethics in rehabilitation: A clinical perspective.* Thorofare, NJ: SLACK Incorporated.

REFERENCES

American Occupational Therapy Association (AOTA). (2010). Enforcement procedures for the occupational therapy code of ethics and ethics standards. *American Journal of Occupational Therapy, 64*(Suppl.), S4-S16.

American Occupational Therapy Association (AOTA). (2010). Occupational therapy code of ethics and ethics standards. Retrieved from https://www.aota.org/-/media/Corporate/Files/AboutAOTA/OfficialDocs/Ethics/Code%20and%20Ethics%20Standards%202010.pdf

Austin, D. (2006). *Ethical considerations when occupational therapists engage in business transactions with clients.* The American Occupational Therapy Association Advisory Opinion for the Ethics Commission. Bethesda, MD: AOTA Press.

Fowler, R. (2007). Are you following your state's supervision regulations? *OT Practice Online.* Retrieved from http://aota.org/pubs/otp/1997-2007/columns/capitalbriefing/2001.aspx.

Jacobs, K., & McCormack, G. (2011). *The occupational therapy manager.* Bethesda, MD: AOTA Press.

Johnstone, M. (2008). *Bioethics: A nursing perspective* (pp. 102-103). Philadelphia, PA: Elsevier Health Sciences.

Kornblau, B., & Starling, S. (2000). *Ethics in rehabilitation: A clinical perspective.* Thorofare, NJ: SLACK Incorporated.

Levinson, D. (2012). *Inappropriate payments to skilled nursing facilities cost Medicare more than a billion dollars in 2009.* Washington, DC: Department of Health and Human Services, Office of Inspector General.

Lo, B., & Field, M. (2009). *Conflict of interest in medical research, education and practice.* Washington, DC: National Academies Press.

Mongello, M. (2007). State disciplinary provisions. *OT Practice Online.* Retrieved from aota.org.

Morris, J. (2007). Is it possible to be ethical? *OT Practice Online.* Retrieved from http://www.aota.org/pubs/otp/1997-2007/features/2003/f_022403.aspx.

Ozar, D., Berg, J., Werhane, P., & Emanuel, L. (2000). *Organizational ethics in health care: Toward a model for ethical decision making by provider organizations.* Chicago, IL: American Medical Association.

Purtilo, R. (2005). *Ethical dimensions in the health professions.* Boston, MA: Elsevier Saunders.

Slater, D. (2006). *Ethical issues around payment for services.* AOTA Advisory Opinion for the Ethics Commission. Bethesda, MD: AOTA.

U.S. Department of Health and Human Services (HHS). (2012). *Medicare fraud & abuse: Prevention, detection and reporting.* Washington, DC: Medicare Learning Network, Department of Health and Human Services, Centers for Medicare and Medicaid Services.

SECTION II

GETTING READY FOR YOUR JOB SEARCH

Chapter 10

Creating a Resumé to Get You Noticed

As you prepare to graduate and consider the options for your first paying position as an occupational therapist or certified occupational therapy assistant, you need to invest thought and time into the preparation of your resumé and cover letter. Your resumé and cover letter represent your first introduction to a potential employer. It can make the difference between getting called for an interview or getting filed with the rejects. For employers, interviews are time consuming—and time is a precious commodity. To get your foot in the door, it is crucial that you provide the clues to your targeted audience that you are worth the time and effort that an interview requires. This chapter provides a concrete approach to preparing your resumé to ensure that it will open doors for you, leading to your first professional position.

CREATING YOUR RESUMÉ

Creating your resumé is an important first step in your job search process. The resumé is a written profile of your accomplishments, starting from your pre-occupational therapy life, followed by a description of your clinical experiences and skills learned in the course of your occupational therapy education. The resumé serves as a document that is intended "to brand, package, market,

Davis L, Rosee M. *Occupational Therapy Student to Clinician: Making the Transition (pp 133-148).*
© 2015 SLACK Incorporated.

and pre-sell" you, the candidate (Ensign, 2012, p. 1). As your career evolves, you will need to update your resumé, but for your first job, it will primarily reflect your academic schooling, degree earned, and fieldwork encounters, along with applicable prior work and life experiences.

Which resumé format is most appropriate for the new graduate occupational therapist to use? In reality, there are many different formats for resumés, and no one format is correct. The most important element to consider is that your resumé is clear, concise, easy to read, truthful, and error free, and that it portrays all of the positive experiences you bring to your potential employer. Since we are in a serious profession, it is suggested that the resumé be conservative and follow a very professional and easy-to-read format.

INFORMATION GATHERING AND SELF-ASSESSMENT

Before tackling your resumé, it is a good idea to sit down and start listing your pre-occupational therapy work history to determine if any of your prior jobs, volunteer experiences, or work skills might enhance your resumé. For example, serving as a restaurant hostess for 10 years indicates customer service skills, commitment, reliability, and a willingness to work hard. Working as a manager for a paper bag manufacturer with responsibility for 10 employees shows that you have communication, organizational, and managerial skills. Serving as a camp counselor for children with disabilities indicates a sense of responsibility, an interest in working with differently-abled children, and an understanding of child development issues. You do not necessarily have to omit a job from your resumé just because it is unrelated to your new profession. Carefully evaluate whether you can put a positive spin on your experiences, which can add depth to your resumé and demonstrate that you come to the job with added value.

After tackling your pre-occupational therapy career, review on paper everything that you were exposed to in your professional education and in your fieldwork experiences. List all of the special populations you have worked with, any special skills you have acquired, projects carried out, or research papers to which you have contributed. Think about how to portray these experiences in your resumé to your maximal advantage.

Why is this important? Because you never know what may be important to a prospective employer. By listing special or unusual skills you learned or were exposed to, you may motivate the reader to meet with you as he or she has a need for those particular hard-to-find skills. For example, you may have led a group for patients with post-traumatic stress disorder in a veterans' hospital or developed and implemented a protocol for a feeding group in a long-term care dementia unit. Those experiences might be of interest to someone serving another population and could give you an advantage for both securing an interview and eventually a position.

ORGANIZING YOUR RESUMÉ

There are several different ways to approach a resumé. The most common types include the following:

◆ *Chronological resumés*: These list your work history with the most recent position listed first, followed by earlier positions (or clinical experiences) in reverse chronological order. Employers usually prefer this type of resumé as they can easily identify what you have done more recently and how long you have stayed at a position. (Note: This could be important as it relates to your pre-occupational therapy jobs if it indicates longevity at a job, which is gener-ally desired and respected). Since a prospective employer will probably be most interested in your occupational therapy experiences, a new graduate will typically list and describe his or her Fieldwork II experiences first followed by Fieldwork I experiences. Often, unrelated paid work experiences are in a separate section. These two sections can be labeled "Occupational Therapy Experience" and "Other Work Experience."

- *Functional resumé*: This is an alternative type of resumé that focuses on your skills and experiences rather than your chronological work history. In a functional resumé, you would highlight your accomplishments and experiences rather than the specific jobs you have held. The actual job descriptions and dates are often included as secondary data, placed in a less obvious place in the resumé. This format is often used when there has been a gap in one's employment history. This would not be the best choice for the new graduate but might work well for someone who is returning to the job market after a hiatus.

- *Targeted resumé*: This resumé is customized to highlight certain specific experiences that are relevant to a particular job or specialty area on which you are focusing. For example, if you complete an affiliation at a hand clinic and are applying for a job in a hand surgeon's office, it would benefit you to highlight that experience on your resumé (while still including all of your other experiences). You would only use the "hand specialty" resumé when applying to that type of specialized job. You would also prepare another more general resumé to cover less specialized positions. For example, Alex completed a fieldwork experience at an acute care hospital and at a school for children with learning disabilities using a sensory integrative focus. When he sent out his resumé to preschools, he emphasized his pediatric experience, elaborating more on the standardized tests he administered, the treatment interventions he devised, and the special documentation skills he mastered. Furthermore, his cover letter to pediatric placements highlighted that experience to get the reader's attention in order to increase his chance for being called in for the interview.

- *Using a candidate profile or objective on the resumé*: A candidate profile presents a brief summary of an applicant's skills, experiences, and goals as they relate to a specific job opening. A resumé objective simply states the type of position you are seeking and is an attempt to demonstrate to employers that you know what you want in a job. A profile explains what you have to offer the employer and helps to sell your candidacy. The profile serves as a stronger statement to prospective employers, describing what you have to offer, not just what you are seeking. The profile or objective statement is typically at the top of the resumé, right under your identifying information (name, address, etc.).
  - ◇ As an example, a resumé objective might state:
      Objective: New graduate occupational therapy assistant with an interest in brain injury rehabilitation seeks stimulating position.
  - ◇ A profile might state:
      Professional Profile: New graduate occupational therapy assistant with experience working with brain injuries and cognitive rehabilitation seeks to promote independence and optimize function for effected individuals in a progressive setting.

Customize the language found in a job listing you are interested in to create your resumé profile. That way, you are enticing the reader to call you for an interview, by demonstrating an interest or knowledge regarding the population it is serving (Doyle, n.d.).

The Layout

There are many ways to format a resumé. The most important element to consider is that the format be easy to read with the most important facts sensibly organized, accessible, and highlighted.

- *Font*: The font size should range between 10 to 12 points. Smaller type can make your resumé difficult to read. Larger font sizes may indicate to the reader that you have little to promote and are attempting to compensate for a lack of substance by filling up the page with large type. We recommend using a conservative font (such as Calibri or Times New Roman) as they portray a serious image.

♦ *Writing style*: Since resumés are supposed to be brief, the descriptions should be written in short phrases. Sentences are generally not used in a resumé. Bullets often work well in succinctly describing work experiences.

Do not abbreviate words, dates, or addresses. This can lead a reader to think you are lazy and haphazard. Remember, not everyone is familiar with acronyms (such as ADLs or ROM), so their use can be confusing. Spell out everything.

All material must be truthful. If there are lapses in the dates, you can explain specifics in the cover letter. Never lie on a resumé!

Using Templates to Create the Best Format

In today's technological world, it is fairly simple to produce a professional-looking resumé. In pre-computer days, people often sent their resumé out to a graphic designer to give it a crisp, professional look. Today, you do not have to look any further than the Internet or to Microsoft or Apple software to find a template that will work for you. Template software provides the user with numerous design choices and the ability to build a resumé to ensure a professional product.

Some question whether templates help or hinder the job search. A templated resumé can result in a product that is common and predictable. For more creative fields, this may be a problem, but in the health professions, the content and clarity of the resumé is much more important than the design. A clear and consistent format, even if it is commonly used, will be appreciated by the reader and will improve the odds that it is looked at.

There are many options for using templates, so where do you start? Tried and true classics like Microsoft will give you bare-bones templates with which to work. Keep in mind that the Microsoft templates are the ones most commonly downloaded, so your resumé might look just like the next person's. However, you can customize a template to make your resumé stand out. Some suggestions for customizing when using a template program include the following:

♦ Do not necessarily stick with the format. Formats are customizable. Use the parts you like and feel free to make changes in the font, borders, and margins.

♦ Go off the beaten path. Since Microsoft is the most used resumé template software, consider investigating some lesser used programs such as Google, or simply search for "resumé templates." There will be numerous programs to choose from.

♦ Create your own. After reviewing a variety of templates, feel free to mix and match elements to create your own design. Make sure that your resumé is consistent and cohesive and that you do not use too many different fonts.

♦ Use resumé builder options offered with most resumé templates. After filling out informational fields, your text is automatically formatted to fit into the template design of your choice. From there you can customize.

♦ Use online profiles. Social media profiles can give you an extra edge when prospective employers are looking at your resumé. This gives the employer the option to find out more about you. Sites such as LinkedIn and About.Me are great professional platforms to represent yourself. Be sure that the profile you are making accessible to a prospective employer is professional and not personal in nature. You do not want an employer to identify any negative information about you from personal social media sites.

♦ Provide a link to your professional portfolio. In later chapters, we go into some depth about developing your professional portfolio. Establish instant credibility by creating a Web portfolio that is fast loading, is visually appealing, and contains well-written information showcasing your accomplishments, mission statement, core values, career progression, and leadership aptitude (Olson, 2012).

Some sample resumés and reference lists are included in Figures 10-1, 10-2, and 10-3 for your review.

LEAH YEATER

9 Mayflower Drive, Belmont, CA 02159
Home: (555) 429-9789–Cell: (917) 467-9391–E-mail: lyeater@gmail.com

Objective

To acquire a position as an occupational therapy assistant that uses my knowledge and skill to provide efficient treatment and emotional support to clients.

Education

LaGuardia Community College, Long Island City, NY

Associate in Applied Science February 2012

Major: Occupational Therapy Assistant

Cumulative GPA: 3.96

Honors: Dean's List

Clinical Experience

Fieldwork II

January 2012 to February 2012

Queens Center for Rehabilitation and Nursing – Queens, NY

- Carried out intervention plans developed by occupational therapist for clients diagnosed with total hip and knee replacements, lower and upper extremity fractures, cerebrovascular accidents, general deconditioning, lower extremity amputations, peripheral nerve injuries, shoulder arthroplasty, laminectomy, and arthritis.
- Assisted in development and implementation of clients' treatment and intervention planning, short-term goals, discharge, and follow-up procedures. Skilled interventions provided include neurodevelopmental techniques, therapeutic exercises, activities of daily living training, cognitive/perceptual retraining, and teaching compensatory techniques, as well as the fabrication of assistive devices.
- Participated in the rehabilitation of a patient with upper extremity prosthesis.
- Experience in measuring for Jobst garment for a patient with burns.
- Provided documentation in compliance with Medicare and Medicaid regulations proving that treatment is reasonable, necessary, and skilled.

Fieldwork II

November 2011 to January 2012

Manhattan Psychiatric Care – New York, NY

- Interacted and provided interventions for patients with a variety of psychiatric disorders, including schizophrenia, bipolar disorders, depression, and eating disorders.
- Led group activities focusing on community living skills, cognitive skills, social learning, cooking, and money management.
- Worked individually with patients on social skills and activities of daily living in preparation for discharge. Participated in team meetings.

Fieldwork I

June 2011 to October 2011

NYC Board of Education – New York, NY

- Observed standardized evaluations and school-based interventions for students diagnosed with pervasive developmental disorders, juvenile rheumatoid arthritis, intellectual and developmental disabilities, and hydrocephalus.

Figure 10-1. Sample resumé (*continued*).

- Assisted the occupational therapist in preparing for treatment and participated in delivering treatment sessions. Reviewed charts and Individualized Education Programs.
- Attended Individualized Education Program meetings.

Fieldwork I

April 2011 to May 2011

Seaside Therapeutic Riding Inc – New York, NY

- Observed equine training sessions for clients with an array of developmental disorders, including pervasive developmental disorders, developmental disabilities, and cerebral palsy.
- Provided physical and emotional support during therapeutic riding sessions to clients and family members.

Other Work Experience

Mayfair Care Center – New York, NY

Transporter

February 2008 to July 2011

Transported more than 80 patients per day to ensure timely attendance for occupational, physical, and speech therapy sessions.

Skills

Strong computer and carpentry skills.

References

Will be provided upon request.

Figure 10-1 (continued). Sample resumé.

Organizing the Content

Whether you use a template or you create your own resumé from scratch, the basic content and organization of your resumé should be as follows.

The Header

The heading should always include your name, home address, daytime and/or mobile phone number, and e-mail address. Do not list a number that blocks unfamiliar calls or list an e-mail address with an offbeat e-mail name (i.e., beermaven@gmail.com, iwhisper@aol.com, glittergirl@yahoo.com). Give an address that is permanent, not a dorm room that you may be vacating soon. (Note: Make sure that your voicemail message is professional. Avoid music, cute messages, or children's voices. An unprofessional outgoing message could portray the wrong impression about you to a potential employer.)

Schools Attended

List your professional education first, followed by other college-level experiences. If you have a particularly high grade point average, won any awards in school, participated in honor societies, or have any other exceptional school-related accolades, include them here.

Fieldwork Experience

A great fieldwork experience can get your foot in the door to your first job. It is imperative that you portray your fieldwork in a manner that makes you stand out from other applicants. Be specific about things you have been exposed to and any special skills learned. For example, if you worked in a burn unit and fabricated splints to prevent contractures for acute burn patients, the experience should be described. Any special skills learned should be included in this section,

LEAH YEATER

9 Mayflower Drive, Belmont, CA 02159
Home: 212-429-9789 – Cell: 917-467-9391 – E-mail: lyeater@gmail.com

References:

Eve Cleveland, OTR
Director of Rehab
Queen's Center for Rehabilitation and Nursing
57-34 45 Street
Elmhurst, NY, 11412
718-896-2437
EveCleve@qcr.com

Jennifer West, OTR
Senior Occupational Therapist
Manhattan Psychiatric Care
168-05 Haven Boulevard
New York, NY, 11121
212-874-3763
jenniferw@manpsych.com

Professor Stefanie Fisher, PhD
LaGuardia Community College
31-10 Thomson Avenue
Long Island City, NY, 11101
718-436-7337
SFisher@lcc.com

Figure 10-2. Sample reference list.

including skills such as stump wrapping, constraint-induced therapy, upper extremity prosthetics, Jobst garment measurement, special evaluation tools learned (such as the Allen Cognitive Test, Sensory Integration and Praxis Test), or leading a group exercise program for recent lower extremity amputees. Do not just talk about the population you worked with, describe what you did with them. All of the descriptions you provide should begin with an action verb. These verbs are listed in the next section and create a positive portrayal of you to the resumé reader. (Note: Keep in mind that this is the most important section of your resumé. Since you do not yet have paid work experience, this is your equivalent. Do not miss the opportunity to sell yourself.)

Using Action Verbs to Market Yourself to Prospective Employers

As you compose the body of your resumé, consider your language and choose active and positive words. All of the descriptions you provide should begin with an action verb. These verbs are listed in this chapter and create a positive impression for the resumé reader. Example: "Initiated" a parent/student play group once a week. Some words to consider include the following: *assisted, collaborated, composed, directed, developed, demonstrated, expanded, formalized, generated, handled, gained, interfaced, launched, maintained, initiated, managed, negotiated, provided, reported, reviewed, supplied, trained,* and *wrote.*

These are only examples. You can come up with hundreds more to describe your clinical and educational experiences.

SIMON DAVIS

36-36 33rd Street, Long Island City, NY 11106 | H: (212) 323-7749 | C: (917) 567-9891 | sdavis@gmail.com

Objective

To obtain a position as an occupational therapist in a well-established rehabilitation setting where I can use my strong clinical skills to optimize function, promote independence, and improve quality of life for the individuals I work with.

Education And Honors

Master of Science in Occupational Therapy

Columbia University, College of Physicians and Surgeons, Program in Occupational Therapy

Graduated October 2012

Magna Cum Laude

Pi Theta Epsilon - Honor Society

Bachelor of Arts in Special Education

New York University, New York, NY

Graduated August 2008

Clinical Experience

Outpatient Hand Therapy   07/2012 to 10/2012

Brooklyn Hand Rehabilitation

- Evaluated and treated patients with diagnoses including amputations, arthritis, burns, complex regional pain symptoms, cumulative trauma disorders, fractures, lacerations, and tendon repairs.
- Fabricated a variety of static and dynamic splints for specific hand impairments and post-surgical conditions including tendon repairs, carpal tunnel syndrome, and arthritis.
- Trained to work with and monitor physical agent modalities, including the application of hot/cold packs, electrical stimulation, paraffin baths, and ultrasound.
- Prioritized and treated numerous walk-in and urgent care cases professionally, promptly, and satisfactorily. Responsible for cleaning and organizing rehabilitation equipment to ensure proper daily working conditions.

In-Patient Rehabilitation   04/2012 to 07/2012

Sands Point Rehabilitation and Nursing

- Provided treatment and care for individuals with amputations, cardiovascular accidents, chronic obstructive pulmonary disease, dementia, myocardial infarction, neurological disorders, Parkinson's, and orthopedic conditions such as total knee and hip replacements.
- Administered formal and informal evaluation tools.
- Collaborated with other health disciplines to provide client-centered interventions and to formulate appropriate recommendations for discharge.
- Developed and implemented treatment strategies that are evidence-based to improve patients' occupational performance.
- Provided all required documentation, including daily treatment notes, treatment plans, weekly goals, reassessment notes, and discharge summaries.
- Familiar with all Medicare and Medicaid reimbursement case mix systems and the MDS tool.
- Developed and implemented protocol for skilled feeding group (which is still being followed).

Acute Mental Health Rehabilitation   **01/2012 to 04/2012**

Hillside Hospital

- Administered initial assessment and treatment planning with patients ranging from late adolescence through early 80s.

Figure 10-3. Sample resumé (*continued*).

- Developed and implemented therapeutic activities to improve functional skills and community living skills with patients diagnosed with bipolar disorder, depression, personality disorder, schizophrenia, and suicidal behaviors.
- Therapeutic interventions focused on cognition, coping skills, activities of daily living, interpersonal and social skills, self-awareness, stress management, self-sufficiency, and time management.
- Reported on clients' progression and discharge recommendations at weekly interdisciplinary treatment team meeting.

Geriatric Setting   11/2011 to 12/2011

Seaview Rehabilitation and Nursing

Level I Fieldwork

  Led multiple group activities to promote cognitive enhancement. Co-led fall prevention group.

Pediatric Setting   09/2011 to 10/2011

United Cerebral Palsy

  Assisted occupational therapist supervisor in developing appropriate treatment activities to effectively enable children to reach developmental milestones and engage in meaningful activities.

Psychiatric Setting   06/2011 to 07/2011

Bowery Settlement House

  Collaborated with Level II occupational therapy students in creating appropriate groups for patients to enhance their activities of daily living, money management skills, occupational engagement, self-care, and social skills.

Related Work Experience

Community Rehabilitation Counselor   10/2008 to 06/2012

Harlem House

- Provided individualized life-skills training to a 14 year old with Down syndrome and a 12 year old with mild mental retardation.
- Created activities and outings to help clients achieve goals in self-care, socialization, and community integration.

Rehabilitation Assistant   11/2011 to 05/2012

Genesis Health Care

- Assisted therapists as needed during patient treatment sessions (i.e., gait training, therapeutic exercises, modalities, activities of daily living, functional activities, range of motion, splinting/adaptive equipment fabrication, wheelchair adjustments, etc.).
- Worked with adult patients in a sub-acute and skilled nursing facility with various diagnoses, including traumatic brain injuries, strokes, dementia, Parkinson's disease, hip fractures, knee replacements, and arthritis.

Skills

Technical

  Microsoft Office Suite

Language

  Fluent in Russian (written and spoken)

Reference

  References are available on request.

Figure 10-3 (continued). Sample resumé.

Workshops Attended

In this section, you should list the names and dates of workshops you attended, the lecturer's name, and continuing education credits received.

Participation in workshops tells prospective employers that you are interested in your craft and are committed to improving your skills. As you gain more experience and your resumé expands, you might omit this section or simply state the name of the course attended. However, at this early point in your career, since your resumé is fairly thin, information about an interesting course could serve as a conversation starter during your interview and indicates a deeper knowledge in a particular area.

Related Work Experience

Oftentimes, new graduates are advised not to list prior employment if it is not related to the profession. However, as discussed previously, prior employment can tell a prospective employer a lot about an applicant. You do not need to describe the job in detail—the fact that you held a responsible job and had longevity there can be a selling point for your candidacy.

You may have held a job in the past that relates to your profession and provides the employer with more insight into your integrity, interests, and commitment. For example, positions such as working at a summer camp for children with disabilities or serving as a baby sitter for a child with autistic spectrum disorder adds strength to your resumé.

Volunteer Experience

Although not a paid position, volunteer experience related to your profession can also provide helpful insight into your commitment, interests, and integrity. List any volunteer experience you have had. If it impacted your decision to pursue a career in occupational therapy, share how it led to your decision. Do not forget to include detail about how skills learned as a volunteer could contribute to your professional career.

Honors and Awards

You worked hard to win awards and you should highlight them to demonstrate to prospective employers your determination and commitment to your new profession.

Special Skills

If you have special skills that relate to your profession, include them. Because occupational therapy is such a holistic profession, many skills can apply. Examples include a knowledge of sign language, carpentry, advanced technology, and nursing skills. You never know when one of these skills could provide you with an advantage in your job search. For example, an occupational therapy department has just added documentation software and everyone is struggling to learn the new system. A candidate appeared who had very strong computer skills, he or she immediately got an edge on the job as it was perceived that the techie could probably learn the system more quickly and could be helpful to the non-technical people in the department.

Languages Spoken

We live in a country filled with individuals from around the globe. Frequently, we are faced with patients and clients who speak languages other than English. Any languages spoken can prove helpful to a facility. In addition, it indicates a determination and commitment in mastering another language. At a facility where the patients speak multiple languages, this can provide you with an advantage in an otherwise even playing field. For example, a skilled nursing facility in Brighton Beach, Brooklyn, NY, has a population that is 75% Russian. Two certified occupational therapy assistant graduates of equal abilities are interviewed for the position. One speaks Russian; the other one does not. Clearly, the Russian-speaking certified occupational therapy assistant will be the preferred candidate because he brings an important skill into the equation.

OTHER RESUMÉ CONSIDERATIONS

Proofread, Proofread, Proofread

With all of the advice and direction provided in this chapter, proofreading your documents is the most important piece of advice we can offer. You have dedicated many years to get to this place and hopefully put a lot of time and energy into creating your resumé. Do not get lazy with the proofreading! After proofreading the document, give it to a friend—or even better, give it to five friends—to read for content, grammar, and typographical errors. Nothing will turn off a potential employer faster than errors in a resumé and cover letter. It speaks volumes about you as a professional.

Prepare Your Resumé for Mailing and E-mailing

With increased reliance on e-mail as a primary form of communication, you should prepare two resumés: one to be mailed and another to be e-mailed to prospective employers. Make sure that your resumé is presentable in both formats. Put the e-mail version in a PDF format to make it user-friendly for the recipient. Test your e-mail versions by sending them to yourself or to friends to be sure that the integrity of the document translates well in the transfer process.

When mailing the resumé, be sure to print it on white or cream paper (no colors). Use a heavy stock, preferably a minimum of 24 pounds, again to indicate the seriousness of your profession and commitment.

TOP 10 RESUMÉ MISTAKES

1. Typographical and grammatical errors. Spell check and proofread carefully. Mistakes jump out from the page and tell the reader that you are someone who does not pay attention to detail.
2. Poor format. The resumé should be clear and easy to read.
3. Not customizing the resumé to the job posting. If you are applying to a specific job opening, try to customize the resumé so that the keywords the screener is looking for jump out at them.
4. Including too much information. No one wants to skim through a long resumé to find the important information. The reader will most likely quit before the information comes to light. Focus on personal or career highlights that are related to the job you are applying for.
5. Writing an objective that does not match the job. Do not write an objective to secure a job working in hand rehabilitation if the job you are applying for is in pediatrics. Again, customize your resumé and cover letter to fit the position.
6. Leading with mundane or irrelevant duties. There are certain things we all know how or should know how to do as occupational therapists, such as document, provide treatment, evaluate (for occupational therapists), and fabricate assistive devices. It is much better to write active statements that showcase important skills and accomplishments to ensure the employer sees that he or she will be getting extra value if they hire you. Consider framing responsibilities in the following manner: Fabricated splints for flexor tendon repair injuries (if applying to a hand clinic); administered and interpreted the Peabody Developmental Motor Scales; or participated in research study relating to effectiveness of constraint induced therapy with post stroke patients. These statements show specific and unusual skill sets that every new graduate might not have.
7. Being too modest. If you have accolades and awards, or have had major accomplishments, include them. This is the time to show off a little.

8. Poor paper quality.

9. Too much white space on page.

10. Font size that is either too small or too large.

Gathering References

It is always important to have references lined up when you create your resumé. Provide names and contact information on an addendum to your resumé, using a similar format (and the same paper) as used in your resumé and cover letter. The contact list will prove helpful to your interviewer and demonstrates that you have organized the process to make it easier to access necessary information.

References should include supervisors at your clinical placements, a professor from your professional school, and possibly people from jobs unrelated to the profession of occupational therapy if the references can provide insight into your work ethic and reliability. Realize that if you are unable to provide references from one of your clinical experiences, it will raise a red flag about your performance at that placement. You might then try to preemptively identify someone at the placement who had a positive experience with you and could provide insight into your performance. Keep in mind that giving the director of nursing as a reference rather than the director of occupational therapy will raise questions as well, but it is better than no reference at all.

HINT: Always try to secure a written reference from your supervisors on facility letterhead while you are still at the placement. People move around a lot and you can often lose track of the people who were in a position to give you a reference. If you secure a written reference, you can bring it to your interview and include it in your portfolio. This gives the prospective employer instant insight into you as a professional. Although the prospective employer can always elect to contact the reference to corroborate the information provided in the letter, the interviewer is often satisfied with the letter in hand.

Composing Your Cover Letter

The cover letter introduces you to the prospective employer. If framed skillfully, it can act as an incentive to the reader to go further and review your resumé. Employers often use the cover letter as a screening tool to determine if you are someone they want to meet. The purpose of the cover letter is to convince the reader that your skills and experiences are applicable to the job you are applying for. Rather than rehashing what is in your resumé, the cover letter should give the reader a feeling of who you are and how you might contribute to the facility.

The cover letter is written in a professional, yet friendly tone with full sentences. It is recommended that it be formatted in three paragraphs.

- Begin with a header, which should be the same as the one on your resumé (and includes your name, address, daytime telephone or mobile phone number, and e-mail address).

- The salutation should say "Dear Mr. or Ms." (if you know the same of the recipient). If responding to a blind advertisement, the salutation can say "To whom it may concern." Unless you have familiarity with the recipient, do not use a first name in the salutation.

- The first paragraph indicates why you are sending a resumé. Example: "I am responding to your ad in the *New York Times* on January 26, 2014, for an occupational therapy assistant."

- The second paragraph should communicate the purpose of the letter. This is where you try to convince the screener that his or her department can benefit from your set of skills. This is also where you can mention special skills you have. Example: "As my resumé indicates, I

SADIE SPINOZA

456 Baltic Street
Brooklyn, NY 11215
Cell: 917-763-8978
Home: 718-863-9675
E-mail: Sspinoza@gmail.com

Ms. Helen Lopez
Director of Occupational Therapy
Beth Israel Medical Center
345 First Avenue
New York, NY 10012

Dear Ms. Lopez:

I am sending you my resumé in the hopes that you have an open position at your facility.

I am a recent graduate of New York University with a Masters Degree in occupational therapy. I have a strong interest in neurorehabilitation, and my dream has always been to work at Beth Israel upon graduation because of your unparalleled reputation in this area. I completed my affiliation at New York Hospital, working with Dr. Glen Grishom, who specializes in both cognitive rehabilitation and neurodevelopmental approaches to treatment. I have had some experience administering the A-One and the AMPs assessment tools.

I would be very interested in meeting with you to discuss any opportunities you might have at Beth Israel. I believe that with my strong commitment, enthusiasm, and work ethic, I could make a contribution to your department. Please contact me at any time if you would like to meet for an interview.

Sincerely,

Sadie Spinoza

Figure 10-4. Sample cover letter.

speak three languages and can be an asset to your department as both a qualified clinician and department translator."

- The third paragraph, which should only be two to three sentences long, indicates where you can be reached and when you would like to come in for an interview. Example: "I am eager to meet with you and I hope that we can arrange a meeting within the next week."

See Figure 10-4 for a sample cover letter.

TIPS FOR FANTASTIC COVER LETTERS

- Make sure that the letter is well written, is grammatically correct, and has no typographical errors. Always use complete sentences.
- Use simple language and be clear and concise.
- Keep the letter positive, providing insight into what you have to offer and why you should be hired. Do not forget to highlight the special skills you have gleaned that might be applicable to the setting.
- Whenever possible, address the letter to a specific person (do the research) and show that you have insight into the facility and the population served.

- Keep it brief—you should be able to convey the important points in three paragraphs.
- Use the same paper and stock that was used for your resumé.
- Do not forget to sign your letter and attach your resumé.

See Figure 10-4 for a sample cover letter that you can use as a guide.

SUMMARY

Your resumé and cover letter are your first introduction to a potential employer. Make an impact by selling your skills. Before starting to tackle the resumé and cover letter, perform a self-assessment and document all of your special skills and experiences to ensure that you do not forget anything when composing the resumé.

Identify a format that is neat, professional, and concise. Make sure your resumé is easy to read and that the highlights are obvious. Make sure that the entire document is well written. This gives a picture of your writing skills, which will be important to a potential employer. Get comfortable with using technology to send your resumé and cover letter. Do not make unnecessary mistakes that may turn off a reader such as poor grammar, typographical errors, poor design, flimsy paper, or a font that is difficult to read.

Organize references ahead of time and prepare an addendum listing their contact information in an easy-to-read format. Get a written reference whenever possible for future use. Be sure to create a cover letter that is designed to convince the prospective employer to go further and review your resumé.

DISCUSSION QUESTIONS/ACTIVITIES

1. List 10 action words that would describe your experiences at your fieldwork sites.
2. Using one of the formats presented in this chapter along with the resumé writing tips, create a resumé for yourself. Identify ways to sell yourself and the skills you have acquired both in your professional education and in your life history. Share and critique resumés with your classmates.
3. Rewrite this cover letter so that it reflects the person in a more positive light and motivates the reader to call the applicant in for an interview.

To Whom It May Concern:

I am interested in the open occupational therapy position you have advertised. I enjoy working with children and would like the chance to work at your preschool. Please call me for an interview.

Sincerely,
Cindy Todd

4. Identify one professional and one work reference with whom you have had contact. Write a letter of recommendation for yourself based upon what you think they would say about you.
5. The resumé in Figure 10-5 has many inconsistencies and errors. Organize with classmates in groups of three and critique the resumé, identifying all mistakes and inconsistencies. Then, revise the resumé to make the candidate more marketable.

LAURE JANE CAMILLORIA

Phone (555) 698-2134
E-mail: LJCdynamicgal@pb.com
1100 Longview Terrace
Pottsville, PA 16722

OBJECTIVE

Seeking an occupational therapy position in a pediatric facility with a concentration of feeding and oral motor focus.

Summary of Qualifications

- *Knowledge of evaluations for pediatrics and geriatrics*
- *Knowledge of treatment theory for oral motor sequential*
- *Excellent interpersonal skills*
- *Highly skilled with technology*
- *Bilingual in Italian/English*
- *Excellent documentation skills*
- *Certified in sensory integration*

Education

Harper College, Binghamton, NY, Graduated BA 2010

Long Island University, Brooklyn, NY, Graduated MA, 2013 Occupational Therapy

Work and Volunteer Experience

01/11-Present-Regal Entertainment Group, Postvill, CA

Ticket Sales-Responsible for selling tickets and candy for a movie theater. Answer customer inquiries. Collect and count ticket stubs.

6/12-8/12-Counselor

HY Daycamp, Ollie, CT

Responsible for caring for 5-6 year old girl campers. Led music groups playing flute.

Fieldwork II

9/2012-12/2012 - Tillie Circle Nursing Home, Marcy Avenue, Bronx, NY

- Under the supervision of an OTR, provided rehabilitative service to clients with various physical disabilities
- Participated in writing treatment goals and progress notes
- Provided treatment for neurological and orthopedic problems
- Educated family members and patients upon discharge

Fieldwork II

January 2013-March 2013-Elissger Long Term Care Health Center, Hastings, NY, 10456

- Responsible for collaborating with team members to decide on patient care.
- Providing OT services to patients with cognitive and mental health disorders including Alzheimer's, TBI, senility, and CVA
- Administered adaptize equipment when necessary
- Documented treatment and progress daily
- Educated staff on techniques to use for facilitating function for patients, as follow-through care

Figure 10-5. Sample resumé (*continued*).

Fieldwork I-

- Worked under OTR supervision
- Mental health facility, 1 day a week

Fieldwork I-

- Played with children ages 3-5
- Attend family meetings with COTA.
- Observed COTA treating children.

References

- Rena Lippin, MSW, RN. 631-518-4110
- Gail Pamichelio, OTR. 631-212-1450
- Susan Hangracgoo, COTA. 631-843-7120

Figure 10-5 (continued). Sample resumé.

REFERENCES

Anderson, L., & Bolt, S. (2011). *Professionalism: Skills for workplace success.* Upper Saddle River, NJ: Pearson Education.

Doyle, A. (n.d.) Top 10 resumé mistakes. About.com. Retrieved from http://jobsearch.about.com/od/resumé tips/a/top-resumé -mistakes.htm.

Doyle, A. (n. d.) Resumé profile vs. resumé objective. About.com. Retrieved from http://jobsearch.about.com/od/resumés /a/resumé -profile.htm

Ensign, R. (2012). Selling yourself in 45 seconds or less. *Wall Street Journal*, June 11.

Olson, L. (2012). 5 essential tips when using a resumé template. Retrieved from http://money.usnews.com/money/blogs/outside-voices-careers/2012/04.

Chapter 11

Proactive Job Search Techniques

LEARNING OBJECTIVES

At the end of this chapter, the reader will be able to:
- Identify personal job-related preferences.
- Develop job search strategies using seven different techniques.
- Understand how to identify the needs of targeted facilities to tailor your marketability.
- Identify the most effective way to respond to job leads.
- Create strategies to make a good first impression.
- Create a portfolio.

Now that your resumé is prepared, you are ready to focus on your job search. To be successful, you must identify a job search strategy. This strategy begins with you. By performing a self-assessment, you will determine your clinical interests along with geographic and scheduling preferences. Taken together, this information is your first step in determining your job search strategies.

Your strategy should be broad-based to yield the greatest number of leads to explore. There are many sources for job leads and different ways to research facilities to target. Job sites, social media, printed advertisements, staffing agencies, and direct mail campaigns are all viable means to identify potential open positions.

That is just the beginning. After identifying openings, you have to market yourself to the identified facilities, initially using the tools you developed in Chapter 1. Those tools alone are not enough. An interview must be earned and your pre-interview strategies and behaviors are what will get you in the door. Success will be yours through preparation that demonstrates your superior communication and organizational skills.

This chapter will cover marketing strategies that will help to develop job leads along with the subtle skills and techniques that will earn you an interview.

Davis L, Rosee M. *Occupational Therapy Student to Clinician:*
Making the Transition (pp 149-159).
© 2015 SLACK Incorporated.

IDENTIFYING YOUR PERSONAL PREFERENCES

The field of occupational therapy is growing and expanding, with many opportunities available for the new graduate. Because the job market is so strong, you as a new graduate have opportunities not available to graduates in other fields. As you start to look for a job, you have choices to make. This is the time to assess your interests and lifestyle preferences to prepare your job search strategy. Before developing your personal marketing plan, consider your preferences and needs related to the following:

- *Population*: After completing fieldwork experiences, many new graduates have developed strong population preferences. Other new graduates may enjoy working with a number of different populations and seek the broadest possible experience before choosing a specialization area. The decision about what population you prefer and whether you want to stay general or seek something specific is a very important first step in determining your job search strategy.

Personal Preference Checklist

As you review the populations you have been exposed to, you can begin to identify what population or type of setting you would prefer. The following are some sample questions that may help you determine your preferences.

- Do you like working with an adult or pediatric population?
- Do you like a fast-paced work environment or do you prefer a slower pace?
- Do you prefer to receive supervision and feedback or do you like to work autonomously?
- Can you work well in a crowded, disorganized environment or are you the kind of person who needs external order to function?
- Do you prefer working in a large setting with many other therapists or do you work best in a smaller environment with perhaps one other therapist?

Personality Assessment

- Write down four words that describe your personality.
- Write down one value that you feel is important in a workplace situation.
- List four strengths that would be useful in a workplace environment.
- Identify two or three weaknesses that may limit your success in a health care setting. What could you do to turn that weakness into a strength?

Based on your experiences, you can ask yourself many more questions. The answers will give you a clue to your personality and how you work best. This will help you to choose which opportunity would work best for you.

- *Location*: A job that is convenient to your home makes life much less stressful. Consider where you want to live and how much of a commute would be acceptable. Determine what neighborhoods are accessible to you. Will you be driving or taking public transportation? These variables must be considered when deciding where to focus your job search. While ease of commute is important to you, it may also be a consideration for your potential employer. When a commute is too onerous, the employer may have concerns that you will not have longevity in the job and will leave when a more convenient position comes along.
- *Scheduling*: Positions in occupational therapy can offer the opportunity for flexibility. This is the time to assess your lifestyle and determine what kind of schedule works for you. If you

have young children, a position in a school might blend in well with your parenting responsibilities. You may be someone who prefers not to get up early, and a flex time position that extends into the early evening (such as an outpatient orthopedic facility) might accommodate your lifestyle.

- *Salary requirements*: Starting salaries for new graduates vary within a fairly narrow range. Some new graduates may decide on their job preferences based on the population that they prefer, without considering salary. Others, especially those with student loan burdens, may want to choose a position based on immediate or future earning potential or special benefits being offered, such as loan forgiveness policies or sign on bonuses.

Review the Personal Preference Checklist on p. 150 and create your own profile before beginning your search. This will help you narrow down your marketing plan based on location, population, and other variables.

JOB SEARCH STRATEGIES

Whether you plan to stay close to where you went to school or decide to move to another community, the techniques used to identify potential employers are the same. They include exploration of the following resources:

- Contacts you have developed through networking
- Internet job and social media sites
- Staffing agencies
- Direct mail marketing
- Specialized periodicals
- Help wanted advertisements
- School job boards

Let's review each of these potential sources of job leads and determine how each of them can be used to uncover valuable job leads.

Networking

Networking involves making connections with people in your sphere who may then connect you to other people and opportunities. In Keith Ferrazzi's (2005) book *Never Eat Alone*, he shares an important insight. To achieve your goals in life, it matters less how smart you are, how much innate talent you're born with, where you came from, or how much you started out with. These are important but they mean little if you do not understand one thing—you cannot get "there" alone. Reaching out to people is a way to make a difference in their lives, as well as a way to enrich your own. Networking is probably the most effective way to secure a job. By talking to people and sharing personal and professional aspects of yourself, you may establish contacts who may lead you to a position—maybe now or down the road. It is never too early to network. Begin on the first day of school and never stop. One of the best ways to network is during your fieldwork experiences. Very often, a successful fieldwork will lead to a paid position. One of the great advantages here is that after working as a student, the facility knows you, knows how you interact with staff and patients, and has a sense of your skills. In addition, you understand the culture of the facility, its patient population, and the growth potential. When an entry-level position opens up in a facility, former students will often have an edge over outsiders submitting a resume. Be sure to stay in touch with former supervisors and let them know your status. If they do not know you are seeking a position, they may not think to contact you.

In addition to fieldwork experiences, your professors often are aware of available positions. Stay in touch with your professors. E-mail makes this much easier to accomplish. Although a phone call with someone who is in a position of power can be awkward, an e-mail is a very easy and non-threatening way to keep in touch. Initiate contact whenever possible. A contact missed could be an opportunity missed. Whether you are looking for a position or comfortably settled into a job you love, continue to attend conferences, workshops, and alumni events. This will keep you visible and in the information loop. Remember that networking is important throughout your career.

Today, social media presents a great source of networking possibilities. The online occupational therapy community offers opportunities to discuss clinical issues, connect with therapists in other countries or in your own geographic area, access important information, uncover new trends in the profession, and, importantly at this junction in your career, help you to identify job openings.

Some tips for professional networking using social media include the following:

- Know the platform and its applications. Mixing business with pleasure is not recommended. Although some social network sites such as LinkedIn focus on the development of professional networking, other sites such as Facebook are more informal and personal. When adding professional contacts to your Facebook friends, be aware that they will be privy to your vacation pictures, news about the new puppy, and other tidbits that they may not be interested in and should not be party to. If you are using Facebook as a networking tool, refrain from using it as a personal communication system geared toward your friends. Keep in mind that employers may gain access to your Facebook page—many often look to Facebook to uncover information about a prospective employee. Do not post anything you would not want an employer to see.

- Customize your communications. If you are trying to make meaningful connections, avoid sending out generic messages meant for everyone on your connection list. Instead, use your communications wisely and try to connect around something that is important to the person you are connecting too. Everyone receives so many e-mails, texts, and social media updates that these communications are routinely ignored, unless they are customized for the targeted audience. For contacts that are well-established, do not just ask for information or favors, ask them about themselves and what they are doing. See how you can be of help to them. For new connections, communicate why you wish to connect to them. Demonstrate an understanding of who they are and what they do, and explain the common interests that will motivate them to allow you in as a connection.

- Ask something specific. People often do not understand the point of social networking sites such as LinkedIn. Everyone is connecting, but no one is bringing anything to the table. If you want to connect, be specific about what you are looking for. For example, you may have an interview at a particular facility and want to know more about their occupational therapy department or may be seeking a critique of your resumé. By asking specific questions, you are more likely to get helpful responses.

- Try to take it offline. Social media allows us to communicate with people near and far; it makes it easy to reconnect and establish new relationships. However, it does not replace face-to-face meetings or telephone conversations as a way of making a connection and building a bond. Ask people about their preferences for communication and, whenever possible, try to make a direct connection.

- Say thank you. When people go out of their way to answer a question or respond to a query, be sure to thank them for their time. While you may be seeking help at one moment, be generous with your time and knowledge when others seek help from you (Klamm, 2010).

Besides the generic sites, there are now many social networking sites and blogs related to occupational therapy that can be useful in your quest to network, make connections, and identify additional sources for open positions in your geographic area. The list of new sites grows each day. If you would like to discuss clinical issues, there are numerous blogs available, or you can even establish your own on Blogspot, Wordpress, or a number of other sites. For identifying pictures or videos or to upload your own videos, refer to YouTube, Google Video, or Flickr (Dobyns, 2008).

Keep in mind that this is an area that is evolving very quickly, with new sites and concepts for networking developing on an ongoing basis. Be aware of what is going on so that you can connect with the latest technology.

Internet Job Sites

Today there are endless Internet job sites that list positions for occupational therapists. In addition to the obvious such as Monster and Craigslist (which do not specifically focus on our profession), there are numerous specialized sites geared specifically toward the occupational therapy professions. These sites are evolving and growing. To find them, simply search for "occupational therapy jobs" in your Web browser and see what comes up. Then, explore the various sites, register with them, and revisit them on a frequent basis while you are searching. Although many of the postings are placed by agencies, facilities often turn to online job sites to fill their openings as well.

Staffing Agencies

Because it is often difficult for employers to find therapists to fill their open positions, they often turn to staffing agencies to recruit qualified therapists. Frequently, these facilities do not bother to advertise their open jobs and turn directly to their agency when an opening occurs. In those cases, you may not hear about the position unless you are registered with the agency that has the position listing. Agencies typically receive their fees from employers to carry out the search, so there is no cost for you to register with them (typically the placement fee is based on a percentage of the first year's salary). An established agency can help you hone your resumé, provide you with helpful information about the local job market, refer you to open positions, and participate in the negotiation process on your behalf. Although there is little downside to signing up with an agency, do not make this your only strategy as some jobs never make it to the agency's roster. By listing yourself with an agency, you cover all bases and open yourself to more possibilities.

Direct Mail Marketing

This method is very proactive and can be customized to your personal geographical and population preferences. Start by researching facilities in your area that serve the populations for which you are interested in working. After you have created a database of facilities, identify the ones that meet your job search criteria. Whenever possible, send your resumé and cover letter addressed to a specific person, such as the Director of Rehabilitation, Chief Occupational Therapist, or the rehabilitation recruiter in the human resources department. It will greatly enhance the possibility of reaching the decision maker rather than the garbage bin. With a little detective work, you can figure out the contact person's e-mail address, making it even easier to send the resumé and/or follow-up to determine if the resumé reached the intended person.

Specialized Periodicals

Because the demand for our services exceed the supply, a number of newspapers and periodicals have been developed that are geared toward the employer's search for therapists. These publications are free to the subscriber and often contain interesting articles, continuing education offerings, and job listings. Try to identify all of the periodicals that cater to your professional geographic region and enter into a free subscription. These magazines can be found at job fairs and conferences, and are usually sent to professional schools for distribution. Because print advertising is being replaced by digital publishing, many of these periodicals are now available online.

Researching Facilities to Target

With so much information readily available on the Internet, it is relatively simple to gather all the information you need to carry out a successful direct mail marketing campaign. Some examples of sources for your job search include facility lists from your health insurance network, long-term care facility lists, the Centers for Medicare and Medicaid Services website (which compares and shares information on all long-term care facilities), or special education school lists from your state education department. Additionally, you can identify facilities by carrying out a Google search related to your specific interest areas such as "hand rehabilitation occupational therapy practices in Brooklyn, NY" or "spinal cord rehabilitation centers in Pittsburgh, PA."

E-mails for people you want to target can be identified with a little detective work. When going onto a facility website, you can often find a few specific contacts. Generally, e-mails follow a pattern. If you find out that the director of nursing can be e-mailed at ajones@abc-carecenter.com, you can probably deduce that Susan Smith (who you found out is the Director of Rehabilitation) probably has an e-mail address that follows the same pattern—ssmith@abccarecenter.com. Today, e-mail is often more effective than direct mail as it is easier for the recipient to respond to an inquiry.

Use your creativity to uncover a wealth of information.

Help Wanted Advertisements

The old-fashioned way of job searching still works, although the number of advertisements in printed newspapers has greatly diminished over the years. It is still worth a try to look in your local newspaper for help wanted ads, especially when they have special health care recruiting editions.

School Job Boards

Local facilities often send job postings to schools in an effort to recruit new graduates. Check the board at your school for interesting openings. In addition, schools now have online job sites that may also contain open positions.

There are many methods of identifying a position and you may wonder which method to try. The answer—try all of them. Do not limit yourself to one search technique. The more aggressive your job search, the greater the odds of you finding a great position.

RESPONDING TO ADVERTISEMENTS AND JOB OPPORTUNITIES

All of your work to identify open positions will invariably result in viable job leads. What you do next may depend upon the source of the lead.

Personal Leads

If you are diligent in your networking initiatives, you will develop job leads based on personal contacts. These are the most effective kind of leads, as you start off with the name of someone to contact who is either a gatekeeper or a decision maker and you have the name of the person who provided you with the lead. If handled properly, a personal lead can get your foot in the door where a blind lead might not.

When given a personal lead, you want to act quickly and professionally, both to take advantage of the opportunity and to prove yourself worthy to the person who has provided the lead. Remember that your worthiness as a candidate is also a reflection on the person who recommended you or provided the lead. If you behave professionally, you reflect well on your source. Even if you do not get the job, the person might be a source of other leads in the future. Do not forget to communicate back to your lead source, thanking him or her for the lead, sharing the steps you took to follow-up and the end result.

Non-personal Leads

When a job is identified through an Internet search or help wanted ad, you can be sure that there will be many responses and a good chance that you will not receive a call back from the potential employer. An employer may receive dozens to hundreds of responses to an ad. After reviewing the first bunch of resumés, if viable candidates are identified, the employer may lose motivation to sift through the rest. If you are really serious about following the lead, you will not stop with just sending the resumé—you will take it a step further. If you know the name of the facility but have no contact information, do a little detective work to identify the contact person. Usually, the contact is either someone in human resources or the director of the rehabilitation department. By making a few calls, you can identify contact names and attempt to reach the contact via phone or e-mail. You will generally get a voicemail when you call, but you can leave a message such as "Hi, I'm Sandra Seigle. I just responded to an ad you placed and I'm very interested in your position, since I did an additional clinical rotation to study hand rehabilitation. I hope you get a chance to review my resumé." Although you may not get the person on the phone, you have demonstrated initiative that could potentially spark interest, giving you an edge for a call back when the resumé crosses his or her desk. You can also try to identify an e-mail address by either calling in and asking for it or using the previously described technique.

KEEPING LINES OF COMMUNICATION OPEN AND PROFESSIONAL

This might seem obvious, but when you are searching for a job, think about how people are going to respond to the way you handle inquiries. Make sure that your outgoing telephone message is professional and brief and that you check your messages frequently. As mentioned previously, make sure you have a professional-sounding e-mail address. Check your e-mails often so that you can quickly respond to any inquiries.

MAKING A LASTING IMPRESSION AT FIRST CONTACT

You have networked and responded to ads. Now the moment comes when you have the opportunity to speak to a potential employer. This is a very important turning point in your job search. Often, the initial phone contact is used as a screening tool to determine whether to grant an interview. The employer may have liked your resumé, but if you fail to communicate effectively on the screening phone call, you may not get the interview. Be prepared for this moment.

- Keep track of all of the jobs you applied to so that when you get callbacks you are prepared with all of the information you need about the facility.
- Research all of the facilities that you have applied to so that you have an understanding of the population, number of beds, and location. It demonstrates an interest and commitment to the process, which gives the employer a sense of what kind of employee you may be. It might

also help you to ask appropriate questions on the initial call and it will certainly help on the interview.

◆ Think of things you could state about yourself on this brief call that might leave an impression on the potential employer. You want to be remembered.

◆ Be friendly but professional.

◆ Have calendars on hand so that you can easily schedule an interview with a minimum of waiting time for the caller.

FOLLOWING UP

Once you have submitted your information, whether through a want ad, Internet ad, direct mail, or agency listing, it is important that you consider your follow-up plan. More often than not, you will not receive any confirmation that your resumé was received. If there is no interest in you as a candidate, most employers will simply place your information in a file.

Although it is difficult to overcome rejection of you as a candidate, you may devise a follow-up strategy that could still get your foot in the door.

For advertised positions, consider sending a follow-up letter. Remind the recipient that you had previously submitted a resumé, restate why you are particularly interested in the position, and explain why you would be a good candidate (such as special skills you have that meet the stated needs of the facility). This might be enough for them to give you a second look. Many times, the first response to an advertisement may be overwhelming. The employer will review the resumés and call in who they perceive as the best candidates. Occasionally, they will fail to hire from the first batch of resumés and may turn to other sources or place another advertisement rather than looking back on the resumés they have already received. This is an opportunity for a rejected applicant to get back in the game by reminding the employer that he or she is still interested and is an attractive candidate worth considering again. That extra follow-up may be the thing that snags the interview. It is better to be their second choice than to not be chosen at all.

For direct mail follow-up, remember that timing is everything. You may have sent in your resumé at a time when there were no openings at the facility. Your resumé may have been tossed or placed in a folder and filed away. Two months later, an opening occurs and no one bothers to go back to the submitted resumé file. In this instance, a well-timed reminder letter might jolt the employer into recognition. You may want to resubmit your resumé with a letter explaining that you had sent it previously and that you are still searching. Add a statement asserting why you think your skills would be useful in that particular setting. With a little luck and good timing, you might get the interview that you missed when the original resumé gets lost in the files.

PREPARING YOUR PORTFOLIO

In preparation for your interview process, we recommend that you consolidate all of your important documents into a portfolio. The professional portfolio is a compilation of your best work, with documents that prove your capabilities, skills, knowledge, and academic accomplishments. In this portfolio, you can compile letters of reference from supervisors, fieldwork grades, documentation samples, submitted papers with grades and teachers' comments, seminars you attended (along with the certificate of attendance), and any other school projects that are worth noting.

All of the material collected in the portfolio should have small notations attached that summarize or identify each document. These notations make it easier for the reader or interviewer to understand what he or she is reviewing.

The portfolio can be presented in an electronic version with all materials scanned into a PDF format that can be uploaded, or it can be created using a hard copy format in a three-ring binder with different sections that are separated by dividers with titles such as "Seminars Attended," "Grades," "Professional Papers," and "Fieldwork Evaluations." Each document should be encased in a clear plastic sheet that creates a neat, organized, and dramatic presentation. Have multiple copies of certain documents such as your resumé and references encased in the plastic should your interviewer(s) want a copy. Do not put the originals in binder. Be sure to present the portfolio to your interviewer for his or her review during the interview process.

Electronic Portfolios

Many apps are available now that can help you create and maintain your ePortfolio. Using an app may help you professionalize and share the product. These apps allow you to include photos and videos and add links to share online work and content.

The portfolio is a reflection of you, so be sure to include only your best work, grades, and examples. Make sure the finished product is neat and clean. Do not present a portfolio that is messy, ripped, stained, or showing wear. It will reflect poorly on you and might indicate that you do not pay attention to details or take care with your work.

The portfolio is another tool you should use to "wow" your interviewer. Be proud of your accomplishments and show them off.

In Chapter 15, we will provide more detail about the development of a portfolio.

EMPLOYMENT APPLICATIONS

Most employers require you to fill out an employment application prior to your interview. These applications often ask the same questions that typically relate to past education, residences, references, and prior jobs held. You will be able to fill out the application more efficiently if all of the information has been compiled beforehand. (Note: Often, the employment applications will require permission to perform a variety of background and reference checks, including criminal background checks. Make sure you understand what the employer has in mind before you sign the document—and keep in mind that refusal to allow background checks might eliminate you as a potential candidate.)

If in doubt about what might turn up on a criminal background check, perform one on yourself to identify any issues that may be uncovered. That way, you will be prepared with explanations, should they be necessary.

STAYING POSITIVE THROUGH THE PROCESS

Looking for a job can be a demoralizing and discouraging process. You are forced to put yourself in a vulnerable and powerless position. It can be uncomfortable to sell yourself to prospective employers. Remember that you are not alone. Everyone looking for a job or who ever looked for one has had the same insecure feelings.

Some advice to keep yourself positive, centered, and productive during the job search process include the following:

◆ Keep active. Do not sit around waiting for something to happen. While searching, find things to do that will enhance your employability status. For example, use this time to volunteer to get some extra experience (and possibly an additional reference) or call your school to see if there are any projects being worked on that you could help with.

◆ Keep networking. Stay in touch with people—your supervisors, classmates, and teachers. You never know who might provide a lead for you.

◆ Stay focused. Keep at the search. Keep doing your research to identify new facilities to apply to. Keep checking all of the online job sites. Do not get discouraged. Right now, your job is to get a job. It is hard work. Stay with it.

Summary

Finding the right job may take work. After putting so much time into completing your education and creating your resume, it is now time to develop your self-marketing strategy. The first and most important step is identifying what you want in a job, be it population, location, schedule, or convenience. You should be prepared to decide which job-related factors are negotiable and which are not (e.g., "I must work with pediatrics, but I am willing to travel and be flexible with my schedule").

After this step, you can begin to use all of the resources available to search for open positions. The search should involve networking, which is the best way to get introduced to a job opportunity. Make a list of any possible connections who can be of help and enlist them in your job search. Beyond that, begin reviewing Internet job sites, consulting with placement agencies, doing your own direct mail campaign to selected facilities, responding to advertisements, and conferring with your school placement office and job board.

After making contact with potential employers, make sure that your mechanisms for receiving and sending messages are professional and reliable and that you follow-up on any leads you have responded to. Do not assume if you have not heard back that your resume was rejected. A reminder e-mail, note, or phone call might be just the push that gets you the interview.

In preparation for your interview, have your portfolio ready to go, both in a hard copy and electronic format. Some interviewers prefer a high-tech approach whereas others prefer good old paper. Be ready for either preference.

Most importantly, do not get discouraged by rejection. Nobody said it would be easy to find a job, but by following the outlined recommendations, you will find the job you were hoping for.

Discussion Questions/Activities

1. Make a list of your personal preferences in relation to population, location, scheduling, and salary needs.

2. In groups of four students, source at least four jobs from periodicals, online job sites, agencies, and job boards. Have each group share their findings.

3. Create your job search portfolio with all appropriate documents. Place multiple copies of each document in protective covers in preparation for your interviews. Bring it to class and share with the other students and seek their feedback.

4. Perform a role playing exercise with classmates in which you are conversing with a facility contact about whether your resume was received and the possibility of an interview. Have fellow students observe and critique the conversation.

5. Identify four online job sites that include occupational therapy positions together in class in groups of two. Create a log of all of the jobs you want to apply to. Include addresses, contact information, and the dates of the advertisements.

REFERENCES

Dobyns, K. (2008). Enhancing practice through online social networking. *OT Practice, 17*(21), 7-9.

Ferrazzi, K. (2005). *Never eat alone: And other secrets to success, one relationship at a time.* New York, NY: Crown Publishing.

Klamm, D. (2010). *5 rules for professional social networking success.* Retrieved from http://mashable.com/2010/07/02/professional-social-networking/.

Chapter 12

Acing the Interview

LEARNING OBJECTIVES

At the end of this chapter, the reader will be able to:
- ➤ Describe the work skills that are most important to employers.
- ➤ Outline steps to prepare for a successful interview.
- ➤ Demonstrate the ability to answer practice interview questions.
- ➤ Define behaviors that are appropriate during a job interview.
- ➤ Compose a post-interview thank you letter.
- ➤ Name five questions that are considered discriminatory under federal law.

You have taken the steps outlined in previous chapters that will lead you to the moment that will determine the path of your new career as an occupational therapist. Through all of your diligence in preparing your resumé and carrying out your job search strategies, you are now getting call backs to schedule a personal interview. Before this point, you were someone whose skills and suitability were measured by how you presented yourself on paper. Now, you will be judged based on how you actually perform in person. This can be an intimidating process, but with proper preparation, you will convince prospective employers that you are the best person for the job.

WHAT DO EMPLOYERS WANT?

With many therapists to choose from, employers are generally looking for professional and personality traits that they believe will contribute positively to their therapy department. New graduates are not expected to be experts in the field. The employer hiring a new graduate expects to invest in the graduate's professional growth. Some of the interpersonal, clinical, and work skills considered most important to an employer include the following:

Davis L, Rosee M. *Occupational Therapy Student to Clinician:*
Making the Transition (pp 161-173).
© 2015 SLACK Incorporated.

- Strong communication competencies—the ability to listen, write, and speak effectively
- Analytical and research skills—the ability to assess a situation, seek multiple perspectives, and identify solutions
- Technical literacy—a basic understanding of computers, word processing, e-mail, and documentation software
- Flexibility, ability to multitask, and adaptability
- Strong interpersonal skills—the ability to relate to coworkers, inspire others to participate, and deal with conflict (see Chapter 6)
- Team work skills, such as being helpful, respectful, pleasant, and able to compromise (see Chapter 5)
- Multicultural sensitivity and awareness toward other people and cultures (see Chapter 7)
- Honesty, integrity, and morality
- Strong work ethic and dedication
- Dependability, reliability, and responsibility (Hollaran, 2012)

Take note of the traits listed previously. Ask yourself if you possess them, how you can improve upon them, and how you might demonstrate them during the interview process.

THE INTERVIEW PROCESS FROM BEGINNING TO END

The Interview Starts at the First Contact

As discussed in the prior chapter, the impression provided to the potential employer begins at your first contact. That contact generally takes place via phone or e-mail. To ensure you make a good first impression, follow these steps:

- When actively looking for a job, check your e-mail and phone frequently. This ensures that calls and e-mails from prospective employers are returned promptly.
- Show professionalism by supplying an appropriate e-mail address and outgoing telephone message. For example, having loud rap music or a small child recording the message might create an impression that could negatively impact your professional image. It could also provide information that you may want to keep confidential such as your marital status or whether you have young children.
- Keep an updated calendar handy so that you can efficiently schedule a meeting should a prospective employer call.
- During your initial conversation (or in your e-mail), you may ask a few pertinent questions that will prepare you for how the interview will be conducted. For example:
  a. Is there a time limit for the interview?
  b. With whom will you be interviewing?
  c. Will it be a group (multiple candidates) or an individual interview?
  d. Will there be time for a tour?

DEALING WITH PHONE OR TELE-INTERVIEWS

Some facilities like to schedule phone interviews prior to a personal interview. This saves the interviewer time by weeding out candidates who do not sound as though they would be appropriate for the job. Make sure that you are not eliminated during this process by ensuring that your environment is free from distractions, noise, and interruptions. Because the interviewer cannot see you, your voice and inflection must demonstrate confidence and interest.

If you are applying for an out-of-town-job, tele-interviews are often used to avoid the need to travel—especially on a first interview. In the case of a tele-interview, practice using this technology with a friend so that you know where to look and how to compose yourself. It might be helpful to have your friend tape the mock tele-interview so that you can correct any habits or mannerisms that might negatively impact the interview.

Scheduling Strategies

When scheduling your interview, the best strategy is to be flexible and follow the lead of the caller. If given some choices, you may have the opportunity to improve your chances of making a positive impression. Morning interviews are often preferable to afternoons as the interviewer is fresher and more willing to listen and engage. On the other hand, when someone is interviewing many candidates in a day or over a span of time, he or she starts to forget prior interviews, giving the last interviewees an advantage over the earlier ones. That being said, do not worry too much about the timing of your interview. Often this decision will not be up to you anyway. The most important thing is the impression you leave.

Preparing for the Interview

Once the interview is set up, it is time to prepare for the big day. Here are some steps to take that could impact the impression you make.

Check Directions and Arrive on Time

There is nothing more likely to turn off an interviewer than being late for the first meeting. It sets an impression that will be difficult to undo. Always get directions for the facility and leave plenty of time to get there. You might even try a dry run so you have a sense of how long the commute will take. Do not take any chances. However, if you are delayed, be sure to call to let the interviewer know that there is a problem.

If you arrive too early, kill time before entering the interview site. When an interviewee arrives too early for their assigned appointment, it can create stress for the interviewer, who feels they must accommodate the early bird. You may think it is wonderful that you are early, but it could be construed that you have poor time management skills. Avoid this by coming in no sooner than 10 minutes before the agreed upon time.

Research the Facility

Before coming in for your interview, find out as much as you can about the facility, the population it serves, the organization of the department, staffing patterns, and affiliations. Speak to your school's placement director, who might have insight into the facility. Speak to students who have affiliated there, as well as former employees, and check out the facility's website. During your interview, try to weave your knowledge of the facility into the conversation. For example, "I understand your facility is rated No. 1 in *U.S. News and World Report for Orthopedic Rehabilitation*. You must have been proud to get that distinction." This demonstrates that you did your research and are resourceful, thorough, and interested.

Creating Your Job Search Portfolio

A comprehensive professional portfolio is an important asset in your job-seeking endeavors. We will go into more detail on portfolio preparation in Chapter 15.

What to Wear to the Interview

It is crucial that you exude professionalism when interviewing, but choosing your wardrobe for the interview can be tricky since you are interviewing for a position where you need to show that you are willing to work and get down on the floor to fix a wheelchair foot pedal while also demonstrating that you are a professional with good judgment. Being too casual or too dressy can portray the wrong impression. For a more in-depth discussion of appropriate professional appearance, refer to Chapter 6.

Preparing to Answer Questions

It is a good idea to prepare for the interview by thinking about how you want to present yourself and what questions might be asked.

Since you are going into the interview armed with a lot of information and knowledge about the facility and the job you are applying for, you will be able to present an image of yourself that is tailored to the position. During the interview, you will want to discuss your familiarity with the population, how your fieldwork experiences apply to this setting, and why you are well-suited to a particular work environment. Always remember that you are selling yourself. Dig deep and identify all of the skills and traits you possess that the facility will value.

Be ready to think on your feet by practicing answers to typical interview questions. Have a friend or family member set up a mock interview where sample questions are asked. That will help you develop interesting answers to challenging questions.

SAMPLE INTERVIEW QUESTIONS

Questions may be designed to elicit information about your interpersonal and communication skills, temperament, and ability to participate in a team setting, as well as to provide insight into your clinical skills.

Typical General Questions

- Tell me about yourself.
- What are your strengths and weaknesses?
- What are your career goals?
- What clinical affiliation did you enjoy the most? Why?
- What do you like to do in your spare time?
- Describe your ideal position.
- What is your pet peeve?
- What do you feel passionate about?
- Tell me about other interviews you've been on. Why did the facility appeal or not appeal to you?

Interpersonal Questions

These types of questions demonstrate your core values, ethics, and interpersonal skills, as well as illustrate your team orientation and ability to communicate.

- Can you describe a conflict you have been involved in and how you resolved it?
- Can you give me an example of a team project you worked on in school and your role in the process?

- In a new work setting, how do you go about forging relationships with coworkers and supervisors?
- Can you describe an ethical dilemma you have faced in the past and how you handled it?
- How do you go about making decisions?
- How would you handle a supervisor whom you feel is not adequately communicating with you?
- Have you ever worked with someone you disliked? How did you manage the interaction?

Keep in mind that when answering questions, you want to put yourself in the best possible light. Answering a question with a rote or predictable answer does not help your chances of making a good impression. Answers should be thought out with examples to demonstrate who you are and how you respond in different situations.

The Best Answer to Typical Questions

1. *What is your greatest weakness?*

This is a very common question. The answer should acknowledge a weakness (since we all have them) that the interviewer will see as a strength or a weakness that you have worked on and corrected.

- Bad answer: "I really don't have any weaknesses I can think of" or "I have a bad habit of being late a lot."
- Good Answer: "I can be very hard on myself and get upset if I am less than perfect" or "I am shy and at times I do not speak up, even though I have something important to say. But I've gotten a lot better lately from having to do so many presentations to the class at school."

2. *Have you ever had a situation where you did not get along with someone you worked with?*

- Bad answer: "I always get along with everyone" or "I once had a boss I hated. He was a complete idiot and didn't know what he was doing. He really annoyed me."
- Good answer: "Yes. One time I was paired up with a colleague to do an in-service at my field-work I placement. While I was working diligently on the presentation, she was not engaged and was depending on me to carry her share. I was so upset at her lack of involvement that I decided to express my frustration with her. The next day I shared (with her) how I was feeling. She apologized and agreed she hadn't been very helpful, but promised to engage in the process going forward. After that, we partnered on the project and became great friends."

3. *Why do you want to work here?*

- Bad answer: "I've heard really good things about the facility" or "I have a few friends who work here so I thought it must be a good place to work."
- Good answer: "I have an interest in neurorehabilitation. I understand you admit a lot of patients needing such an intervention and a number of therapists here with advanced training who like to mentor. I believe this will be a great place to grow and learn."

Interviewers will likely ask questions to identify your clinical knowledge, thought processes, communication skills, and personality. They are trying to envision what it would be like to spend every workday together. Are you someone they would like to "live" with? Although clinical knowledge is important, your likability factor will be an important element in securing the job. For more on this, review Chapter 3.

Remember as you interview that it is not only about whether the interviewer likes you and wants to hire you, it is also about whether you like the facility and staff. Are the staff working there people you want to spend your days with? Is this the job you want? Is the environment one that you could be happy in? By completing your Personal Preference Checklist (in Chapter 11) and preparing your own questions in advance, you will gain insight into the facility that will help you make a decision down the road (see Chapter 14).

QUESTIONS TO ASK A PROSPECTIVE EMPLOYER

In addition to preparing for questions that might be asked of you, you should also prepare for the interview by identifying questions you would like answered. This not only provides you with additional information, but it demonstrates your thoughtfulness and interest. The following are some examples of appropriate questions to ask:

- Can you describe what you are looking for in a candidate?
- What kind of supervision should I expect?
- How does your supervision structure work?
- What kind of productivity do you expect from your treating clinicians?
- How often will I be evaluated? Do you use a standardized evaluation tool?
- Am I given dedicated time for documentation?
- What are the documentation requirements?
- Is there reimbursement for continuing education?
- Do you have a fieldwork student program in place?
- What is the expected dress code at work?

Although it is expected and appropriate to ask questions, do not dominate the interview with questions. Two or three appropriate questions will enhance your candidacy. Four or more might prove counterproductive, making it appear that you are interviewing them.

If you get called back for a second interview, your questions should evolve in sophistication, since you already know the basics about the facility. At this point you may ask more specific questions about salary and benefits, since clearly there is demonstrated interest in you as a candidate.

SAMPLE QUESTIONS FOR A SECOND INTERVIEW

- Could you tell me what a typical day is like?
- What do you like the most about working here?
- Who would I be reporting to in this job?
- If I am offered the job, when would you like me to start?

Do Not Volunteer Information That Could Be Used Against You

Although you may want to share your personal life with your interviewer, we suggest that you not volunteer a lot of personal information during the interview. It is illegal for potential employers to ask questions relating to race, ethnicity, age, sexual orientation, marital status, or family status (see section in this chapter on your rights as an interviewee). That being said, do not accidentally provide information that might be used to discriminate against you. For example, by volunteering that you are engaged and getting married in a few months, the interviewer might surmise that you are going to be distracted, will need to take time off, and might become pregnant in the near future. By volunteering that you love spending time with your young children on the weekend, you provide information that might lead the interviewer to deduce that you will not be available for weekend coverage and may need to take time off when your children are sick. By volunteering your medical history (such as a prior cancer diagnosis, diabetes, or even a learning disability), you might lessen your chances of being hired due to concern that you might be out sick a lot or require additional assistance and support due to your condition. It is very difficult to prove discrimination, but it does happen and you do not want to hurt your hiring chances by disclosing unnecessary information.

THE MOMENT OF TRUTH

There is nothing better than being prepared. By following the steps outlined previously, you are entering the interview confident and ready for anything. Keep in mind that occupational therapy interviews are usually friendly and collegial. No one is out to intimidate you. The interviewer wants to uncover who you really are and how you might fit into the department, so be as real as possible. Follow the suggestions outlined next to ensure that the interview is successful.

Pay Attention to the Unspoken

As you sit in the department waiting for your interview, you will get a good sense of its pace and energy. It is very important that you read the interviewer's signals and identify information from your observation to help you relate in a way that is congruent with the interviewer's style, needs, and preferences.

- Greet everyone you meet in a friendly and professional manner from the moment you enter the door. You never know who the decision makers are. Assume everyone has some influence in your hiring. This includes the security guard, the receptionist, and the people on the elevator. Treat everyone you meet as though they are a decision maker.

- Do not speak on your cell phone or respond to texts or e-mails while you are waiting for your interview to begin. Turn devices off and put them away. Quietly read a magazine while you wait. You do not want to give the impression that you are a social media/e-mail addict.

- Shake hands. A strong handshake is a universal greeting. Be sure your hands are dry and the handshake is neither too strong nor too weak. People will make judgments about you based on your handshake.

- Follow the interviewer's lead. Although you want to get in as much information about yourself during the interview, there are people who prefer to talk about themselves. They may not really want to hear what you have to say. If you have a "talker," let him or her talk. The interviewer will think you are wonderful just because you are listening to him or her.

- If the interviewer seems to be in a rush, keep things short. It is important to read the nonverbal signals, which provide clues that the interview is over.

Upon entering the interviewer's office, you should do the following:

- Look around the room to get a sense of the interviewer's interests. Diplomas, pictures, or even desk trinkets can give a clue about a person and prove to be a conversation starter. For example, Meredith, a certified occupational therapist, noticed that the human resources director had many books on cars and miniature antique cars on his desk. She asked him about the collection and shared with him that her grandfather was an antique car collector. He was pleased that she took an interest in his hobby.

- Take off your coat and face your interviewer. If more than one person is interviewing you, be sure to shift your gaze from one to the other. No one likes to be ignored, and this perceived slight could cost you a job.

- Remove your resumé and references from your folder and provide them to all interviewers. (Be prepared with multiple resumés to distribute, even if you submitted one prior to the interview.) Be sure to have the resumé folder ready rather than searching through your purse or briefcase.

- Offer to show your portfolio and use the information contained in it to support statements you make about yourself and your accomplishments.

- Be alert and calm. Think before answering and converse sincerely. Be sure to use proper grammar and avoid slang.

- Listen carefully.

- Keep answers brief and provide examples to emphasize your points.
- Avoid negativity. Although everyone has had bad work experiences, it is best not to discuss them while on an interview. Never complain about former bosses, supervisors, or workplaces. Complaints about people say more about you than them.
- Always ask if there is time for a tour of the facility. This will give you more time to connect to the interviewer and will provide you with useful information about the environment. While on the tour, you should smile and be helpful when appropriate (e.g., helping pull a wheelchair out of the elevator if you are in position to do so). Often, a patient will start speaking to you. That is a great moment to demonstrate your interpersonal skills—do not be afraid to engage. During the tour, try to say something positive about what you are observing.

   Body language says a lot about what you are feeling, sometimes conflicting with what you are saying. Be aware of what your body is portraying to your interviewer. Some messages to avoid include the following:

- *Appearing nervous*: While interviews can be nerve racking, it is important that you stay calm and confident. Signals of nervousness can include foot taping, pushing hair back, touching your face repeatedly, or playing with an implement such as a pen (Figure 12-1A).
- *Appearing evasive*: Sometimes in an interview, we are faced with a question that we are unprepared for, do not know the answer to, or would prefer not to reveal. Try to deal directly with such questions by giving yourself time to respond, saying something such as, "That is a good question. I have to think about that." Avoid assuming an evasive stance, which might include averting eye contact; fidgeting; or providing a confusing, long-winded, or unintelligible answer (Figure 12-1B).
- *Appearing arrogant*: It is good to be confident, but overconfidence can read as arrogance. Signs may include speaking rather than listening, providing long-winded answers, or a casual posture (such as crossed legs, arm slung over chair back, expansive hand gestures). This is generally a big turn off for the interviewer as the candidate is acting like he or she is too good for the job and judging the interviewer and the facility. (Even if the candidate is judging, he or she should not look like that.) The "arrogant" candidate may be covering up his or her insecurities but is using a very ineffective technique that is not likely to impress anyone (Figure 12-1C) (Adapted from Hindle [1998]).

Interviewing Do's and Don'ts

What to Do

- Express yourself clearly with a strong voice, good diction, and grammar.
- Pay close attention to your personal appearance.
- Offer a firm handshake.
- Make eye contact with the interviewer.
- Fill out applications neatly and completely.
- Have as much knowledge as possible about the facility with which you are interviewing.
- Take criticism gracefully.
- Have questions prepared about the facility and the position.
- Display a sense of humor.
- Display self-confidence.
- Remember your interviewer's name and use it during the interview.
- Take time to think before answering difficult or unexpected questions.

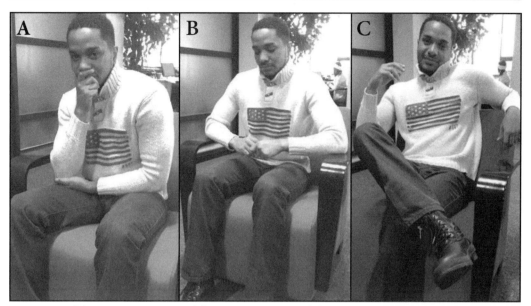

Figure 12-1. (A) Appearing nervous. (B) Appearing evasive. (C) Appearing arrogant.

- Take an extra copy of your resumé and a list of references to the interview.
- Follow-up with a thank you note restating your interest in the position.
- Contact the employer by phone if someone does not contact you within 1 week after the time from which it was indicated that you would be notified about the position.

What Not to Do

- Be overbearing, overaggressive, or conceited.
- Show a lack of interest or enthusiasm.
- Emphasize money as your main interest in the job.
- Make excuses for unfavorable factors in your work history.
- Condemn past employers or institutions of education. (Keep comments positive.)
- Display a dislike for schoolwork.
- Be indecisive.
- Display intolerance or prejudice.
- Be late for the interview.
- State geographic restrictions.
- Contradict yourself.
- Take notes during the interview. Jot them down immediately after.
- Glorify your past experiences to appear ready to assume a job that you are not qualified for.
- Smoke or chew gum, even if your interviewer is doing so.
- Answer your phone or even let it ring. Be sure to put devices on silence mode (Interviewing do's and don'ts, n.d.).

Sometimes the interview process may not be as formal as expected. For example, Vivian was being interviewed for a Director of Occupational Therapy position at a prestigious long-term care facility. The outgoing director was interviewing her and asked if she would like some herbal tea. She then offered to add some of the "energizing, healthful elixir" she got at the health food store. Vivian enthusiastically agreed to both the tea and the elixir, and they proceeded to talk about health food for most of the interview. The director was extremely impressed with Vivian (even though they never got to the subject of occupational therapy). She got the job and never let on that she detested tea because she really wanted to make a good impression.

Sometimes, you need to go where the interviewer is taking you rather than where you want the interview to go. It is important that the interviewer like you, and showing an interest in what interests him or her is the best way to achieve this goal, even if the line of questions and conversation does not make sense to you.

CLOSING THE INTERVIEW

Watch for signals indicating that the interview is over. Typically, the interviewer will look at the clock or ask you if you have any more questions. This is not the time to ask about salary, vacation time, or benefits, as this implies you care more about the financial incentives than you do about the contribution you can make to the facility. As health professionals, the perception is that we are interested in the clinical, not the financial. Keep that perception going at this point in the process. (You can ask about those important financial issued on the second interview, or when being offered the position.)

Now is the time to ask what the next steps are in the interview process, including when the hiring decision will be made. You can indicate that you are interested in the job. As you are leaving, you may ask for the interviewer's business card. This is useful for the thank you letter you will be writing.

POST-INTERVIEW THANK YOU LETTER

After your interview, we recommend that you write a thank you letter to the people who have interviewed you. The letter is meant to express appreciation and serve as a means to strengthen your candidacy. The thank you letter can:

- Remind your interviewer about who you are and why you would be good for the position.
- Set you apart from the competition.
- Give you the opportunity to sell yourself again.
- Reaffirm your interest in the position.
- Solidify the decision to hire you.
- Demonstrate that you are courteous and professional.

The letter can be very simple and straightforward. If you have been communicating through e-mail, you can send your thank you using that medium. Otherwise, it should be mailed. A handwritten note is acceptable, provided it is neat and legible. It should be on a thank you card or on simple stationery. Make sure that your note reflects proper grammar, spelling, and punctuation.

Elements to include in your thank you letter include the following:

- Acknowledging appreciation for the interviewer's time in meeting with you.
- Highlighting something you learned from the meeting or were impressed by.
- Expressing your interest in the position.
- Summarizing why you would be good for the position.
- Supplying any additional information you forgot to mention or promised to provide.
- Clarifying an answer you provided if you believe you messed it up during the interview. (For example: "I've been thinking about the answer I gave about working with children with autism spectrum disorders. Upon further thought, I realized …" [saying something to correct your misstatement]).

Thank you notes should be brief. A neat handwritten note displays a more human and sincere side of you, but a typewritten note is fine as well. If you are interviewed by more than one person, send each person an individualized note (do not send the same note to each person since they may compare them). Use the business cards you collected to address the note to ensure that names are spelled correctly (people can get very insulted by a misspelled name) and titles are accurate. Send the note out within 2 days of your initial interview (Erdlen & Sweet, 1979). The following is a sample thank you note:

Ms. Heidi Pashi
Director of Rehabilitation
Tyler K. Rosewell Rehabilitation Center
123 Apple Court
Hempstead, NY 11965

Dear Ms. Pashi:

Thank you for meeting with me yesterday to discuss the occupational therapy position available at your facility. I was very impressed by your dynamic department. I especially enjoyed observing the treatment session with Ricardo Rosa, your occupational therapy supervisor. He shared a lot of great information about the facility's treatment philosophy and how your supervisory structure has facilitated his professional growth as a new graduate.

I was especially excited to learn about the population you serve. At my Level 2 fieldwork experience at Burke Rehabilitation, I spent six weeks working with patients with brain injuries. This challenging population allowed me to integrate my clinical skills with my keen interest in cognitive rehabilitation. The knowledge I gained through my research project on remediating short- and long-term memory deficits would prove very helpful in this setting as well.

It would be an understatement to say that I am very interested in your position. Please let me know if there is any other information you would need before making a decision. I look forward to hearing from you.

Sincerely,
Lulu Zeldawitz

UNDERSTANDING YOUR LEGAL RIGHTS AS AN INTERVIEWEE

Although most potential employers are fair and reasonable, it is important that prospective employees be aware of the protections afforded them under federal law. Under Title VII of the Civil Rights Act, employers may not discriminate based on race, color, religion, sex, or national origin. Other federal laws also prohibit pay inequity and discrimination based on age, disability, mental status, or pregnancy status. Although employers do not have to hire you based on a protected status, they are not allowed to ask questions that can be construed as discriminatory. It is important that you understand what constitutes a discriminatory question and that you plan on how you might respond should such a question be asked.

Frequently, interviewers are not aware of what constitutes a discriminatory question and, in the course of a casual conversation, may innocently ask an inappropriate question. Obviously, if you want a job and are asked a discriminatory question, you should not confront or address it directly, as this might hurt your chances of getting hired. Rather, you should try to redirect the question to something positive about yourself. The most common questions that are considered discriminatory relate to family life and parental status. Stay away from discussing covered issues to avoid disclosing information that could be used in a discriminatory fashion. The following are all illegal interview questions:

- Anything exploring the interviewee's age
- Exploration of birth place, nationality, ancestry, or national origin
- Exploration of religion and religious observations
- Inquiries about an applicant's marital status, as well as number and age of children
- General questions about arrest/criminal record (Anderson & Bolt, 2011)

Some examples of unacceptable and acceptable questions might include the following:

- "How much could you travel?" (This question does not convey to the applicant the minimum requirements of the job. A better phrasing would be, "The job requires traveling 50% of the time. Would that be agreeable?")
- "What type of discharge did you receive from the Army?" versus the more acceptable, "Tell me about any job-related experience you had in the Army."
- "Do you own your own home or do you rent?" vs "This job will require you to relocate. Is that a problem?" (William Mercer Incorporated, 2000).

SUMMARY

After thoroughly preparing for the interview process, you have now reached the moment that will ultimately determine whether you will be hired. Although some people are inherently more comfortable with the interview process than others, anyone can bolster his or her hiring chances through proper preparation.

The first step is to understand what future employers want in an employee. With all things being equal in terms of education and fieldwork experiences, interpersonal skills will separate the successful from the unsuccessful candidate. The interviewer will be working closely with whomever he or she hires and will want to ensure that the person is someone he or she would want to be with on a daily basis. Although it is difficult for an interviewer to infer whether the interviewee has desired traits, such as work ethic or dependability, judgments about personality and interpersonal skills can be made and will definitely impact the hiring process.

Prepare yourself for the interview by checking out directions and travel time, researching the facility, updating your portfolio, and answering mock interview questions. Also, prepare the questions you want to ask the interviewer about the facility. It can be difficult to think of appropriate questions during the interview, so have some ready in advance.

Remember that the interview process begins at your first contact. Your phone message should be professional and you should respond in a timely manner when you get an inquiry about a job interview. When arriving for an interview, be on your best behavior from the time you walk through the door. You never know who you just held the door for or helped pick up dropped papers—it could be the person interviewing you.

Pay attention to the unspoken clues you give off about yourself. Do not text or have a phone conversation while you are waiting for your interview. Turn off your phone ringer. Sit quietly, and if possible, engage with the person in reception. He or she might put in a good word for you later.

During your interview, concentrate on listening to what the interviewer is saying to you and asking of you. This may clue you in to what the interviewer is looking for in a candidate. Most importantly, do not provide information that could be used against you. Employers are not allowed to ask potentially discriminatory questions, but interviewees often provide such information inadvertently in the course of conversation. Be aware of what you are disclosing and keep it professional.

Following the interview, keep up the contact with a follow-up thank you note. You may not get every job you interview for, but you will learn from every interview you have. It is good practice.

Discussion Questions/Activities

1. Break into groups of three or four students. Together, make a list of the 10 traits considered most important to an employer. For each trait, list examples of how you exhibit these traits. Think about how you could weave these examples into your job interview. Share your answers with the other groups.

2. Perform a check of your personal communication systems. Ask yourself if they are professional and if they portray you in a way that would support your candidacy for a position. How can they be improved?

3. Discuss in pairs what you think would be appropriate attire for a job interview at a public school, long-term care facility, hospital, and private hand practice. Why did you make the choices you did? Compare your answers with other students.

4. Role play with classmates and break into groups of four or five. Choose one student to leave the group while the others devise interview questions for a mock interview. Bring the "interviewee" back for the interview using the questions devised. Critique the answers provided.

5. Identify two interesting vignettes from your work history or during fieldwork that could be used to support your personal and clinical work skills. Share with a classmate to see if your experiences are compelling.

6. Compose a sample thank you letter to be used following an interview and exchange with classmates for critique.

7. Think about how you might respond if asked questions that are considered discriminatory under federal law. Set up a role play situation and ask a candidate some questions to see how these are answered.

References

Anderson, L., & Bolt, S. (2011). *Professionalism: Skills for workplace success.* Upper Saddle River, NJ: Prentice Hall.

Erdlen, J., & Sweet, D. (1979). *Job hunting for the college graduate.* Lexington, MA: DC Heath & Co.

Hindle, T. (1998). *Interviewing skills.* London, England. DK Publishing.

Hollaran, L. (2012). *What are employers really looking for?* Retrieved from http://occupational-therapy. advanceweb.com/student-and-new-grad-center/student-top-story/what-are-employers-really-looking-for.aspx.

Interviewing do's and don'ts. (n.d.). Retrieved from http://www.AcetheInterview.com/interview/othertips. php. 2011, November 4.

William Mercer Incorporated. (2000). *College relations and on campus interview guide.* New York, NY: William Mercer Incorporated.

Chapter 13

Understanding Your Salary and Benefits Package

LEARNING OBJECTIVES

At the end of this chapter, the reader will be able to:

- ➤ Describe the six principles of salary negotiation.
- ➤ Identify three ways to ascertain salaries in a specific geographic location.
- ➤ Name five typically offered employee benefits.
- ➤ Distinguish between a Health Maintenance Organization (HMO) and a Preferred Provider Organization.
- ➤ Name three important considerations when choosing a disability insurance policy.
- ➤ Identify three questions to ask potential employers to clarify benefits offered.

Once the interview is complete and you have wowed your interviewers, you will be faced with the next step—evaluating your offer and negotiating your salary and benefits. It is at this point where you become the decision maker, determining whether this facility is a place where you would like to put down roots. The salary and benefits being offered will be two important factors that will help you decide whether you want to accept the position.

Salary and benefit negotiations can be an uncomfortable part of the job-seeking process. It is often difficult and awkward to ask potential employers for a richer employment package than what is being offered. Asking for more money when faced with a job you want and negotiating with the people you are going to be working with is an intimidating process. Although salary and benefits are frequently not addressed during the "courting" process, it is perfectly appropriate and expected that you address these issues at a second interview or at the time that an offer is submitted to you. This chapter will help you understand what is being offered and your role in securing a package that works for you.

Davis L, Rosee M. *Occupational Therapy Student to Clinician: Making the Transition (pp 175-184).* © 2015 SLACK Incorporated.

NEGOTIATING IS A CHALLENGE

Studies conducted at Wharton Business School reveal what we already suspect—salary negotiations trigger anxiety (Brooks & Schweitzer, 2011, p. 3). Research shows that this anxiety can be harmful to the negotiating process. It was found that people who are anxious get lower first offers, respond more quickly to offers, exit the bargaining situation earlier, and ultimately realize lower salary and benefit outcomes (Brooks & Schweitzer, 2011, p. 3).

The conclusion of this study reports that if an applicant can harness his or her anxiety and feel more comfortable with the negotiation process, he or she will achieve a better outcome. A self-confident mindset helps you to establish yourself in the negotiating process and can translate into more successful salary negotiations (Brooks & Schweitzer, 2011, p. 28).

On the other hand, the new graduate is an untested entity. The facility must invest in the training process and hope that its short-term training investment will yield a strong, skilled, and loyal employee. The negotiation process must be a balance between believing in yourself as a new clinician and requesting a realistic package that is commensurate with your standing as a new graduate (within a particular geographic region and job market).

THE BASICS OF SALARY NEGOTIATION

The purpose of salary negotiation is to understand the parameters of the offer and to determine whether you can improve upon the offer through a give and take discussion.

Miller (1998) outlines some important principles for carrying out salary negotiations:

- *Be prepared*: Understand what the salary ranges and benefits are in your geographic area for similar positions. That way, you will know whether the offer is competitive.

- *Research how the facility you are interviewing with is getting reimbursed for your services*: That will give you insight into what you might be worth to an employer from a reimbursement standpoint. For example, in a long-term care facility, rehabilitation services can drive profitability. The rehabilitation staff and their ability to understand the reimbursement systems are very important to the employer. In another setting, occupational therapy may be a value-added service, in which case your financial contribution may be considered less tangible. Knowledge is power, so find out as much as you can.

- *Recognize that employment negotiations are unique*: Unlike the negotiating skills used when buying a home or a car, when employment negotiations end, you will be working with your former "adversary." Therefore, remember that although you are looking for the best possible package, you do not want to tarnish your image by over-negotiating.

- *Understand your needs and those of your prospective employer*: You must determine your priorities and needs before embarking in the negotiation process. For example, if you know that you need paid family benefits, you might seek out a larger employer who is willing to absorb this significant cost (smaller settings usually do not). Keep in mind that there are often institutional constraints in an organization that might prevent it from giving you the benefits you seek. Due to nondiscrimination laws, an institution must treat everyone equally. Therefore, it usually cannot customize an employment benefit package to woo you. Additionally, when applying for a job in municipalities, there is a typical set salary and benefit package based on experience that cannot be negotiated.

- *Understand the dynamics of the negotiations*: The level of demand in your geographic area will impact on the richness of your offer. If the job market is glutted and you are one among a number of candidates, you will have much less bargaining power. However, if the job market is tight and the facility has been searching unsuccessfully over a long time to fill an opening, you have more negotiating power.

- *Know when to quit bargaining*: There comes a point in the negotiation when you have achieved all you can. At that point, you should thank the person and either accept the offer or move on. If you do not recognize when to stop negotiating, you run the risk of offending your new employer. Most companies want to treat you fairly and make you happy. Being perceived as greedy or unreasonable can taint the deal or do harm to you in the mind of your new employer.

- *Let the negotiation process set the stage for a positive ongoing relationship with your new employer*: The initial negotiations are the starting point for your career with your new facility. They set the tone for the relationship. If you get too little, you are disadvantaged throughout your career. If you push too hard, you can leave a bad impression with your new employer that will last for your tenure there. Only you can identify where the happy medium is (Miller, 1998).

SALARY NEGOTIATIONS FOR OCCUPATIONAL THERAPISTS

Although it is important to understand the concepts behind negotiation, it is more crucial that you understand the rules that apply to the occupational therapy job market.

Understanding Your Market

Entry-level salaries for occupational therapists and certified occupational therapy assistants generally fall into a fairly narrow range. If the position you are seeking does not offer benefits (i.e., vacation, paid time off, sign on bonuses, etc.), the salary will tend to be greater than if a full complement of benefits are offered. (The rule of thumb is that benefits equal about 30% of your salary, so a position without benefits should pay you 30% more than one with benefits.) Salaries are usually presented in a range based on experience. This pay range will provide a boundary for both the employer and clinician to use during the salary negotiation process. As a new graduate, if given a range for a particular position, assume that you will fall in the lower end due to your lack of experience.

Before going out on interviews, do some research on salaries in your geographic area. You can do this in a variety of ways, including accessing AOTA's salary research data (if you are a member of AOTA, this is readily available on its website), conducting discussions with therapy agencies, networking with new graduates and currently employed occupational therapists, seeking out published salary surveys, or having a discussion with academic advisors.

Negotiating Options

It is always difficult to discuss money with a potential employer, especially for a new graduate working in a helping profession. The belief is that we went into the profession to do good and that talking about salary is in poor taste. However, you have worked hard for your degree and deserve a competitive salary. As discussed previously, your employer probably has a range in mind that is based on the economics of its reimbursement and the demand for your services in that particular specialty area, along with the current state of supply and demand for occupational therapists in your geographic region. You must be aware of all of these factors when negotiating so that you have a sense of how great the need is for you. Keep in mind that you will probably be competing with other therapists for the position and that an employer may have a preference for the less expensive candidate.

If you have chosen to engage a therapy agency to help you seek your position, this is the time when you will gain an advantage on the competition. As your representative, the therapy agency will negotiate salary and benefits with the employer. It will advise you on how realistic your salary demands are and can sometimes help in getting you some extras needed to seal the deal.

Be aware that employers will often ask what salary you are looking for rather than offering a range. Try to avoid answering this question directly as the information can be used to identify the minimum amount they can pay you. You are better off countering by asking how much they had in mind to pay for the position or making a statement such as, "At this point in my career, the job is more important to me than the salary." If a range is given, this is a good time to ask about the other benefits. As we stated previously, a job offer is an aggregate of salary and benefits—and the benefits can add immeasurably to the value of a position. For example, if you are planning to go to graduate school and the facility will reimburse much of this expense, it may be worth much more to you than a higher salary.

Understand the Facility's Review Process

The last step after finding out about an offer is to identify the facility's policy on future raises. This can be asked at the close of negotiations in a polite way, such as "Do you perform annual performance reviews? How are raises given? Are they based on performance or time on the job?" By asking this question, it implies that you are confident, believe in your capabilities, and are expecting to be a solid, long-standing employee. By asking about the review process, you can gain insight into whether you can expect increases in your salary over time. If the facility does not have a structure for salary reviews, be wary because that indicates a level of disorganization that will force you to approach the administration for salary increases, giving it all the power and putting you in a vulnerable position. The employer may say that it review salaries annually. You should then ask what kind of raises it has historically given. In a health care setting, everyone usually gets the same increase, which is generally a percentage of salary, such as 3% to 5% per year. Do the math. Your salary potential will be based on the amount you are starting with. Often, new employees that arrive after you could end up making more than you do, even after years of employment, as the base salary offered to new employees can rise faster than the increases you are getting as a percentage of your salary. If down the road you find this is true, approach management about bringing your salary up to the level of the newer employees. They may not want to lose you and might be willing to meet your request.

The Written Offer

It is a good idea to ask for a written offer letter that outlines everything that has been discussed, including salary and benefits. This way, there can be no misunderstanding or confusion down the road. This is especially helpful when you are leaving one job for another. Should the job fall through, you have documentation that the offer was made.

UNDERSTANDING EMPLOYEE BENEFITS

Employee benefits consist of non-wage compensation provided to employees in addition to regular salaries. These benefits support the economic security of the employee and can add between 20% to 50% to the cost of your employment (e.g., if your salary is $50,000, the cost of your benefits could run your employer between $10,000 and $25,000 per year, depending on what is being offered) (Sage, 2005).

Understanding the benefits being offered is as important as finding out about your salary. The problem is that, although your salary offer is straightforward, it can be difficult to understand the benefits and the value of those benefits in relation to your salary. The following information should help you understand these variables and guide you in making an informed decision when comparing offers.

Generally speaking, facilities have an established set of benefits that they offer to all employees. These benefits are typically not negotiable since, under federal law, employers must not discriminate in their offering of benefits and are obligated to offer and pay the same for everyone. Therefore, it is important to understand the employer's benefit plan and use this knowledge when comparing job offers.

Health Care Insurance

Health care insurance is probably the most sought-after employer-paid benefit. Under the Affordable Care Act, all Americans are required to have health insurance. The easiest and least expensive way to secure coverage is through your employer. Today, employees have other options through participation in health exchanges where individual policies can be purchased. If your employer provides this coverage, they will generally make a contribution to your premium. Whether offered through your employer or through health exchanges, it is important that you understand some of the basic elements of health care insurance.

Questions to Ask About Health Insurance

What does it cover? Generally, health plans cover hospitalization, physician visits, and prescription drug reimbursement. Be aware that all health insurance coverage is not alike. When seriously considering a position, it is a good idea to meet with someone in human resources who can provide you with a summary plan description for your review. This will outline the specifics of your coverage. Questions to ask the human resources representative include the following:

1. Does the facility cover your family or do you need to pay an additional premium for this coverage?

2. Does the facility cover the entire premium or are you required to make a copay on your premium?

3. What kind of plan is it? Some facilities offer HMO coverage, which means that you must seek providers enrolled in a particular network or you will have to pay out of pocket for your care. If you have preexisting medical conditions for which you are being treated, you should make sure that the specialists you see are in the employer's network. In a point of service (POS) plan, you can generally see any physician you choose, but financial incentives are offered to keep you within the network. For example, if you choose to go out of network, under the POS plan, you must meet your deductible (the amount of out-of-pocket expense you must lay out before your insurance will reimburse). You will usually pay the physician up front and submit your bills to the insurance company for reimbursement. After submission of your claim, the insurance company will determine how much of your claim will be covered. If it deems the physician charges are out of line based on your geographic region or if you neglected to get a precertification for the visit, you may not get the reimbursement that you expected.

Other considerations include the following:

♦ *Deductible*: An important variable to consider when evaluating a plan is the deductible. This is the amount that you must pay out of pocket before the insurance company starts to assume your medical or dental costs. Some plans offer very high deductibles (such as $2500), meaning that you may have to cover all medical expenses out of pocket until you reach that amount of expenditure. At that point, your coverage takes over. These types of plans are sometimes called "catastrophic coverage," as it will pay for major illnesses but not for common physician visits. If you have a high deductible plan, you should plan to set aside enough money to cover the deductible on a yearly basis.

♦ *Coinsurance*: This is the copayment that must be paid up front when you go to a doctor or the emergency department. Generally, the insurance company will assume a percentage of the charge and you are responsible for the non-covered part. Most often there is an 80/20 or 70/30 split of expenses. Typically, the insurance company assumes 100% of costs once you reach a predetermined maximum.

♦ *Prescription drug benefits*: Does the plan cover prescription drug medications? Many prescription pharmaceuticals today are extremely costly. If you develop or have a significant medical history, could you afford your drugs without this benefit? A good plan generally includes drug coverage, usually with some kind of copay depending on the drug being prescribed.

◆ *Family coverage*: Due to the high cost of health insurance today, most employers no longer pay for family coverage but will offer employees the option to self-pay. If this is an important benefit for you, find out if your prospective employer will pay the premium for your family. If not, what is the premium? Is it affordable? Family coverage can cost as much as $25,000 per year. If a facility is willing to pay for this benefit, it may be worth significantly more to you than a salary differential of $25,000.

Dental Insurance

Generally, this provides a limited amount of coverage, such as $1000 to $1500 per year. Some plans will cover for more than the set amount if you choose an in-network dentist.

Pension Plans

Some employers have established a 401K plan (if working in a for-profit organization) or a 403B plan (if working in a not-for-profit organization). In these plans, the employee makes a set contribution from his or her paycheck. The employee does not have to pay income tax on the amount contributed until it is withdrawn after age 59.5 years. You can usually borrow from the plan for specific reasons, such as the purchase of a home. Some employers make matching or percentage contributions to the plan, increasing its value as a benefit.

Even better, but harder to find in this day and age, is an employer-paid traditional pension plan. In this plan, your employer puts away money that will generate ongoing income for you at the time of your retirement. These types of retirement plans are less prevalent now but can be found, especially if you work for a municipality.

Disability Insurance

What would happen to you if you could not work because you were disabled? This situation occurs more often than most people realize. Unless you do not depend on your income to support yourself and your family, it is important to research the kind of disability insurance offered by your employer. In many states, employers are required to offer mandated coverage. The benefit will usually come into effect after a prolonged waiting period, reimburses only a small percentage of your income, and usually is of limited duration. It is always recommended that you purchase your own supplemental disability insurance that can cover up to 60% of your income, in your own profession, and over a long-term period should your disability be of extended duration. Although this book is not geared toward providing in depth information on this topic, we urge everyone to do research to ensure that personal financial needs are met in case of a permanent or temporary disability.

What You Should Know About Disability Insurance

◆ The definition of disability can vary. Make sure any policy you consider covers you in your own profession. That means that if you cannot perform the tasks of an occupational therapist you will be covered. Some policies cover you based on the fact that you can function in any job. For example, if you have a brain injury from a car accident and can no longer function as an occupational therapist but can work as a supermarket packer, your disability payments will be denied.

◆ Make sure your policy is noncancellable. You want a policy that cannot be cancelled and guarantees renewals as long as your premiums are up to date, regardless of the state of your health. Otherwise, you could potentially be paying for a disability policy for 20 years, which could be cancelled just at the point that you need it.

- Understand that some disability payments are taxed. If you pay for disability coverage with a before-tax payroll deduction (such as one your employer offers), the benefit will be taxed. If you pay for it after taxes (such as a policy you buy privately), the payments will not be taxed.
- Do not count on disability funding from Social Security. It is difficult to qualify for and you would probably need to prove that you cannot perform any job.

Paid Time Off

This benefit can vary widely and is an important consideration when comparing offers. Paid time off consists of paid holidays, sick time, and vacation time. Everyone needs time off to tend to personal issues and to get away from work stresses. To avoid unexpected absences, many employers will combine them or offer to pay for unused sick time. You should expect your vacation time to increase with your years on the job.

CLARIFYING THE OFFER

To understand what is being offered, it is helpful to ask clarifying questions about the benefits you would like to understand better. Some questions to ask include the following:

1. Does the organization combine sick and vacation time or are they separate?
2. Does the employer pay for unused sick time or do you lose what you do not use?
3. How is vacation time accrued?
4. Does the amount of vacation increase over time?
5. Are professional expenses covered, such as association dues?
6. Does the organization pay for continuing education and provide tuition assistance? If so, is there a limit?
7. What other perks do you offer—designated parking spot, free lunch, day care, or group life and disability insurance?
8. Are you expected to join a union?

INDEPENDENT CONTRACTOR VS EMPLOYEE STATUS: UNDERSTANDING THE DIFFERENCES

Thus far in this chapter, we have focused on securing a salaried or employee position. However, in the occupational therapy job market, there are a number of other ways that we can work. This section will explain the different ways we can operate, the definitions and differences between independent contractor and employee status, when each status is appropriate, and what your obligations are under each.

In reality, there are two variables in determining your employment status and billing options—how you are getting paid for services rendered and how taxes are handled for the work you have completed. A brief summary is as follows:

Per diem or *contract* refers to providers who get paid by the hour or the day. When paid this way, you are often considered an independent contractor, but if federal, state, and local taxes are withheld, you can be also be considered a per diem or contract employee.

The term *salaried* applies to someone who is an employee of a facility. He or she will be paid based on an annual salary (rather than by the hour or the treatment). The salaried employee has an ongoing relationship with a facility, taxes are withheld, and benefits (such as paid time off and health and dental insurance) are typically provided.

Fee for service is a way of paying a therapist based on the treatment he or she provides. This is often seen in home- and school-based delivery models where payment is computed by billing unit or visit. Under this scenario, if services are not delivered, there is no payment. Documentation time may not be reimbursed either. When being paid via fee for service, withholding taxes may or may not be taken out, depending on the arrangement made with the organization.

What Does it Mean to Be an Independent Contractor?

In the world of therapy, an independent contractor is a professional who offers his or her services to the general public under a specified agreement or contract. Unlike an employee, an independent contractor generally does not work regularly for an employer. The independent contractor retains control over his or her schedule and number of hours worked, as well as the jobs accepted and performance of a job. The independent contractor is also responsible for maintaining books and records. This individual does not receive fringe benefits; must pay federal, state, and municipal taxes directly; and is responsible for self-employment taxes to cover Social Security contributions.

Kaitlyn, an independent contractor, has put together a caseload that meets her needs as a mother of three young children. In a typical week, she treats five patients referred to her by a home care agency, treats three early intervention cases, and provides Saturday coverage at a local subacute facility. She determines her own schedule, accepts cases when her schedule allows, bills her clients on a monthly basis, and pays all of her own self-employment taxes.

Just calling yourself an independent contractor does not guarantee that you meet the criteria as defined by the Internal Revenue Service (IRS). According to the IRS, to determine whether a worker is an independent contractor or employee, one must examine the relationship between the contractor and the client. Evidence of control and independence must be considered. The IRS examines evidence based on three categories: behavioral control, financial control, and the type of relationship.

Behavioral control refers to whether the referring agency has the right to direct or control how or when the work is done through instruction, training, or other means. Whether a client exerts behavioral control might be determined by whether a therapist can decide what work to accept, that they carry out the treatment unsupervised, and determine their own schedule.

Financial control covers whether the business has the right to direct or control the financial and business aspects of the professional. This may include the following:

- *The extent to which the worker has unreimbursed business expenses (such as staff to perform billing, functions, rent for an office, etc.)*: Does the worker pay for his or her own equipment and supplies used in providing the services, or are they provided by the facility?

- *The extent of the worker's investment in the place where services are performed*: Does the independent contractor have an office that he or she pays for, or is he or she performing services at a facility in which he or she has no financial stake?

- *The extent to which the worker makes his or her services available to the relevant market*: For example, does the independent contractor advertise to the public, have listings in the phone book, or maintain a website?

- *The extent to which the worker realizes a profit or incurs a loss*: For example, is the independent contractor guaranteed payment for work completed, or must he or she wait for reimbursement from the primary payer to ensure their payment?

- *The frequency with which the licensed professional is paid*: Is the person paid on a regular, predictable basis or on a per project basis? Consistency is an indicator of an employee–employer relationship.

The manner in which the parties set up their relationship can determine whether the status is one of an independent contractor or employee. These variables include the following:

- Whether there are written contracts describing the relationship the parties intend to create

- The extent to which the independent contractor is available to perform services for other businesses
- Whether the client provides the independent contractor with employee type benefits, such as insurance, a pension plan, vacation, or sick pay
- The permanence of the relationship—does it go on for years or is it transient?
- The extent to which services performed by the worker are a key aspect of the regular business of the company

Questions to Ask Yourself to Determine Whether You Are an Independent Contractor or Employee

1. Do you offer your services to a universe of clients or do you provide your services primarily to one client?
2. Is your assignment long term?
3. Have you made an investment in your practice that is not reimbursed (e.g., purchasing the equipment you use to perform your duties or hiring an administrative assistant to do your billing)?
4. Do you make independent decisions about how your services are provided or do you receive instructions from the facilities you serve? Does the facility tell you how to document, bill, and treat?
5. Is there a contract for services between you and the client? Does the client outline the manner of your performance in this contract?

It is important to evaluate the issues relating to whether you are truly an independent contractor. It is recommended that you secure an accountant and lawyer to guide and advise you in the process (Internal Revenue Service, 2013).

SUMMARY

Negotiations are difficult and can be awkward, but it is the last step in landing the job. When making the decision about what job to take, you must seriously evaluate your needs and your family's needs. After considering the professional advantages of one job vs another, the benefits and salary being offered become important factors in the decision-making process. For some, benefits may be the most important consideration. For others, it is the salary. Critically evaluate what is important to you and weigh the relative values of each. Then, make the decision that works best for your circumstances.

DISCUSSION QUESTIONS/ACTIVITIES

1. In class, students should initiate a salary and benefit research project to understand what salaries to expect in your geographic region. Include the following:
   a. Published salary surveys
   b. Interviews with working therapists
   c. Meetings with therapy recruiters
   d. Other sources

   Use these data to establish where your baseline salary should be and share together with the class.

2. Research the disability insurance market. Develop an understanding of important elements, such as definition of disability, cancellation clauses, length of coverage, taxable vs nontaxable benefits, and computing benefit needs.

3. Research the health insurance market. Develop an understanding of important elements, such as deductibles, coinsurance, out-of-pocket expenses, lifetime maximum, exclusions, preexisting conditions, exchanges, and how the Affordable Care Act impacts our choices.

4. Ask three friends or family members for an illustration of their health care plans. Compare the illustrations to determine differences amongst classmates. Research any unfamiliar terms.

5. Invite a placement agency recruiter to the class and have students prepare questions to ask regarding job openings, salary ranges, benefits, and the differences between independent contractors and employees.

6. Have students gather in pairs and role play how they would negotiate a higher salary following 1 year of working at their first placement. Choose a couple of groups randomly to role play their scenario in front of the class. Have students respond whether they would be inclined to give the raise and benefits or, if not inclined, why not.

REFERENCES

Brooks, A., & Schweitzer, M. (2011). Can nervous nelly negotiate? How anxiety causes negotiators to make low first offers, exit early and earn less profit. *Organizational Behavior and Human Decision Processes, 115*(1), pp. 43-54.

Internal Revenue Service. (2013). Independent contractor (self employed) or employee? Retrieved from http://www.irs.gov/business/smallbusiness&self employed.

Miller, L. (1998). Principles for negotiating: The ten commandments of employment negotiations. From: *Get more money on your next job.* New York, NY: The McGraw-Hill Companies. Retrieved from http://careers.scs.illinois.edu/wp-content/uploads/2014/09/Principles-for-Negotiating.pdf.

Sage, B. (2005). What does that mean? Understanding Health Insurance terms. Retrieved from http://www.personalinsure.about.com/od/health/a/aa032805a.htm.

Chapter 14

Finding the Perfect Job Fit
Assessing Organizational Culture

LEARNING OBJECTIVES

At the end of this chapter, the reader will be able to:

➢ Define the concept of organizational culture.

➢ Identify five benefits of a strong organizational culture.

➢ Understand the four concepts that contribute to happiness in the workplace.

➢ Identify eight characteristics of a healthy organizational culture.

➢ Name 10 items to consider when assessing whether an organization is a good fit.

So far, we have outlined techniques and strategies to help you develop your job search materials, identify open positions, and impress your interviewers to secure an occupational therapy position. In earlier chapters, we focused on assessing your personal preferences, such as population, location, salary, and benefits, when considering a position. However, it is also important to determine which position works well for you based on your needs and priorities. What represents a good fit? Where will you be the happiest? It is not just about what the employer wants in you; you also need to figure out what you want in an employer.

In this chapter, we will discuss the concept of organizational culture. What types of organizations work with your particular personality and learning style? How does the culture of a workplace impact job satisfaction? What organizational priorities are important to you? How can you uncover the culture of a workplace to ensure you make the right decision about which job to accept?

Davis L, Rosee M. *Occupational Therapy Student to Clinician:*
Making the Transition (pp 185-196).
© 2015 SLACK Incorporated.

WHAT IS ORGANIZATIONAL CULTURE?

Everyone wants to enjoy going to work. They seek to be part of something meaningful and want to be comfortable, be accepted by their colleagues, feel camaraderie, and sense that their supervisors respect them and that administration is supportive and appreciative of their efforts.

The concept of organizational culture can be described as the collective personality of an organization. It is woven from an organization's attitudes, expectations for members' behavior, and stated and unstated values, beliefs, collective memories, customs, and rituals. Individuals base their daily work behaviors on these learned, shared assumptions. These eventually become habitual, patterned, and integrated. Reinforced over time, these behaviors and traits manifest as "the way we do things around here," thereby creating the organizational identity (Kimball, 2005, p. 3).

To succeed in any workplace, you need to adapt to the way things are done. However, before you start a position and make an investment in your future, it is important to uncover whether the culture of the workplace is congruent with who you are, your values, your goals, and your learning style. If not, the position will not be a good fit.

UNDERSTANDING THE COMPONENTS OF AN ORGANIZATION

Every organization is composed of various rules, values, and unspoken behaviors that reflect the organization, its staff, and management. Organizational culture represents the personality of the facility that you are considering. This personality is formed by a number of components, which include the following:

- *Rituals and ceremonies* include things such as new hire trainings, welcome lunches, annual holiday events, and company-sponsored educational events.
- *Symbols and slogans* are usually more abstract reflections of the culture. They may reflect the organization's goals and include awards or incentives that symbolize preferred behavior, such as an Employee of the Month award. Slogans are linguistic representations of preferred actions or behaviors, such as "we put our patients first" or VNS of New York's slogan: "We're here to help—whenever you need it." These slogans not only impart information to customers and clients, but they also provide cues to employees about how they should perform their jobs.
- *Stories* are narratives based on true events, which are often exaggerated when passed along from old to new employees. They may be about the organization's history, challenges that had to be overcome, or heroes of the organization. At Therapeutic Resources, we often share with the staff how we started the business by working in a nursing home full time while identifying clients, making calls on pay phones during our lunch hour, and interviewing therapists in our apartments at night. These stories became part of our history. Such stories might retell how everyone stayed overnight and took care of the patients during a flood or blackout or the way everyone responded when there was a nursing strike. Those are experiences that say a lot about the facility and the bonds that have formed between colleagues.
- *Values* reflect the conscious desires of the organization. They communicate to employees the kind of behavior the organization wants to promote and reward. Values are often "sold" through written symbols or slogans that are used in marketing campaigns (as mentioned previously). However, true values can only be tested within the organization through an employee's perception and experience of the way the employer handles problems and challenges within the organization. The values of an organization are reflected in its ethics, its commitment to employees, and the manner in which it empowers and controls employees as they carry out their duties and responsibilities.

All of the previous information results in assumptions by the employee about the organization's culture. It provides guidance in determining behavioral expectations of that culture and how he or she feels about his or her job and career (Gupta, 2009).

Every organization has developed its own personality that is based on its leaders' goals and values. These organizational traits evolve over time as leaders evolve and leadership changes. These traits form the framework of the culture in each particular organization. Some important dimensions that impact the culture include the following:

- *Attitudes toward innovation and risk taking*: Does the organization encourage and reward new ways of doing things or does it want to maintain traditional approaches?

- *Patterns of communication*: Is communication, instruction, and reporting set up within formal hierarchies or is it a more informal process? Does the organization seek feedback from employees or does it expect them to carry out orders without question?

- *Internal or external focus*: Is attention more focused on the clients being served or is the orientation more focused on maintaining internal functions (i.e., strict adherence to policies and procedures, such as limiting visiting hours to between 2 and 4 p.m.). Is the organization flexible in meeting the needs of the patients, clients, and customers?

- *Uniformity or diversity*: Do attitudes and expectations within the organization value consistency (doing things the same way) or diversity (adapting and changing based on new situations and challenges)?

- *People orientation*: Does management support and value their human resources? Are they flexible in family emergencies? Do they value work–life balance?

- *Team orientation*: Does the organization encourage and reward individualism or does the structure foster and value teamwork?

- *Aggressiveness/competitiveness*: To what extent are organizational attitudes focused on dominating rather than coexisting, cooperating, and learning from one another (Davies, Nutley, & Mannion, 2000).

THE IMPACT OF ORGANIZATIONAL CULTURE ON EMPLOYEES AND CLIENTS

Organizational culture has a strong impact on job performance, financial performance, customer and employee satisfaction, and innovation (Fisher & Alford, 2000). Collins and Porras (1997), in their book *Built to Last*, evaluated the best companies and their prime competitors across a number of industries. They sought to uncover the secrets of firms that enjoyed long-term success. They found that the best companies had a sense of stewardship, vision, and discipline as well as leaders with vision and strong values (Collins & Porras, 1997). In the health care environment, where life and death interventions are provided on a daily basis, organizational culture has been associated with important components of care such as patient safety, improved nursing care, and greater job satisfaction (Boan & Funderburk, 2003). In the United Kingdom, the government takes an activist approach in managing the culture, believing it is one route toward improved health care (Davies, Nutley, & Mannion, 2000). It has even been documented that hospitals known to be good places to work have lower Medicare mortality rates (Aiken, Smith, & Lake, 1994; Boan & Funderburk, 2003).

A strong organization produces many positive end results for the people who work there, as well as for the people being served. These include the following:

- *Attracting better talent*: The best people want to work in the best places. This creates a positive staffing cycle, the opportunity to learn from the best, and a work environment where outcomes are maximized.

- *Retaining talent*: People who like where they work are less likely to leave for another position.
- *Creating energy and momentum*: When people are motivated and excited about what they are doing, they exude energy and excitement, which is contagious and palpable.
- *Changing the way employees view work*: Surrounded by positive energy and enthusiasm, people will look forward to going to work, work harder, and give it their all.
- *Making everyone more efficient and successful:* Employees benefit from having support from their leaders who provide them with the tools to perform their job more effectively.

HOW FINANCIAL PRIORITIES CAN IMPACT ORGANIZATIONAL CULTURE

Typically, occupational therapists are motivated by altruistic goals and a desire to contribute to the well-being of their clients. In the heyday of fee-for-service medicine and a seemingly bottom-less pit of government funding for education, the concept of providing the client with whatever the client needed—without any thought of the financial consequences—was possible, but that model has changed over the past few decades.

During the 1980s, prospective payment systems were introduced to health care, resulting in the adoption of more businesslike practices and behaviors. Cost-cutting measures were undertaken, organizations were restructured to promote efficiencies, and delivery of care was changed with greater oversight over length of stays. Strict documentation requirements were implemented to ensure the services provided were deemed reasonable and necessary. Suddenly, organizational cultures were forced to adopt new practices in response to greater financial pressure to deliver services efficiently and effectively. The focus on financial sustainability changed how we deliver services and has resulted in decreased satisfaction for the clients we serve and providers of care. There is less time to spend with clients, resulting in an impersonal health care system.

However, it is possible to operate a financially sound organization while maintaining a corporate culture that delivers quality care and supports the providers delivering the care. Although financial considerations must now be factored into what we do as occupational therapists, it is still possible to identify workplaces that offer conservative fiscal policies along with a positive organizational culture. Finding the right one will be your challenge.

ORGANIZATIONAL ETHICS

The way an organization manages ethical issues is an important part of its organizational culture. This is an especially important consideration for a licensed health professional who is obligated to practice under the AOTA's *Code of Ethics and Ethical Standards* and state licensure requirements. In today's health care environment, there are constant challenges relating to clinical decision making, policies, political contexts, team structures, and consumer demands (Gallagher & Tschudin, 2010). The organizational pressures that result from these challenges can lead to conflict, frustration, moral distress, and the potential for requests to perform an act that could be considered unethical (Kurfuerst & Yousey, 2012). Organizational ethics refers to the attitudes and standards exhibited by administrative and management leaders within an organization in response to the demands of outside influences, such as third party payers, governmental authorities, and consumers. Occupational therapists can experience pressure from consumers, regulatory bodies, and forces within their own organization. Such pressures may be related to service delivery, therapy plans, inequitable care, inaccurate billing and documentation, or compromises in staffing patterns. Constraints in time and money will continue to exist in health care; therefore, occupational therapy practitioners must understand how to handle these ethical challenges while addressing the needs of the clients and communities being served. The way an organization deals with these pressures has a direct impact on its practitioners and affects what is considered acceptable responses to these pressures.

An ethical workplace climate is impacted by both the services that are delivered to clients, and the overt and covert values that shape the organization and impact decisions being made. Berghofer and Schwartz (2012) stated:

> An ethical organization is a community of people working together in an environment of mutual respect where they grow personally, feel fulfilled, contribute to a common good, and share in the personal, emotional, and financial rewards of a job well done. There is a shared understanding that success depends on a constellation of relationships both internal and external, not all of which are under the organization's control, but which it can influence through the way it operates from a platform of ethical principles. (p. 4)

Winkler, Gruen, and Sussman (2005) identified four key considerations in the development of an ethical organization: (1) providing care with compassion, (2) treating employees with respect, (3) acting in the public spirit, and (4) spending resources responsibly.

The management team at your facility must foster a work environment that supports ethically sound decisions. While this seems obvious and logical, with the pressure to cut health care costs, ensure productivity, maximize reimbursement potential, deal with staffing shortages, and meet the demands of managed care organizations, choosing the ethical highroad can be challenging. Taking shortcuts on ethics can impact the morale of the staff, compromise the safety of patients and staff, and potentially lead to negative organizational and personal consequences. Understanding the ethical culture of an organization is an important step in identifying whether a position is right for you.

Being Happy at Work

In a recent article about Zappos (the online shoe sales website), its CEO noted that he succeeded in creating an environment that emphasized creativity, fun, and happiness in the workplace. It has been proven that happy employees produce more, have better attendance, deliver better service, require less management and monitoring, are more committed to the job, and are less likely to quit (Heskett, Sasser, & Wheeler, 2008).

It has been clearly established that workplace culture has a major impact on whether you will be happy on the job, but what does "happy on the job" really mean? Harvard Business School along with the Ross School of Business' Center for Positive Organization Scholarship has carried out research on happiness in the workplace (Spreitzer & Porath, 2012, p. 4). It came up with one word that describes the mood of the successful workplace—thriving. A thriving workforce is one in which employees are satisfied and productive, as well as engaged and energized in the process. Workers who are thriving demonstrate better overall performance, experience less burnout, are more committed to their organization, and are more satisfied with their jobs (Spreitzer & Porath, 2012, p. 4).

The study identified two components of thriving (Spreitzer & Porath, 2012, p. 4). The first is vitality—the sense of being alive, passionate, and excited. The workplace encourages vitality when it reinforces that the employee is making a difference. The second is the opportunity to learn—the growth that comes from gaining new knowledge and skills. Learning not only bestows a technical advantage and status, but it also sets in motion a positive cycle where professionals believe in their potential for further growth. The two qualities work together. For example, learning without the opportunity to apply newly acquired skills to practice can lead to burnout. Vitality can be deadening when the work environment does not give its workers the opportunity to learn. To ensure satisfaction and happiness, one should seek out employers who will provide the opportunity to thrive and learn (Spreitzer & Porath, 2012, p. 4).

CONDITIONS FOR THRIVING AND LEARNING

How can you determine which work setting will offer opportunities to thrive? Harvard research has uncovered four mechanisms that create the conditions for thriving employees (Spreitzer & Porath, 2012, p. 4). These include providing decision-making opportunities, sharing information, minimizing incivility, and offering performance feedback.

- *Providing decision-making opportunities*: When employees are given latitude in making decisions that affect their work, they feel in control and empowered. Usually, the person with the greatest knowledge of a job is the person doing that job. He or she is the one who understands the roadblocks in the organization and how frustrations impact the ability to perform a job. When a supervisor allows a therapist to identify solutions to problems and implement them, rather than superimposing his or her solutions, it leads to greater autonomy and encourages participation and ownership in the process. For example, Julie, an occupational therapist, was working in a school setting where there was limited space available to provide the sensory-based program that many of the children on her caseload needed. Julie thought about asking her supervisor to provide a solution to the problem. Knowing that her supervisor encouraged her staff to seek their own solutions, Julie decided it might be better if she tried to figure it out on her own. Upon investigation, she noticed that certain large rooms in the school were empty at particular times of the day. She observed and documented when the rooms were empty and did some research to support their usage before presenting the idea to her supervisor that she borrow the rooms when they are empty. Based on her efforts, she was able to use the rooms 3 hours per day, during which time she scheduled the children who required the larger setting. She felt gratified that she was able to solve the problem herself and appreciated the support she received from administration. Her supervisor appreciated the work she put in to identifying a solution on her own.

- *Sharing information*: Employees are much more likely to participate and contribute when they understand why they are asked to do what they do. To encourage participation and motivation, people should understand the impact they are making. For example, in the long-term care arena, reimbursement is based on a complicated formula, combining treatment minutes and treatment days to qualify for high reimbursement categories. If the minute or day requirements are not met, the facility is in jeopardy of losing a significant amount of revenue for that particular patient over a 2- to 4-week period. A supervisor will often tell a provider that he or she has to treat the patient for a specific number of minutes per day but does not explain why or share the ramifications if the minute or day requirement is not met. By not explaining the importance of the time requirement and its impact in dollars and cents, a therapist may not be as diligent in making sure the criteria are met.

- *Minimizing incivility*: An environment where people are not civil to one another can be toxic and can undermine morale and motivation. Research has shown that 50% of employees who experienced uncivil behavior at work intentionally decreased their efforts (Spreitzer & Porath, 2012, p. 7). Two-thirds spent a significant amount of time avoiding the offender and about the same number said their performance had declined because of the behavior (Sprietzer & Porath, 2012, p. 7). Incivility causes unhappiness and prevents people from thriving. The culture of the workplace will determine how uncivil behavior is handled. If the culture has no tolerance for disrespect, the attitude will be contagious. If the culture tolerates uncivil behavior with no attempts to correct it and no consequences for the offender, a spiral of negativity and unhappiness results.

- *Offering performance feedback*: Feedback creates opportunities for learning and a culture of thriving. Feedback is very helpful in resolving uncertainty and keeping people focused on their goals and responsibilities. Feedback that is presented with respect and civility will energize staff and promote growth. Therapists (especially new graduates) should look for positions where they will receive regular constructive supervision, which contributes professional growth and improved performance.

ASSESSING CULTURAL FIT

When interviewing for a job, it is important that you ask questions that will provide the clues to the organizational culture of the facility. If you are observant, you will feel the culture of an organization. As you enter a facility for the first time, observe the environment—the physical layout, the dress code, the manner in which people address each other, the smell and feel of the place, and its emotional intensity (Schein, 1990). Although these clues might seem superficial, they provide insight as to what lies beneath. A tour of patient floors will provide you with insight and information regarding the facility's cleanliness and the staff's attitude toward patient care. A clinic in the basement of a facility with old and neglected equipment might provide clues regarding the administration's attitude about the importance of the department. A facility that places a high value on its rehabilitation department and makes an investment in its appearance and cleanliness will likely be a better place to work.

Unlike observable variables, assessing the values of an organization may be more difficult to uncover on an initial interview. Some information might be gleaned through targeted questions. For example, Roberto, an entry-level therapist, was interviewed at a large pediatric hospital serving fragile children with severe medical conditions. During the interview, Roberto asked the interviewer what kind of supervision he might expect. He was told that he was expected to handle his caseload without any supervision since he should know what he is doing. Roberto was taken aback by the answer, as he had expected that there would be some formal supervision that would help him grow and develop his skills—especially since he would be working with such a fragile population. The answer to his question provided a clue and a warning that this might not be the position for him. When considering a position, think about what is important to you—your values and priorities—and be sure to ask questions that uncover the philosophy of the facility.

IDENTIFYING THE CHARACTERISTICS OF A HEALTHY ORGANIZATIONAL CULTURE

To help you assess a facility's organizational culture, be on the lookout for clues and characteristics that can be uncovered during the interview process. Some of these include the following:

- *Organizational pride*: When employees speak highly of their employer and defend them against criticism, it is usually a pretty good sign of a strong organizational culture. Pay attention to the work environment. Do employees have trinkets on their desk from company gatherings or mementos that recognize the organization? During the interview, do you notice that employees speak positively about their employer? Are you getting the sense that they are giving you negative "veiled" messages about the organization?

- *Always seeking to do and be better*: Does the facility encourage continuing education participation? Is there room for growth and advancement into positions such as senior therapist, student coordinator, or supervisor? Is there a student program? Does the department perform quality improvement activities? Does it proactively plan new programs to meet unmet needs?

- *Strong teamwork and communication*: The more open an organization is to exchanging ideas between employees and management, the more likely it is to promote a positive culture. Do you notice that people are engaging with each other and exchanging ideas? Is there a team approach? Does the interviewer encourage current staff to meet with you so that they can have some input regarding who is being hired?

- *Quality leadership*: Good managers are interested in their staff, are supportive, and seek to offer help so that everyone can succeed. Leaders who communicate well are honest, clear, concise, and consistent; they inspire and motivate their staff; and they build trust. Investigate whether the rehabilitation director seems to care about his or her employee's problems, conflicts, and clinical challenges. Does the staff seem to like their supervisors? Good managers help you to grow. Poor managers can make life very difficult. Find out how long the managers and staff have been there. Longevity of staff is usually a good sign that you are walking into a positive work environment.

- *Good relationships between employees*: When there is camaraderie and teamwork among staff, it is usually an indication of the organization's culture. Do you get the sense that the physical therapists, occupational therapists, and other team members get along? As you tour the facility, do you notice that different disciplines are chatting and greeting each other warmly? Does it seem that it is an "every man for himself" type of environment or does it seem like people are working together for the common good of the organization and its clients? Try to ask questions on your interview that might provide clues.

- *A strong customer service orientation*: When there is an awareness of the importance of treating the client/customer/patient well, it is usually a sign that an organization will also treat its employees well. What is the attitude of the facility toward their clients/patients? If an inpatient setting, are the patient's rooms inviting and clean? Do the patients look well taken care of? Are clothes tidy and clean? Is the environment geared toward the people who live there? Are the aides watching their favorite soap opera in the common room or are they tending to their patients? Is the music appropriate to the age of the clientele? If an outpatient environment, are patients left waiting? Is equipment up to date and well kept? Do you get a sense that there is an orientation toward accommodating clients/patients needs or do patients need to adapt to the facility's needs? As health care providers, our orientation is toward the clients we serve. Most of us will be much happier in an environment that reflects client-centered priorities.

- *Honesty and safety*: It is important to look for an employer who protects the safety of its employees and operates in an honest and forthright manner. You do not want to be part of an organization that supports unsafe practices. For example, if a patient requires maximal assistance for transfers, does the facility provide extra help to ensure that they can be safely performed, protecting both the patient and the employee? Are the wheelchairs well kept or are the brakes slipping and footrests askew? Have you gotten feedback that the facility asks its providers to participate in unethical activities, such as fudging treatment minutes to meet reimbursement requirements, cosigning notes for people never observed or supervised, or changing documentation to accommodate a mistake that was made in the past? See Chapter 13 for more information on this.

- *Education and staff development*: For a fulfilling career, it is crucial that therapists participate in activities to promote professional growth. Facilities who invest in their staff are demonstrating their commitment to their employees and the clients they serve. They know that with improvement in clinical skills comes improvement in clinical outcomes and higher morale.

- *Cutting-edge ideas*: Good organizations are always looking for new ideas and programs. Employers who elicit input from their employees are usually good ones to work for. Encouraging creativity is healthy for an organization. It allows everyone to participate in developing a more effective and productive work environment. Fieldwork students often bring innovations to a department, such as new technology applications. Newly hired employees can bring ideas for programming from their previous employer or fieldwork setting. As an example—Johanna, a new therapist, suggested creating a mini therapy room on the subacute floor to avoid crowding in the therapy department. This improved efficiencies as the patients did not need to be transferred by elevator, and many of them were able to get to the therapy room independently. An open-minded rehabilitation director will listen and implement new ideas. This openness and opportunity to contribute makes for a better work experience.

CULTURAL COMPATIBILITY OBSERVATION CHECKLIST

Keep your eyes and ears open to uncover the clues to the organizational culture of the facilities where you are interviewing.

1. Observe the treatment environment. Is it clean? How does it smell? Is it well kept? Is there enough room for the clients? Is the equipment age appropriate? If in a school setting, are there bright and friendly colors? If in an adult setting, is the music being played appropriate for the population served? Is the equipment clean and new or does it look worn and outdated?

2. Check out the workspaces. Are they cluttered? Is adequate room devoted to each therapist? If using a computerized documentation system, are there ample computer stations?

3. Observe the interactions between staff. Do people seem friendly? Do they seem to get along and like each other?

4. Find out about vacation time and days off. A good workplace considers the needs of its workers for rest, relaxation, and time off.

5. Find out about supervision and continuing education offerings.

6. Does the facility have a student program? Such a program demonstrates a dedication to developing future professionals while giving therapists an opportunity to serve as mentors and teachers.

7. Is the facility participating in any research efforts?

8. Get a sense of how long managerial staff have been working at the facility. The longevity of the staff is always a good sign. Are there a lot of openings at the facility? Staff turnover is usually bad sign.

9. Has the facility experienced difficulty with state and federal surveys? This is public information that can be easily accessed for hospital, subacute, and long-term care facilities. (Note: Check out Nursing Home Compare on the Centers for Medicare and Medicaid Services' website [http://www.medicare.gov/nursinghomecompare/search.html] to find out about a long-term care facility's most recent survey findings.)

10. Does the staff go out socially together? This is usually a sign of a cohesive, happy environment.

11. Is there any information available on the Internet to provide insight into the organization's culture?

SUMMARY

Choosing the best employment opportunity is a crucial first step in your career as an occupational therapist. It is important to understand the concepts of organizational culture when determining whether a particular job is a good fit for you. To do this, you must uncover information about the organization with which you are interviewing. This is done through a variety of methods, such as asking the right questions during your interview, observing the environment during your facility tour, talking to former and current employees, researching on the Internet, etc. Attention to this important concept will go a long way in ensuring you select a position that meets your professional and social/emotional needs.

DISCUSSION QUESTIONS/ACTIVITIES

1. When one enters a workplace, one observes and feels its artifacts. These include the physical layout, the dress code, the manner in which people address each other, the smell and feel of the place, and its emotional intensity. Describe artifacts you observed at one of your fieldwork settings. What do your observations tell you about the setting (i.e., bureaucratic or informal and collective). Share these descriptions aloud with fellow students.

2. Choose a partner in your class. Create a dialogue between a fictitious director of occupational therapy and an occupational therapist he or she is interviewing for an open position. One of you takes the role of the occupational therapy director and the other takes the role of the interviewee. Write down the questions the occupational therapist should be asking and the answers to ascertain the culture of the organization. By the end of this exercise, do you get a feeling about the culture of this made-up organization? Is it a place you would want to work? Why or why not? What else would help you decide whether this is the right fit for you?

3. Ask four members of the class to step outside. Break up the remaining class members into four groups. Each group will determine their organization's culture, including values, rules, and physical environment. Designate roles for the team (such a director of occupational therapy, supervisor, therapists). Once you have established your department, welcome back the four members, assigning each one of them to a group. Using the questions that were created, conduct a group interview in which you try to entice the interviewee to work for your organization.

    At the end of the exercise, have each group discuss the following questions:

    a. Why would you choose (or not choose) to work for this organization?

    b. How did the group work together as a team? Was it a collaborative process or did some members seem out for themselves?

    c. How did the group interact with the interviewee (describe this)? Were they able to sell their organization?

    d. Was there any evidence of the organization's ethical standards during the interview?

4. Complete the Organizational Culture Activity (Figure 14-1).

REFERENCES

Aiken, L., Smith, H.L., & Lake, E. (1994). Lower Medicare mortality among a set of hospitals known for good nursing care. *Med Care, 32*(8), 771-787.

Berghofer, D., & Schwartz, G. (2012). *Ethical leadership: Right relationships and the emotional bottom line.* Retrieved from http://www.ethicalleadership.com/business article.htm.

Boan, D., & Funderburk, F. (2003). *Healthcare quality improvement and organizational culture.* Washington, DC: Delmarva Foundation for Medical Care.

Collins, J., & Porras, J. (1997). *Built to last: Successful habits of visionary companies.* New York, NY: Harper Collins.

Davies, H., Nutley, S., & Mannion, R. (2000). Organizational culture and quality of health care. *Quality in Health Care, 9*, 111-119.

Fisher, C., & Alford, R. (2000). Consulting on culture. *Consulting Psychology: Research and Practice, 52*(3), 206-217.

ORGANIZATIONAL CULTURE ACTIVITY

ORGANIZATION CULTURE SURVEY

As a student in the academic community of your school, you can get a feeling for your program's culture by completing the survey below. After you complete the survey, compare with classmates and note the similarities and differences.

ORGANIZATION CULTURE SURVEY						
In this organization …	1) Strongly Disagree	2) Disagree	3) Neutral	4) Agree	5) Strongly Agree	N/A
The way things are done is very flexible and easy to change.						
The teachers are organized.						
The program director sets the tone for the entire program.						
Attempts by students to create change are usually met with resistance.						
There is a solid feeling that administration and teachers adapt for students individual needs.						
The program's administrative assistants provide a smooth transition for students at every level.						
Teachers are interested in your success.						
The program has tools and treatment equipment that are current and plentiful.						
The classroom environments are conducive to learning.						
We are encouraged to contact teachers, program directors, or administrative assistants whenever we need assistance.						

By answering these questions, you can discuss what the culture of your occupational therapy program promotes. If you were the director, what might you do differently?

Figure 14-1. Organizational culture survey.

Gallagher, A., & Tschudin, V. (2010). Education for ethical leadership. *Nurse Education Today, 30,* 224-227.

Gupta, A. (2009). *Organizational culture.* Retrieved from http://www.practical-management.com/ Organizational-Development/Organization-Culture/html.

Heskett, J., Sasser, W.E., & Wheeler, J. (2008). 10 reasons to design a better corporate culture. Harvard Business School Working Knowledge. Retrieved from http://hbswk.hbs.edu/item/5917.html.

Kimball, B. (2005). *Cultural transformation in health care.* Princeton, NJ: The Robert Wood Johnson Foundation.

Kurfuerst, S., & Yousey, J. (2012). Leading with ethics: Creating an ethical climate in your occupational therapy department. *OT Practice,* CE 1-8.

Schein, E. (1990). Organizational culture. *American Psychologist, 45*(2)109-119.

Spreitzer, G., & Porath, C. (2012). Creating sustainable performance. *Harvard Business Review, 14(*1), 3-9.

Winkler, E., Gruen, R., & Sussman, A. (2005). First principles: Substantive ethics for healthcare organizations. *Journal of Healthcare Management, 50*(2), 109-119.

SECTION III

ACHIEVING PROFESSIONAL TRANSITIONS

Chapter 15

Advancing Your Continuing Competence
Strategies to Build a Better You

LEARNING OBJECTIVES

At the end of this chapter, the reader will be able to:

- ➤ Define the four types of competencies found in all work settings.
- ➤ Name three competency areas that relate to occupational therapy practice.
- ➤ Identify five ways employers assess employee competency.
- ➤ Name the five standards occupational therapists and certified occupational therapy assistants must follow to ensure ongoing competence.
- ➤ Identify and explain the eight components for developing a continuing competency plan.
- ➤ Demonstrate the ability to use the AOTA's Professional Development Tool (PDT) in the development of a continuing competence plan.
- ➤ Name 10 activities appropriate for maintaining continuing competence.
- ➤ Describe the value of the mentor/mentee relationship to foster continuing competence.
- ➤ List 10 benefits of attending professional conferences.
- ➤ Describe 10 ways to improve your conference experience.

As you enter your final fieldwork experiences and plan for graduation and your first job as an occupational therapist or certified occupational therapy assistant, it is important to understand that your education is not coming to an end—it has only just begun. With new technology, improved treatment modalities, and an evolving health care environment, change will be an ever-present variable in your professional life and practice. As the profession changes, the knowledge we acquired in our academic studies can become obsolete. As professionals, we have an important obligation to the public, our employers, and the payers of our services to stay professionally current and competent. This obligation involves the lifelong learning of skills and abilities to ensure we meet and exceed the standards of our profession. This chapter will introduce basic principles

Davis L, Rosee M. *Occupational Therapy Student to Clinician:*
Making the Transition (pp 199-218).
© 2015 SLACK Incorporated.

of continuing competence and demonstrate how you can assess, develop, and implement your own competency plan to ensure that your service delivery skills are optimized.

UNDERSTANDING THE ELEMENTS OF COMPETENCY

In general terms, competence refers to a person's characteristics that are related to job performance. It is determined by a combination of one's knowledge, traits, skills, and abilities (Kak, Burkhalter, & Cooper, 2001). Knowledge refers to an understanding of facts and procedures. Traits are personality characteristics, such as self-control or self-confidence that cause a person to behave or respond in a certain way. Skills refer to the capacity to perform a specific task or action involving both knowledge and the strategies used to apply knowledge. Abilities are the attributes one has inherited or acquired through previous experience that one brings to a new task (Kak et al., 2001, p. 3).

As occupational therapists and certified occupational therapy assistants entrusted by the public to provide occupational therapy services as per our standards of care, we must demonstrate the self-control, knowledge, and skill required to provide competent care. Achieving competency is a lifelong process that only ends when we stop practicing our profession. We must commit to it through a number of processes, which we will be elaborating on in this chapter.

Therapists who are not up to date on clinical and administrative issues and industry standards will lack the knowledge needed to provide appropriate treatment and documentation based on current regulations, clinical pathways, and outcome benchmarks established by third-party payers. This ignorance can impact patient outcomes and reimbursement. By not keeping current and improving your skills, you jeopardize not only the recovery of the clients you serve, but also your job, your license, and your career.

As a professional, there is an expectation in any workplace setting that certain types of competencies will be mastered. According to Decker and Strader (1997), they include the following:

- *Generic competencies* represent abilities that anyone in a work environment would be expected to have. For example, every employee, regardless of the job description, is expected to take responsibility for being at work on time, adhere to an assigned schedule, complete work assignments, and show respect for clients and fellow workers.
- *Management competencies* relate to the skills expected of someone at a managerial level such as hiring, supervision, training personnel, managing work flow, and administering budgets.
- *Threshold or minimum requirements* involve the skills that are expected at the entry level of any position. For example, a newly graduated certified occupational therapy assistant would be expected to know from day one how to independently provide treatment and documentation, perform wheelchair positioning tasks, or identify the need for and fabricate adaptive equipment. Although it is understood that the newly graduated occupational therapist's competency will be basic, he or she is still expected to perform at a reasonably skilled level.
- *Job-specific competencies* are more advanced and usually involve a higher level of knowledge and skill than that expected of an entry-level practitioner. For example, an occupational therapist working with hand injuries would be expected to have high-level specialty skills with (preferably) an advanced certification in hand therapy.

As an entry-level therapist, you will be expected to possess generic and threshold competencies from day one. No one expects a newly graduated therapist to have developed advanced job-specific competencies. You can be sure that performance expectations will increase as you become more seasoned on the job. The development of job-specific competencies will determine your success on the job, the opportunity for promotion, or the chance to move on to another more challenging and higher paying position.

Example of New Graduate Competency Expectations

Chase is a new graduate working with two different populations within one setting—adults needing short-term rehabilitation and children with learning disabilities. He possesses the generic competencies of an entry-level therapist with job-specific competencies in administration of the Sensory Integration and Praxis Test (SIPT). That competency is what helped him to get hired. Even though Chase is an entry-level therapist, he was expected to perform SIPT evaluation tasks at higher than an entry-level competency level, as he sold himself as someone who had achieved competency in test administration in his fieldwork. As a student, he was allotted much more time to administer and interpret the test than he would be allowed as an employed therapist. His competency quickly improved due to the pressure he felt from his supervisors to be productive. Had he not gotten up to speed quickly, he probably would not have survived on the job.

Even though you may be performing at a threshold level at the end of your final fieldwork experience, once you are being paid to perform occupational therapy services, expectations will quickly increase. In the interest of patient outcomes, it will be expected that you exhibit the competencies related to the population and equipment you are working with, specific procedures you are expected to carry out, or advanced practice skills that are part of the environment in which you work, including the following:

* *Age-related competencies*: Occupational therapists and certified occupational therapy assistants must be able to demonstrate competency with the population they are working with. For example, if working in an adult orthopedic population, you must understand the contraindications of certain actions (such as too much hip flexion following hip replacement surgery), the principles of therapeutic exercise, and the ability to apply activities of daily living training within the restrictions of the condition. Without age-specific competencies, you increase the risk of doing harm to your patients, or at the very least, not assuring best outcomes.

* *Equipment-related competencies*: If you are working with equipment, you must be able to demonstrate competency in its use. For example, many occupational therapists and certified occupational therapy assistants use modalities such as ultrasound, paraffin, or hot packs. Since significant harm can result from improper use, competency must be established before using any modalities in a clinical setting.

* *Competencies related to specific skills or procedures*: When working in a specialized setting, you must demonstrate competency in the skills needed to ensure best outcomes for your patients. For example, while working in a hand practice, you must be able to demonstrate the ability to fabricate splints or apply the appropriate treatment protocol following a tendon repair. If working in a traumatic brain injury setting, you must be familiar with the progression of brain injuries, understand and be able to evaluate cognitive and perceptual deficits, and develop and implement appropriate treatment plans based on levels of function (Braverman & Gentile, 2003).

HOW EMPLOYERS ASSESS COMPETENCY

Although much of this chapter will focus on developing continuing competency, ongoing professional development, and lifelong learning, we must also focus on the important issue of competence that relates to an individual's capacity to perform job responsibilities in the here and now (Braverman & Gentile, 2003).

As described previously, it is expected that we are ready to meet the challenges of providing standards of care when a patient is referred to us for treatment. As one of our professional obligations, we are responsible for ensuring our own competency in all areas that relate to our practice. Additionally, our employers have an obligation to ensure that the occupational therapists they engage are capable of effectively performing the specific skills expected of them. This is important for many reasons—to ensure best outcomes, to protect against liability, and to meet accreditation requirements.

This can be difficult when employers come from different professional backgrounds and do not understand what occupational therapists are expected to know and how we must perform our clinical job responsibilities. Employers must develop assessment tools that can accurately measure the competencies needed for the job. Typical methods of assessing competency include the following:

- *Post-tests*: These can be used effectively when concrete information must be learned and integrated. Post-tests are appropriate to assess our understanding of such concepts as fire and safety regulations, privacy rules, or infection control procedures.

- *Demonstration of a skill set to another skilled observer*: This may include demonstrating the administration of a standardized test, fabrication of a splint, or application of a modality. This approach is often used when preparing for an accreditation survey to prove and document staff competency. Typically, a series of skills are identified and a set of standards to perform the skill are established. The provider is then observed performing the activity and is deemed either competent or in need of further instruction. For example, if transfer training from wheelchair to bed is the skill being assessed, the facility may develop a "Wheelchair Transfer Competency Test." The tool would list the steps required to safely perform the task, such as proper positioning of chair, removal of leg rests, locking brakes, proper clinician body alignment, etc. The test result is placed in the therapist's file. It may be reviewed by the Joint Commission on Accreditation of Healthcare Organizations (JCAHO) (or other accreditation bodies) during a survey or perhaps used as evidence in the case of litigation.

- *Observation of treatment sessions*: As part of the supervision process or the annual review, a therapist may be observed to determine if his or her interventions meet or exceed standards of care. If not deemed competent during the observation, a plan of correction would be developed with a follow-up plan to ensure competency is reached.

- *Case studies*: Here, individuals are presented with situations to analyze in order to demonstrate their evaluative and clinical reasoning skills. This would be useful in cases where the provider is expected to interpret standardized evaluation results. The case presented might provide the raw scores and the practitioner would be expected to convert the data, draw inferences from the results, and develop the treatment plan.

- *Peer-review process*: Therapists treat side-by-side with their colleagues all day. These colleagues are in a good position to provide feedback to their coworkers in either a formal or informal basis. We will write more about this later.

- *Self-assessment*: As professionals, we must take the time to self reflect and critically assess our skills and areas in need of improvement. More about this will be discussed later in this chapter (Braverman & Gentile, 2003).

CONTINUING COMPETENCE STANDARDS

Once you graduate and attain a registered or licensed status (depending upon your state's regulations), it is assumed that you are competent to practice occupational therapy. However, as discussed previously, this level of competence is only the first step. Evolving and improving professional competencies becomes part of our lifelong practice, assuring successful outcomes for our patients, a high regard for our profession, and a satisfying career. The AOTA defines continuing competence as:

> a process involving the examination of current competence and the development of capacity for the future. It is a component of ongoing professional development and lifelong learning. Continuing competence is a dynamic, multidimensional process

in which the OT and OTA develop and maintain the knowledge, performance skills, interpersonal abilities, critical and ethical reasoning skills necessary to perform current and future roles and responsibilities within the profession. Continuing competence is maintained through self-assessment of the practitioner's capacities in the core of occupational therapy, which reflects the knowledge of the domain of the profession and the process used in service delivery. (AOTA, 2010a, p. 1)

To this end, the AOTA has developed five standards that occupational therapists and certified occupational therapy assistants must follow to ensure their ongoing competence:

1. *Standard 1—Knowledge*: occupational therapists and certified occupational therapy assistants are expected to possess a comprehensive understanding of any and all information required to master the core of occupational therapy concepts associated with one's primary responsibilities. This includes integration of relevant evidence, literature, and epidemiological data related to one's primary responsibilities and populations served; integration of current association documents and issues; and the ability to anticipate new knowledge to acquire and meet the needs of the population being served.

2. *Standard 2—Critical Reasoning*: Occupational therapists and certified occupational therapy assistants are expected to develop critical reasoning skills needed to make sound judgments and decisions. These skills include deductive and inductive reasoning, problem solving, and the ability to reflect on one's own practice and management and synthesis of information from a variety of sources in support of decisions made.

3. *Standard 3—Interpersonal Skills*: Occupational therapy professionals are expected to develop the skills necessary to maintain professional relationships with others within the context of their responsibilities and roles. Such skills include the ability to communicate appropriately with consumers and others from diverse backgrounds; use feedback from multiple sources; modify professional behavior; collaborate with clients and professionals to attain optimal consumer outcomes; and develop, sustain, and refine team relationships.

4. *Standard 4—Performance Skills*: This is the expectation that all therapists will demonstrate their expertise, aptitudes, proficiencies, and abilities to competently fulfill their roles and responsibilities. This includes competency in their practice, the therapeutic use of self, the therapeutic use of occupations and activities, the ability to integrate current practice techniques and technologies, updating performance based on current evidence-based literature, and quality improvement processes that prevent practice error and optimize client outcomes.

5. *Standard 5—Ethical Practice*: Occupational therapists and certified occupational therapy assistants are required to identify, analyze, and clarify ethical issues or dilemmas and make responsible decisions within the changing context of his or her roles and responsibilities. This includes understanding and adhering to our profession's code of ethics, laws, and regulations; the use of ethical principles to understand complex situations; the integrity to make and defend decisions based on ethical reasoning; and the integration of varying perspectives in the ethics of clinical practice (AOTA, 2010a, p. 1).

DEVELOPING A CONTINUING COMPETENCY PLAN FOR PROFESSIONAL DEVELOPMENT

As professionals, we have an important obligation to further our skills and education to assure the public that we are competent to deliver the services we were licensed to provide because treatment philosophies, strategies, and technologies change over time. To stay current so that we provide the best possible interventions to our clients and patients, we must develop a plan for ourselves to continuously improve upon our professional competencies. This process is different for everyone and is based on where and how we practice, how we learn best, and what we need to master to provide the best levels of care.

To this end, the AOTA has developed a document entitled the "Continuing Competence Plan" (AOTA, 2010b), which identifies critical elements for professional development as well as performance and outcomes. This plan has eight components, which form a continuum that can be entered at any point, depending on the situation. The components include the following:

1. Triggers
2. Examination of responsibilities
3. Self-assessment
4. Identification of needs
5. Development of a plan
6. Implementation
7. Documentation of professional development and change in performance
8. Implementation of changes and demonstration of continuing competence

Although we suggest you refer to the original document (Hinojosa et al., 2000) for a complete summary of the process, we will briefly outline some of the basic tenets as an introduction to the document so that you can begin to think about developing your own continuing competence plan.

Triggers

Triggers represent changes in practice, regulation, and reimbursement that require a practitioner to master new skill areas. Triggers are inevitable and actually make our professional lives more interesting and challenging.

- **Example:** In 1998, Medicare changed the skilled nursing facility reimbursement system from a flat cost based rate to a prospective payment system based on the amount of resources used by each individual patient. As an occupational therapy director at the time, Simon took an interest in the new system, studied it, and developed a strategy that would allow his facility to take advantage of the reimbursement opportunities that were available in the new system. By being proactive in mastering this change and applying it to practice within the rehabilitation department, Simon was able to improve reimbursement for the facility while increasing patients' access to occupational therapy services.

In addition to reimbursement changes, triggers can include changing into a new practice area, returning to practice after a long absence, employer-mandated process changes, an unsatisfactory job performance rating, or one's own personal interests and need to grow and change (Hinojosa et al., 2000).

Once we recognize a trigger that requires us to expand our knowledge base, we must move on to the next step.

Examination of Responsibilities

We enter our profession with basic skills learned in our academic training and fieldwork settings. Thereafter, we must continuously reassess and improve these skills to meet clinical challenges presented. For example, 10 years ago, all documentation was performed manually in longhand. Today, most documentation is performed through the use of software programs, requiring therapists to master technical skills and the ability to type efficiently. That is just one of unlimited changes we must address and master. For example, a therapist getting promoted to a managerial position must learn a new set of managerial skills in order to succeed. A therapist wanting to start his or her own private practice may have mastery over practice skills but will need to learn a new set of sub-skills related to business management, accounting, law, marketing, and personnel management. Although it may seem obvious that with change, new skills may be required, it takes insight to identify the new skills we need to master to ensure competency in our positions.

Self-Assessment

By understanding our responsibilities, we can begin to "assess our performance, analyze the demands and resources of the work environment, and interpret information about our consumers' outcomes" (Hinojosa et al., 2000, p. 4). Some of this information is gathered informally using feedback regarding our performance from colleagues, supervisors, and clients. It can also be gathered using formalized methods such as self-assessment tools, treatment observations, patient satisfaction surveys, and performance reviews.

Identification of Needs

It is not always easy to assess our own strengths and weaknesses. Feedback from outside sources who we respect and who are in a position to observe our professional skills can be very helpful in identifying areas in need of improvement.

In AOTA's (2003a) Professional Development Tool (PDT), self-assessment is defined as a formative and dynamic process that facilitates the practitioner to move through various stages of professional improvement or development. The primary purpose of the PDT is self-assessment and self-appraisal (Moyers, 2004). Self-assessment involves asking the question "What can I do to prepare or increase my capacity for the competency demands of the future?" (Moyers, 2004). Self-review is an outcome-oriented process that asks the question, "What can I do in a controlled situation and how well does my performance conform to standards?"

Two sources of information regarding our competency include the following:

1. *Annual employment review*: The review will usually assess both interpersonal and clinical skills. It is a good idea to have access to the form your employer uses to assess performance beforehand so that you understand how others will assess your performance. Your own self-assessment should be compared to the feedback received from your supervisor. Large discrepancies between the two may indicate that your insight into your performance may not be accurate. A thoughtful performance evaluation can help you identify areas in need of improvement. Your supervisor can assist in the development of your goals and plans for continuing competency.

2. *Peer-review*: One of the most accessible ways to get a sense of professional performance is through peer review. Peer review can provide objective feedback that can help you to identify strengths and weaknesses that may be difficult to uncover on your own.

   The process involves the following:

   - Identify a peer whom you respect and is willing to serve in the role.
   - With the chosen peer, plan which professional roles you would like to have assessed.
   - Use open-ended questions to give and receive feedback, including, "What do I do best?" or, "What aspect of my performance needs improvement?"
   - Comments should be specific, constructive, positive, and supportive. These rules should be established from the beginning of the process.
   - Feedback should be presented verbally and in writing so that there is documentation that can be referred back to.
   - All feedback should be confidential.

   Discussions should include how performance improvement can be achieved (AOTA, 2003a).

After gathering the self-assessment information, it should be synthesized to identify areas that need improvement. The results of this self-assessment will be used to develop your continuing competence plan.

Development of a Plan

Based upon our self-assessment of skills, we can create a continuing competence plan. This involves four steps:

1. Prioritize needs based on the self-assessment. Identify the key areas that require development and make them a priority in your plan. For example, if your position requires you to master documentation software and your notes are due on Friday, clearly this is a competence that needs mastery fairly quickly vs a new treatment skill you would like to learn, but is not essential in your day-to-day practice.

2. Review (or develop) goals and objectives. Consider what your expected outcomes should be. For example, you expect that by the end of the month, you will be able to complete a progress note in 10 minutes (based on improved typing skills and improved knowledge of the software).

3. Identify resources and options to improve your skills. Here, the options are endless. You may choose to take a course, secure a mentor, self study, or go back to school.

4. Modify goals and objectives based on your current situation. For example, if you want to return to school but do not have the funds to pay tuition, you might consider an alternate, less costly approach to acquire the knowledge you seek, such as a distance learning program or seeking a mentor. Plan development is a dynamic process. The plan should take into consideration professional priorities, preferred learning styles, lifestyle considerations, timeframe, and available resources (Hinojosa et al., 2000).

Part of the process when developing your continuing competence plan is determining your professional goals. This may be confusing as you must determine whether to concentrate on where you are now or plan for the future when you may be working in a different setting. To orient yourself, it is a good idea to start with a professional mission statement that incorporates short-term (1 year) and long-term (3 to 5 years) goals. Hinojosa (2004) lays out certain criteria that can help in goal development. Goals should be as follows:

- Specific and measurable behaviors, skills, attitudes, or actions
- Personally and professionally important
- Consistent with your mission
- Attainable
- Challenging
- Feasible, taking into considering personal obligations, professional duties, and institutional resources
- Performance focused
- Observable
- Verifiable (Hinojosa, 2004)

Once the goals are developed, competencies needed for each goal should be identified. Goals can have one or more competency and should be realistic and practical. All competencies should include specific knowledge, critical reasoning, performance skills, interpersonal skills, and ethical reasoning needed to demonstrate the competencies under specific circumstances.

Example of the plan development process: As a student, Eileen was interested in pursuing her certification in the administration of the SIPT. At that time, she wanted to focus on mastering sensory integration as a treatment approach. After identifying her goal, she developed a plan for the next 2 years to achieve the goal. The plan included the following:

- Securing an affiliation that would expose her to the appropriate population and give her the opportunity to learn about sensory integration. She wanted to learn how to administer the test and understand theory to help to secure a paid position where she could apply her skills.
- Taking courses simultaneously with her affiliation to start the certification process.

- With a strong and thorough preparation, attempt to secure a position where she would be able to use, enhance, and develop her skills using a sensory integrative approach.
- Continuing to pursue activities to improve her knowledge, understanding, and skills. To that end, she identified a study group where she could interact with peers to discuss treatment methodologies, test administration, and interpretation.
- Identifying a mentor to help enhance her skill set.
- Once qualified, taking and passing the certification exam.
- Achieving respectable competency in this practice area.

When Eileen reached the point of competency, she changed and enhanced her goals based on the next steps she wanted to take in her career (which turned out to be totally unrelated to the original plan).

Example: Patrick was working for 2 years treating adults in a subacute setting. His supervisor asked him to take an occupational therapy student for a Fieldwork I assignment. Patrick was suddenly anxious that he did not have the competencies in fieldwork supervision to adequately perform the job. To clarify what skills were needed and whether he possessed them, he asked himself the following questions:

- What are the responsibilities of the role?
- What knowledge, interpersonal, and performance skills are needed?
- What critical and ethical reasoning skills are needed?
- What expectations do others have?
- Are there situations (personal or otherwise) that may affect performance in this role (Jacobs & McCormack, 2011)?

As the right questions are asked, one can identify whether the competencies are present or they need to be developed. If the goal is to be able to provide effective supervision to a Fieldwork I student, one can then identify the competencies that he or she needs to develop to be able to do the following:

- Understand the requirements needed to be a supervisor
- Provide appropriate professional feedback to a Fieldwork I student
- Observe the student's clinical skills
- Document the students' progress effectively (Jacobs & McCormack, 2011)

The next step is to identify how to meet established goals and develop the competencies needed. For Patrick, this might include meeting with his supervisor to discuss Patrick's obligations as a supervisor, identify a mentor within or outside of his facility, or review the literature.

Implementation

By now, you have identified areas to work on to improve competence and figured out how you want to approach the process. Now it is time to go into action and implement the plan. The implementation plan should not be static; it should evolve as situations change. For example, you may choose to study for an advanced degree because your employer offers tuition assistance. If you decide to leave the employer, you might reconsider the plan due to the cost of the degree and decide to take a different route toward acquiring the knowledge.

As you are implementing the plan, you should identify the expected outcomes and how you will measure them. Hinojosa et al. (2000) suggest three methods:

1. *Examination*: This involves testing your competence in the area you are working on, if such a test is available. For example, *OT Practice*, a publication of the AOTA, offers continuing education articles that always include multiple choice final exams. Successfully passing these tests demonstrates knowledge and competency in the area being studied.

2. *Portfolio*: This represents a compilation of your practice experiences, including performance observations, case studies, peer ratings, consumer feedback, specialty certifications, advanced practitioner recognition, and documentation of professional activities such as publications and presentations.

3. *Outcome education*: This involves evidence of completion of academic and continuing education activities (Hinojosa, 2000).

Documentation of Professional Development and Change in Performance

As you participate in activities that contribute to your continuing competence, it is important that you develop a documentation system that confirms competence and maintains information needed for certification, licensure, and employment. In addition to meeting the requirements of accrediting organizations such as the Joint Commission (formerly JCAHO) and Commission on Accreditation of Rehabilitation Facilities (which require competency information on all providers working in an organization seeking accreditation), you will also need documentation when audited by the National Board for Certification in Occupational Therapy and state authorities to maintain your license or certification to practice in your state (AOTA, 2003c). Documentation methods may vary based on one's practice area and may include credentialing through the AOTA's Specialty Certification and Advanced Practice programs, post-testing following an advanced practice course, or development of a portfolio that allows the practitioner to compile all of his or her evidence of continuing competence in one document.

Implementation of Changes and Demonstration of Continuing Competence

As professionals, we must continuously monitor and assess our performance, in order to evolve our continuing competency plans. Continuing competence is demonstrated behaviorally as one improves in areas identified through the self-assessment process. Competency status is ensured through ongoing attendance at continuing education programs, portfolio development, and self-reflection. The process ensures a satisfying career and the best level of performance in whatever practice area we choose to enter (Hinojosa, 2000, p. 7).

DEVELOPING YOUR PORTFOLIO

Portfolio development is a process that results in a product that contains a record of the activities you have identified to meet your current professional development needs. It also holds your self-assessment and professional development learning plan, which can be updated and amended as activities are completed and goals met (AOTA, 2003b). Because individual career paths are variable, credentialing agencies and licensure boards consider a well-constructed portfolio to be a valid method for demonstrating competence.

Reflection is an important part of your portfolio development. As you complete and document various professional development activities, you should assess the personal meaning and significance of each activity and apply this new knowledge, understanding, or skill to your practice. It is often helpful to include a written reflection or summary of impressions for specific activities or competencies in your portfolio.

You may decide how you want to document your professional life, but typically the structure of the portfolio includes the following:

◆ *Credentials*: education, certifications, licenses, and professional memberships

- *Documentation* of work experiences, workplace service, quality assurance activities, letters from consumers, patient satisfaction survey results, peer-review evaluations, and annual performance reviews
- *Honors*, recognitions, awards, and achievements; scholarships, residencies, fellowships, etc.
- *Professional service*: National, state, local, and community
- *Scholarly activities*: publications, research activities, grants, teaching activities, and creative activities
- *Educational activities*: formal learning, independent study, learning opportunities, and incidents
- *Sample documentation*, such as progress notes, evaluations, and discharge plans
- *Samples* of exceptional school papers or assignments (PDT/Portfolio) (AOTA, 2003b)

USING THE AOTA'S PROFESSIONAL DEVELOPMENT TOOL TO DEVELOP YOUR CONTINUING COMPETENCE PLAN

If all of the previous information seems complicated and overwhelming to implement, the AOTA has made it much easier for its members by creating the PDT. This tool is downloadable (for members) from the AOTA website (AOTA, 2003a, 2003b). It lays out an in-depth organizational format that includes a review of the processes, descriptions, definitions, as well as a number of forms that are designed to do the following:

- Assess your professional development needs and interests
- Create a professional development plan
- Document your professional development in a portfolio format

The tool provides an in-depth outline for performing your self-assessment, which includes reflection, identifying areas for professional development, providing a guide for gathering relevant data to plan professional development, laying out a structure for creating the professional development plan that includes identifying competencies, selecting strategies, developing the plan, and creating a portfolio.

The PDT includes a variety of templates that can guide you in your self-assessments, professional development plan, portfolio structure, and organization as well as tools that can be used for peer review and client satisfaction evaluations.

ACTIVITIES FOR ACQUIRING COMPETENCY

In the AOTA (2003c) document "Model Continuing Competence Guidelines for Occupational Therapists and Occupational Therapy Assistants: A Resource for State Regulatory Boards," a template is provided to be used by regulatory boards when addressing participation in continuing competence activities. This model can be used by professionals to identify what kinds of activities can be effective in contributing to continuing competence, as well as which activities will count toward your certification. Requirements vary from state to state, so it is important that you are aware of your state's continuing education requirements.

Note: Depending on the state you reside in, continuing competency can be defined differently. Additionally, the points allotted for various activities can be vastly different. For example, in New York, continuing education units are labeled continuing competency units (CCUs). The NBCOT labels continuing education units as professional development units (PDUs). Most continuing education credentialing organizations allot units for different activities, such as mentoring, volunteering, lecturing participation in professional panels, holding an office in an occupational therapy organization, teaching, or performing research. All are considered avenues to gain competency. Check your state's association for its definitions of continuing education and the types of activities that can count toward them.

Qualified activities for maintaining continuing competence include the following:

* *Continuing education courses*: This would include attendance and participation in live events, such as a workshops, seminars, conferences, or in-services that may or may not involve a formal assessment of learning. Documentation of participation would include a certificate of completion naming the course, date, instructor, sponsoring organization, location, number of hours attended, and number of continuing education credits earned.

* *Academic coursework*: In addition to traditional academic studies, this may include onsite or distance learning academic courses from an acceptable institution. Documentation should include a transcript indicating successful completion of the course, date, and description.

* *Independent study*: Includes reviewing books, journal articles, and videos. Documentation should include the particulars about the publication read and a statement describing how the activity relates to the licensee's current or anticipated roles and responsibilities.

* *Mentorship*: This involves serving either as a mentor or mentee. Documentation should include the name of the mentor and mentee; a copy of a signed contract outlining specific goals and objectives; designating the plan of activities to be met by the mentee, dates, and hours spent on mentorship activities; and outcomes of the mentorship agreement.

* *Fieldwork supervision*: Participation as a clinical fieldwork educator qualifies the supervisor to receive credits toward continuing competency requirements. Documentation should include verification by the student's program director regarding the student's name, school name, dates of fieldwork, or the signature page of the completed student evaluation form.

* *Professional writing*: Publication of a peer-reviewed or non–peer-reviewed book, chapter, or article can be accepted for credit toward continuing competency requirements. Documentation will consist of a reference for the publication including title, author, editor, and date of publication or a copy of acceptance letter if not yet published.

* *Providing professional presentations and instruction*: This includes a first time or significantly revised presentation of an academic course or peer-reviewed or non–peer-reviewed workshop, seminar, in-service, electronic, or Web-based course. Documentation may consist of a copy of the official program/schedule/syllabus including presentation title, date, hours of presentation, and type of audience.

* *Performing research*: Qualifying activities may consist of development of or participation in a research project. Documentation would include verification from the primary investigator indicating the name of the research project, dates of participation, major hypotheses or objectives of the project, and the licensee's role in the project.

* *Development of grants*: Successful submission of grants may count toward continuing competence requirements. Documentation would include the name of the grant proposal, name of the grant source, purpose and objectives of the project, and verification from the grant author regarding the licensee's role in the development of the grant (if not the author).

* *Participation in professional meetings and activities including board or committee work with agencies or organizations*: If an activity is professionally related to promote and enhance the practice of occupational therapy, then it can be counted toward continuing competence requirements. Documentation would include the name of the committee or board, name of the agency or organization, purpose of service, and description of the licensee's role. Participation must be validated by an officer or representative of the organization or committee (AOTA, 2003c).

USING THE MENTOR/MENTEE RELATIONSHIP TO FOSTER CONTINUING COMPETENCE

As students, we take for granted that our supervisor will focus in on our professional needs and growth, provide guidance and advice, review our evaluation and treatment plans, observe our treatment interventions, provide feedback on our performance, and assume responsibility for what we do. As you enter the job force and assume a paid position, there is a good chance that no one will assume this role. You may have a supervisor, but his or her job is not dedicated to overseeing you and your work. Now you are on your own and may want to seek out a seasoned practitioner to take you under his or her wing to help you grow professionally.

Work places have differing philosophies regarding the supervision process. With productivity pressures evident in all settings, the new graduate is assumed to be competent enough to perform independently, albeit with entry-level skills. Supervision may be provided but on an occasional and informal basis. It probably will not resemble the supervision you received as a student clinician. After a very brief honeymoon period, the new therapist will be expected to carry a caseload and provide evaluation and treatment duties within the same time frame as more experienced staff. If a new therapist cannot get up to speed relatively quickly, he or she may not make it in that setting. The problem is that at this stage in your professional life, you have a lot to learn and no one is dedicated to showing you the way. One solution is to identify a mentor.

(Note: All certified occupational therapy assistants are required to be supervised. The specific supervision requirements are based on individual state regulations. For more information about what your state requires, consult the AOTA website or your state's professional education department.)

The terms *mentoring* and *supervision* are sometimes used interchangeably but are actually different functions. They are definied as follows:

> Mentoring is a relationship between two people in which one person (the mentor) is dedicated to the personal and professional growth of the other (the mentee). The relationship is often mutually beneficial and collaborative and both parties participate willingly and knowingly in the development of the mentee. A supervisor, on the other hand, functions more as a monitor or gatekeeper of performance. (Urish, 2004, p. 1)

(Note: For the purpose of this chapter, we refer to the mentor/mentee relationship as a mechanism for ensuring competency. Pursuing the mentor/mentee relationship is an encouraged activity. Supervision, on the other hand, is a requirement of certification.)

The mentor is identified as a person with the knowledge, skills, and attributes to inspire and push a person to his or her greatest potential (Shrubbe, 2004). Mentors are able to share their wisdom and organizational skills with others who they see as willing and enthusiastic receivers of knowledge who are open to change and eager to learn.

For the relationship to work and flourish, there needs to be a fit between the mentor and the mentee. Both need to have similar philosophies, compatible professional interests, and complimentary communication styles (Kram, 1985). A good mentor must be interested in the person he or she is mentoring and possess self-awareness, empathy, and relationship building skills (Kram, 2004).

Although it may seem as though the mentoring relationship works only one way, it actually is mutually beneficial. For the mentor, benefits include personal satisfaction, strengthened professional reputation, increased influence, and development of a supportive relationship (Urish, 2004)—in addition to skill enhancement through the instruction process. For the mentee, benefits include improved clinical competence, increased professional satisfaction, possible career mobility, increased knowledge and skill, improved professional self-confidence, development of a supportive relationship, support in developing new skills, and increased awareness of strengths and limitations.

Over a career, one can shift roles from mentor to mentee and back again. While the new graduate clearly benefits from the mentoring process, the experienced therapist may benefit as well as new roles are assumed. For example, Eve, a therapist working in a long-term care facility, was promoted to director of the department. Although the clinical skills Eve used in her prior role as staff therapist were well developed, she now had an entirely different set of responsibilities she needed to master—including supervision, budgeting, financial oversight, and human resources. To facilitate growth and improve competence, Eve sought out a more experienced colleague with managerial experience who helped her develop the new skills she needed for the position.

Establishing and Maintaining a Mentoring Relationship

When establishing a mentor relationship, participants should begin by identifying their vision and goals for the relationship. The goals should be mutually agreed upon and consistent with the strengths of both members. The AOTA's *Professional Development Plan* (available on the AOTA website) can be used as a tool to develop goals and measure outcomes (AOTA, 2003b). You can use the "Professional Development Plan Worksheet" to hone in on goals, strategies, resources, success indicators, and target dates. You can also use the "Peer Review Check Off Form" and "Open Ended Questions Form" to provide feedback from the mentor to mentee (AOTA, 2003a). Whether these tools or other less formal methods are used, it is important to document goals for the relationship and outcomes (behaviors that demonstrate role integration and increased competence) (Jacobs & McCormack, 2011). By documenting the process, the mentee can identify when he or she has accomplished objectives, indicating that either new objectives need to be established or the relationship has accomplished its goals (Jacobs & McCormack, 2011).

Types of Mentoring Relationships

Since the mentoring process is so effective in promoting professional and personal growth in both the mentor and mentee, such relationships should be fostered throughout our careers. Typically, mentoring relationships can take various forms, such as the following:

- *Formal and informal mentoring*: In formal mentoring situations, mentors and mentees are assigned to one another by the management of the organization in an attempt to improve performance, job satisfaction, and success. Informal relationships are naturally occurring pairings that are based on mutual interests or interpersonal connections. Informal relationships are found to be more long lasting and productive since they are based on the free will of the participants. Formal mentoring relationships often work well when they are short term and meant to meet an immediate need, such as tutoring on a specific skill, learning a new software system, or receiving guidance and orientation when starting a new position.

- *Group mentoring*: The group mentoring process presents some advantages and disadvantages over individual mentoring. Although the relationship is less intense and not entirely focused on the individual mentee's needs and goals, the group process can bring a wider perspective and greater interaction between members. For example, for a group of newly hired occupational therapists in a public school setting where all are grappling with the demands of an environment that provides little support, a group mentoring process with an experienced therapist would be helpful. Such a group could provide emotional support through the transition to a new setting and promote the development of long-lasting work and personal relationships.

- *Peer mentoring*: This is an extension of group mentoring. The difference is that there may not necessarily be an expert member or mentor to guide the group. Rather, the group members have the same level of experience. Through participation in a group process, they are able to problem solve, share solutions, and support one another in a way that is helpful and meaningful. Examples of this may include a local occupational therapy association's special interest group meeting or groups of therapists who come together to present cases, review the literature, or share experiences.

- *Virtual mentorship.* Interactive technology can be used to bring people together to establish mentor/mentee relationships. Web-based technologies can now expand access and meeting time options. It also allows people who are geographically separate to work together. Opportunities to connect virtually are increasing with forums using chat rooms, webinars, and Skype, with many more opportunities to come (Jacobs & McCormack, 2011).

ATTENDING CONFERENCES TO FOSTER CONTINUING COMPETENCY

One of the most exciting and stimulating opportunities available to the entry-level therapist in his or her continuing competence program is attending professional conferences. In addition to meeting NBCOT and state licensing continuing education requirements, conference participation is a great way to stay current, learn new information, make new contacts, and enhance professional stature.

Benefits of Attending Conferences

- Opportunity to learn new and innovative interventions and best practice guidelines designed to improve your skill level
- Exposure to educators who are presenting the most current theories and practices
- Interaction with other professionals who share information, as well as data and clinical advances in particular practice areas
- Opportunity to network with colleagues
- Exposure to vendors and the opportunity to interact with the latest merchandise related to our profession
- Opportunity for on-the-spot interviews from recruiters (Note: Always have your resumé and/ or business cards on hand)
- Compilation of continuing education credits to support your licensure and NBCOT membership
- Exposure to new software, textbooks, and authors
- Opportunity to attend student or school mixers
- Feeling like a real professional (Jackson, 2010)

To ensure the best possible conference experience:

- *Register early*: Conferences often sell out and there are usually discounts offered for early registration. Take advantage of the savings.
- *Emphasize your student status*: If still in school, check to see if a student discount is offered. If not evident in the published information, call before registering. If there is no student discount available, ask the organizers if you can get one. They will often make an exception if asked, especially if registration is low.
- *Try to take a friend*: Multiday conferences can be much less lonely and more enjoyable when going with a friend. At the end of the day, you can discuss what you've learned.
- *Find out if there will be handouts provided at the conference*: The handouts are often posted online for downloading beforehand. If that is the case, be sure to download and bring them to the course.

- *Dress professionally*: Since conferences provide a great opportunity to network, it is important that you look professional. Although business attire is not necessary, a clean polished look is appropriate. Always wear your name badge as it helps with networking opportunities.

- *Participate*: If you have an opportunity to speak or present a poster session, go for it. It will look great on your resumé and provides networking opportunities along with additional continuing education units (CEU) credits. As a participant, do not be afraid to ask questions and be noticed. It can facilitate networking following the event.

- *Stay at the official conference hotel*: That is where the action will be, where you will have the greatest chance to run into colleagues and former professors and have the opportunity to network.

- *Behave professionally*: You never know who is noticing your behavior and who is around you. Acting rowdy at the bar might get you noticed by the person who is going to be interviewing you next week for your dream job. Even when waiting in line for the bathroom or in the cafeteria, think about the impression you are making. Do not talk loudly on your cell phone or conduct inappropriate conversations. You never know who is listening in. Remember, you are always "on." This is business.

- *Show up on time for conferences*: It can be distracting and annoying for other participants and the speaker when people come late for sessions. Being on time is part of being a professional.

- *Network*: Exchange information with people you meet. Get e-mails and make contacts. This is your opportunity to meet fellow professionals who work in different geographic regions doing different things. You never know when the contact will come in handy. Remember, Bill Clinton collected business cards from his college days onward. Many of those contacts helped him become president. The same could be true for you.

- *Never miss an opportunity to speak to someone*: An extension of networking is that you never know who is next to you and how he or she might be able to help you in the future. Not making conversation is a lost opportunity (Lampton, 2011; Singleton, 2011).

Two Examples of How Attending Conferences Have Benefitted the Authors

Many years ago, we attended our state association conference. During a break, we ran into a classmate who we had not seen in many years. During our conversation, she mentioned that her private practice was booming and she had a backlog of children needing a therapist. As we were just starting our staffing agency, we offered her a therapist to help treat the backlog of referrals. She paid us an hourly rate for the "use" of one of our therapists. That helped us launch Therapeutic Resources.

Several years ago at the AOTA convention, we ran into a colleague who we knew from our local occupational therapy association. She mentioned that she had written a book, so we went over to the publishers' booth to take a look at the display. She then suggested that we write a book based on what we have learned over the years about the job-seeking process, professionalism, and the effect of social skills on career success. That suggestion prompted us to pursue a publisher and was the beginning of this book project!

ACHIEVING ADVANCED COMPETENCY

Board Certification and Specialty Certification

These certifications provide formal recognition for practitioners who have engaged in a process of ongoing, focused, and targeted professional development. Certification is validation by your professional organization and to your dedication to continuing competence and quality service delivery (AOTA, 2013). Clinicians seek out specialty certification for personal accomplishment, professional recognition, and career advancement. Achievement of this status bestows on you the ability to add credentials to your title, giving you further validation as a professional.

Board certification is offered by the AOTA to occupational therapists in the areas of gerontology, mental health, pediatrics, and physical rehabilitation. Specialty certification is offered to occupational therapists and certified occupational therapy assistants in driving and community mobility; environmental modification; feeding, eating, and swallowing; low vision; and school systems.

To obtain this certification, recipients must develop portfolios highlighting related ongoing professional development, in addition to meeting minimal experience requirements in the area being certified and direct delivery in the last 5 calendar years of services in the certification area being sought.

In addition to specialty certifications, occupational therapy students are encouraged to participate in research to promote the field through the American Occupational Therapy Foundation (AOTF, 2012a). The AOTF was established to support research and educational initiatives that strengthen the profession of occupational therapy, promote the use of technology to improve practice, enhance quality of life for the populations we serve, and improve the financial stability of the organization. The student division of the AOTF is Pi Theta Epsilon (AOTF, 2012c). Students applying for membership must meet rigorous requirements, including authorship of scholarly written work and submission of a short essay along with an acceptable grade point average. Following completion of one full academic term, students may apply for admission. Among other benefits, membership assures graduation with honors, provides an additional credential indicating an interest in research, and demonstrates a commitment to excellence (AOTF, 2012c), which can never hurt when seeking a position.

Note: If interested in attaining more information about board and specialty certification, refer to AOTA certification on the AOTA.org website. Additionally, there are other non-AOTA certifications that therapists can pursue in their specialty areas.

CONTINUING COMPETENCE AND ITS IMPACT ON LEGAL PRACTICE REQUIREMENTS, PROFESSIONAL CREDENTIALING, AND CERTIFICATION

By graduating from an educational program that is accredited by the Accreditation Council for Occupational Therapy Education and passing the NBCOT initial certification examination, basic competency is established for the occupational therapist and certified occupational therapy assistant. However, this is just the beginning as different regulatory bodies will require the practicing therapist to continuously demonstrate his or her competency to practice. These requirements will vary from agency to agency and state to state.

State regulatory boards are public bodies created by state legislatures to protect the public from harm caused by incompetent or unqualified health care practitioners. These boards determine whether therapists have the proper credentials to practice. These state licenses or certifications are renewed on a regular basis. In a majority of states, the renewal process requires evidence of CEUs or PDUs (depending on the terminology used in a particular state), as a prerequisite for license renewal. These CEUs can present themselves in various forms such as publication of a professional article, professional presentation, self study, mentoring, and attendance at a professional conference (AOTF, 2012b).

In addition to state licensure requirements, the NBCOT, a private credentialing body, has a mission to protect the public (NBCOT, n.d.). Its primary responsibility is to develop, update, and administer the initial certification examination that is used by state regulatory boards to determine whether to allow the practitioner to practice as an occupational therapist or certified occupational therapy assistant in his or her state. Passage of the NBCOT examination is what allows occupational therapists to use the initials OTR and for the certified occupational therapy assistant to use the initials COTA. Once the examination is passed and a therapist is allowed to practice in his or her state, he or she is not required to maintain NBCOT certification, but therapists who do not maintain their certification with NBCOT cannot use the insignias OTR and COTA. To renew certification, practitioners must obtain 36 PDUs during a 3-year renewal cycle (NBCOT, n.d.).

SUMMARY

Graduation is only the beginning of the learning process for the occupational therapist and certified occupational therapy assistant. To experience a satisfying and successful career, the new graduate must make a commitment to continuing his or her education to ensure competency in the delivery of care.

This chapter provides a model for achieving continuing competency throughout one's career. As professionals with an obligation to the populations we serve, we must improve and evolve our skills as our careers progress and we face new challenges. We are responsible for developing a plan for our continued competency. The process begins with an understanding of the basic concepts of competency and applying them to our profession and practices. The first step is to determine our own competency using a variety of assessment techniques. Based on this assessment, we can identify our own strengths and weaknesses and begin to develop a lifelong plan of continued growth in clinical, managerial, and interpersonal skills. This continuing competency plan will be a cornerstone of our professional life, which will guide us in our educational endeavors.

Our roadmap can be created using the AOTA's Standards for Continuing Competency, Continuing Competency Plan, and PDT. The plan should be dynamic, changing and evolving as careers change. By committing to this process, we assure that our skills are up to the standards of our profession, fostering pride in our abilities to provide the best possible levels of care to the populations with whom we are working.

DISCUSSION QUESTIONS/ACTIVITIES

1. List your career goals for the next year and for the next 5 years. Then, create a plan for achieving them.
2. Outline the competencies you would need to achieve the above goals.
3. Download the AOTA PDT (http://www/aota.org/pdt/index.asp). Familiarize yourself with the tool and fill it out.
4. Form into groups. Imagine you are a supervisor. What kind of competencies would you expect from a first-year clinician in the following settings?
   - Preschool
   - Acute care hospital rehabilitation department

- ♦ Early intervention center and home-based agency
- ♦ Home health care agency

5. Identify a fictional character who you think would be the perfect mentor.
   a. What traits does this person have that would contribute to your psychosocial development?
   b. What traits would contribute to your career development?
   c. What personality traits make this person a good mentor for you?

   Share your answers in a classroom discussion.

6. Break into groups of two for the following role-play experience:

   Scenario: Lenore has been assigned a new fieldwork student, Diane. Lenore is new to supervision but is eager to hone her mentoring skills. In Diane's second week of fieldwork, Lenore is approached by the head nurse on the medical/surgical unit, who complains to her that her student was speaking disrespectfully to patients and staff and was then seen sitting on the edge of a patient's wheelchair armrest while waiting for the elevator.

   With your partner, choose who will play Diane and who will play Lenore. Then, engage in a 5-minute dialogue in which Lenore mentors Diane by providing productive feedback based on the information received from the head nurse.

   As a class observing this interchange, note what you thought was positive about the exchange. How would you feel if you were getting that feedback? What did you specifically observe about the approach, including the words chosen and the tone and body language of both participants in the exchange?

REFERENCES

American Occupational Therapy Association (AOTA). (2003a). AOTA professional development tool. Retrieved from http://wwwa.AOTA.org/pdt/index.asp.

American Occupational Therapy Association (AOTA). (2003b). AOTA professional development plan. Retrieved from http://www.AOTA.org/pdt/p3_3.htm.

American Occupational Therapy Association (AOTA). (2003c). Model continuing competence guidelines for occupational therapists and occupational therapy assistants: A resource for state regulatory boards. Retrieved from http://www.AOTA.org/-/media/Corporate/Files/Advocacy/State/Resources/ContComp/modceguidelines.pdf.

American Occupational Therapy Association (AOTA). (2010a). AOTA standards for continuing competence. Retrieved from http://www.AOTA.org/-/media/Corporate/Files/Secure/Practice/officialDocs/Standards/Standards%20for%20Continuing%20Competence%202010%20Revision.pdf.

American Occupational Therapy Association (AOTA). (2010b). Standards for continuing competence. *American Journal of Occupational Therapy, 59,* 661-662.

American Occupational Therapy Association (AOTA). (2013). Board and specialty certification. Retrieved from http://www.aota.org/Practitioners/profdev/certification.aspx.

American Occupational Therapy Foundation (AOTF). (2012a). Vision, mission goals & strategic plan. Retrieved from http://www.aota.org/aboutaota/visionmissiongoals.asps.

American Occupational Therapy Foundation (AOTF). (2012b). State continuing competency requirements. Retrieved from http://www.aota.org/-/media/Corporate/Files/Practice/OTAs/ContComp/CC%20Requirements%20Full$20Final%202012.pdf.

American Occupational Therapy Foundation (AOTF). (2012c). Pi Theta Epsilon, member orientation handbook.

Braverman, B., & Gentile, P. (2003). A guide for managers and supervisors to develop a system for assessment of competencies, administration and management special interest section. American Occupational Therapy Association.

Decker, P.J., & Strader, M.K. (1997). Beyond JCAHO: Using competency models to improve healthcare organizations. Part I. *Hospital Topics, 75*(1), 23-8.

Hinojosa, J. (2004). Developing personal professional competencies. *OT Practice Online.* Retrieved from http://www. ot.phhp.ufl.edu/files/2011/12/hinojosa.pdf.

Hinojosa, J., Bowen, R., Case-Smith, J., Epstein, C.F., Moyers, P., & Schwope, C. (2000). Self initiated continuing competence. *OT Practice, 5,* CE 1-8.

Jackson, D. (2010). Make sure you attend professional conferences and conventions. Retrieved from http://www.GradSchool.com/article-detail/conventions-conferences-1563.

Jacobs, K., & McCormack, G. (2011). *The occupational therapy manager,* 5th ed. Bethesda, MD: AOTA Press.

Kak, N.,Burkhalter, B., & Cooper, M.A. (2001). Measuring the competence of healthcare providers *USAid Quality assurance project, 2*(1) pp. 1-28.

Kram, K. (1985). *Mentoring at work.* Glenview, IL: Scott Foresman.

Kram, K. (2004). The making of a mentor. In D. Clutterbuck & G. Lane (Eds.), *The situational mentor: An international review of competencies and capabilities in mentoring* (pp. xi-xiv). Burlington, VT: Gower.

Lampton, B. (2011). Professional conferences—a few things to keep in mind when planning to attend. Retrieved from http://www.businessknowhow.com/growth/conf10.htm.

Moyers, P. (2004). *Self assessment and discoverability: Part II.* Bethesda, MD: American Occupational Therapy Association. Retrieved from http://www.aota.org/Pubs/OTP1997-2007/columns/contcomp/2004/.

National Board for Certification in Occupational Therapy (NBCOT). Mission statement. Retrieved from http://www.nbcot.org/public. 22, October 2014.

Shrubbe, K. (2004). Mentorship: A critical component of professional growth and academic success. *Journal of Dental Education, 68,* 324-328.

Singleton, T. (2011). How to get the most out of your first professional conference experience. Retrieved from http://www.accountingweb.com/blogs/accountingweb/ima-young-accounting-pros/how-to-get-the-most-out-of-your-first-professional-conference-ex.

Urish, C. (2004). Ongoing competence through mentoring. *OT Practice Online.* Retrieved from http://www.aota.org/practitioners/resources/OTAs/OTA-Leadership.

Chapter 16

Moving Up, Moving On
Making the Right Career Choices

LEARNING OBJECTIVES

At the end of this chapter, the reader will be able to:
- Identify ways to stand out in the workplace.
- Describe how to ask for a raise or promotion.
- Identify how to deal with staff and former peers after receiving a promotion.
- Predict how to deal with not getting a sought-after promotion.
- Estimate how to size up a new team he or she is supervising.
- Identify six reasons that indicate it is time to leave a job.
- Identify the best methods of looking for a new job while still working.
- Describe the proper steps to take when leaving a job.

Although the general theme of this book relates to your first job as an occupational therapist—getting it, keeping it, and thriving in it—there inevitably comes the point where you start thinking about what is next. Are you still growing in your current job? Are there other populations you would like to work with that you are not currently exposed to? Is there a higher position in the organization that you are seeking? The variations on the theme are endless, but as professionals, we are always seeking growth and change. In this chapter, we will dissect the process of moving up and moving on and identify your strategy to help you transition successfully to your next job.

DETERMINING WHEN IT IS TIME TO MOVE ON OR UP

As entry-level occupational therapists, your first paid position represents the culmination of your dreams and hard work. You have achieved your educational goals, completed your professional training, and are actually getting paid to do what you love. This transition from student to clinician is a period of intense learning, training, and growth. Getting paid as an occupational

Davis L, Rosee M. *Occupational Therapy Student to Clinician: Making the Transition (pp 219-234).* © 2015 SLACK Incorporated.

therapist creates a much different level of expectation than performing at a student level. This first professional work experience is where you will learn to live up to greater expectations and work on your interpersonal skills, team building skills, and clinical skills.

Although it may not seem possible now, the day will come when you are so comfortable at your job that you determine to seek new challenges and experiences. This is the moment when you realize it might be time to move up or move out.

Keep in mind that it is typically expected that a new therapist remain in his or her first job for at least 1 year before seeking a change in position. If you start making position changes too early (and too often) in your career, you may get branded as uncommitted, unreliable, and scattered. Too many moves reflected on your resumé will serve as a warning to potential employers that you do not stick things out and that you might be a bad bet as a new hire.

GETTING PROMOTED

If you love where you work but are getting stale in your position, the logical direction for continued growth is to seek a promotion. Many larger facilities offer opportunities to move up into senior-level management or even corporate positions within the organization.

Typically, a promotion does not just happen automatically; it has to be earned. We discussed in an earlier chapter the importance of marketing yourself as a student. These same marketing techniques should continue as you progress to a working therapist. To move up in an organization, you need to "show your stuff" in a way that is productive and professional. You should let people hear and see the constructive contributions you are making. Some steps to make yourself stand out in the workplace include the following:

- *Delivering a consistently great performance and expanding beyond your job expectations (without being asked)*: This includes professional behaviors such as punctuality, dependability, efficient use of time, and team skills (to name a few).

- *Take initiative/create new opportunities at work*: It goes without saying that you should perform whatever work tasks are expected of you in an efficient and professional manner. However, when you take on extra work, which can enhance the department or the reputation of the facility, you get noticed by your supervisors and higher ups.

  ◊ **Example:** Marcy is working in an acute care hospital while pursuing a more advanced occupational therapy degree. As part of her academic program, she designs a research study that she would like to carry out in the facility. Marcy presents the project to her superiors, who approve its implementation. The study is later published in a professional journal, shedding a positive light on the facility. Marcy gets noticed for her extra efforts, and the facility benefits from her work.

  ◊ **Example:** Etta, a certified occupational therapy assistant, is dissatisfied with the documentation tool being used at her long-term care facility. It does not easily capture all of the technical information needed for reimbursement. Without being asked, she decides to take on the project of redesigning the form. When she presents the new form to the staff, it is so well received that it gets adopted in other departments as well. She not only makes herself look good, she makes her manager and her department look good as well.

  ◊ **Example:** Ella is a recent occupational therapy graduate working at a residential facility for adults who are intellectually disabled. She and the recreation therapist receive permission to start a program that takes selected clients out to community restaurants for lunch on a weekly basis. The goal is to build and improve upon activities of daily living skills, including communication, money handling, and community living. During client care meetings, Ella and the recreation therapist were able to describe the progress and challenges of each client in the new context. The team was impressed with the results. The program was expanded to a larger number of clients and became an integral part of the facility. Ella wrote up her experiences, which were published in a local newspaper. She was able to add her achievement to her resumé and received wide recognition.

- *Volunteering for a committee*: Often, a problem or issue is identified at a facility and a committee is formed to develop solutions. Sometimes the committee is specific to the department or may be interdisciplinary. For example, a department determines that its documentation tools are now obsolete. They decide to form a documentation committee to review the forms and redesign them. In another example, a facility is planning the renovation of a floor that contains the recreation department and the rehabilitation department. The administration has asked them to come together to make recommendations about the use of the space. Volunteers from each discipline participate.
  - ◊ In both cases, volunteering increases one's exposure and stature in the facility. You not only get the opportunity to network, but you also make yourself known as an active participant, a doer, and a leader. Your reputation for participation can help when a promotion possibility comes along.

- *Develop mentoring relationships*: We covered the benefits of the mentoring relationship in length in the previous chapter. One of the major benefits of a mentor is that he or she often spreads the word about you to higher ups. The more respected someone is, the more credibility the person can lend to your reputation. In the case of a promotion opportunity, if a well-regarded mentor recommends someone from in-house, management may readily accept the recommendation and not look to the outside for talent.

- *Communicate the great work you are doing in a professional manner*: Some believe it is good to be self-effacing. Although this may be true in certain circumstances, in a work setting, it is always a good idea to let people (especially higher ups) know about the contributions you are making. For example, Lindsay, an occupational therapy consultant in a nursing home, takes the initiative to improve the facility's revenue by creating reimbursable programs that did not exist before. Rather than just quietly carrying out the task, she summarizes all she has created and includes the information on her monthly statistics, which are submitted to the administrator each month. The report serves as a marketing tool for her to demonstrate to the administrator, who might not otherwise notice, that she was going above and beyond in her job responsibilities. When he decides to hire a rehabilitation manager to oversee the department, she was the first one he contacted to interview for the position.

- *Make friends with the boss*: Your boss can be a great ally and can help you guide the way in the organization to understand the politics, the people you need to know, and the path toward promotion.

- *Make friends with the support staff*: The security guard, the occupational therapy aide, the nurse's aides, and unit clerks can all be instrumental in helping you succeed on the job. Value and nurture your relationships with them (Hansen, 2013).

ASKING FOR A RAISE OR PROMOTION

Asking for a raise or a promotion is difficult for most people. The problem is that if you do not communicate your desires, you may be passed over. Remember that managers are usually not thinking about you and your needs—they have larger issues to consider. The assumption on their part may be that if you do not ask for something, you are satisfied with the status quo. If you believe that you have made contributions to your facility and are important to your employer, you might consider making a formal presentation requesting a rate increase or, if an opening occurs, requesting the opportunity to be promoted. Some suggestions for successfully attaining a raise or promotion include the following:

- Revisit your job description and identify the tasks you have mastered and added onto your responsibilities so that you can clearly articulate your growth and progress.

- Before making any requests, make sure you have an understanding of the current market and salary trends in your area. Speak to as many people as you can and check with your local association and with the AOTA regarding salary survey information. By being armed with salary information, you can demonstrate with data that your salary is below market. If your employer wants to be sure to keep you, current data may help to sway him or her to see your points.

- Choose the best time to speak to your employer. Having an offer in hand, which has not yet been accepted, is a good time to speak to the appropriate person about an increase or a promotion. Everyone wants what they cannot have, and the fact that you have an offer may increase your current employer's motivation to give you what you want. This will give you the added confidence to ask for the salary you want. (Note: Sometimes going to your employer with an offer will backfire as the employer may be upset to find out that you are looking. Be prepared that this could happen, in which case you may be escorted to the door and forced to take the offer at the alternate site. Do not bluff—only come in with an offer if it is real and you are truly interested in it.)

- Maintain a positive attitude during the discussion. Do not give any negative or desperate vibes. The fact that you are having a hard time paying your rent should not factor into your logic. Go in knowing that you deserve the raise (or promotion), not that you need it. Having control over your emotions is a sign of maturity, which further supports your request for more responsibility and higher pay (Reed, 2010).

Another option is to request a promotion or a raise using e-mail. Although it is not the most direct way, it does create a paper trail and documentation of your request and may also be more effective when dealing with a very busy manager who may not have time to sit and talk. Additionally, the e-mail can be easily forwarded to other parties who may be involved in the decision-making process. In the e-mail, outline all of the reasons why you think you deserve the promotion. Specify how you have contributed to the department and provide information on any unique skills you have and any additional education that can contribute to your role in the new position. Write with confidence and have an outside party proofread and edit your e-mail to ensure its clarity and to avoid errors or confusing language. Send the e-mail on a less busy day. Follow-up within 72 hours to discuss the content of the e-mail with your supervisor (Stoval, 2013).

It has been well documented that women often have more difficulty than men do in asking for what they want in a work situation. Women who make demands are often characterized as being aggressive or selfish. To avoid that perception, when women ask, they may present themselves in ineffective ways, such as using speech that is tentative and indirect. Rather than commanding confidence, women sometimes retreat to indirect phrases such as "I'm not an expert, but…" or "I know this is a bad time to ask for a raise, but…" or "I'm not sure this is a good idea, but…." Many women adopt an upward vocal inflection at the end of sentences, turning a declarative statement into a question, which conveys weakness, uncertainty, and a need for approval. The article states it is helpful if women remain bold and straightforward when stating what they need (Klaus, 2011, p. 7).

You Got the Promotion, Now What?

You have worked hard, done all the right things, and are now being rewarded with a promotion. You should be proud. A promotion is a validation of what you have accomplished in your current job, your strong interpersonal and clinical skills, and how much potential your managers believe you have to contribute going forward. Often, the person rewarded with the promotion may not be the best performer in the department. A lot of variables besides who is the best are considered when moving someone into a more responsible, managerial position. People skills may trump clinical skills if the position relates to supervising staff. Or, your initiative, independent studies, or research projects may have weighted the decision. While you are reveling in your great fortune, others at work may be joining forces to discuss the inequity of your getting the promotion over them. Some of your coworkers may be disgruntled but willing to accept the inevitable. Be aware that there may be others who are motivated to undermine your ability to perform in your new position. They may feel that they deserved the promotion or question whether you deserved it. Whatever the reaction, you need to be ready to address possible negative attitudes and behaviors as you prepare to lead. As you embrace your new responsibilities, be prepared to prove yourself in your new position.

- *Give up the idea of still being one of the gang*: You are now the boss. Some of the group may be happy for you, some may be resentful, and some may not care. Regardless, your job now is to assume a leadership position to do the job you were promoted to do. Keep in mind that your peers may not accept you as their boss until you accept yourself as their boss (Halter, 2011).

- *Do not go in like gangbusters*: Although new managers often want to prove themselves and make immediate changes that they believe will lead to improvements in the department, it is important to hold back. You need to set the stage for changes and get the staff on your side, otherwise they will likely sabotage your efforts. Change can and will come, but implementing the change needs to be done delicately and with finesse. For example, Raul was promoted from occupational therapy supervisor to department director after 3 years on the job. He was very excited about his promotion and immediately wanted to make changes he thought were necessary to improve certain functions. One problem he identified was the way adaptive equipment was handled by nursing. On his second day in the new position, he compiled the list of all adaptive equipment out on the floors and made index cards with colored markers providing detailed instructions on their use. Raul laminated the cards and, on his third day, he proceeded to post them over the patient's beds. On day four, he came to work to find a pile of his laminated cards with a note from the director of nursing saying "see me." He was very upset and went to see her to find out why she took down his cards. The director of nursing proceeded to challenge his contention that the signs were necessary. She said her staff knows who has devices and how and when to put them on and take them off. She felt the signs were not only unnecessary, but also insulting to her department. She was angry that he initiated this change without consulting with her. Although Raul tried to explain his side of the story, he saw there was no convincing her. From then on, she became a formidable adversary. He realized later that he should have worked on developing his relationships with the other department directors and communicate his ideas before taking unilateral action. The damage could not be undone, and he experienced difficulty with the nursing department from that day forward, but he did learn a valuable lesson.

- *Make sure you understand your new duties*: Sit down with your supervisor to get clarity about what you are supposed to do. Some duties you may be familiar with, such as assigning a caseload, clinical supervision, and reimbursement oversight. However, there may be some managerial tasks you have never been responsible for before, such as budgeting, preparing payroll, and approving vacation time. Try to secure a job description outlining all of your responsibilities. Then, meet with your direct supervisor to establish what his or her policies and procedures are regarding these responsibilities. For instance, if you need to hire new therapists, what is the procedure? Are you responsible for recruiting new staff or does the human resource department handle this? Are you aware of all of the benefits when interviewing candidates? Are you knowledgeable about employment law? As discussed in previous chapters, certain actions on your part regarding employment and hiring can create legal liabilities for your facility. Become familiar with the law and what your constraints are.

- *Make sure the announcement of your promotion is handled well by administration*: Although this may be out of your control, when a promotion is about to be announced, the way the announcement is handled can impact staff reactions. If there are multiple internal candidates for the job, out of respect, the other candidates should be informed before the rest of the staff. The announcement should go out simultaneously to all involved parties in the form of an e-mail or other appropriate forms of communication. By controlling the message delivery process, the facility may avoid the gossip and rumor mills, which can often impact morale.

♦ *Immediately establish a dialogue with your team*: A great leader knows how to communicate and is open and honest about staff expectations. Find out about staff frustrations (you may know firsthand as a member of the department), what they think can be changed, and how it can be changed. Often, people look to supervisors for all of the answers when they have the answer themselves. A great technique is asking someone what he or she would do to handle a particular problem. It takes the pressure off of you for coming up with all of the answers and empowers the staff to become part of the solution.

♦ *Size up your team*: As you assume your new position, you will start to get a sense of the team, people's roles, and relationships and who your supporters are vs who will be resistant to your leadership. Former friends may be difficult to manage, especially if they see your new responsibilities as getting in the way of your time with them. Often, the people you anticipate having the most difficulty with can become your greatest supporters. Staff can be divided up into supporters, apathetic, and dissenters (Halter, 2011). *Supporters* are on your side. They believe in your mission and goals and are willing to help you achieve those goals. The *dissenters* are the naysayers who want to avoid change and hope that you fail so that things can stay the same. They will challenge your authority as a manager and sabotage your efforts. The *apathetic* are considered harmless, but actually, in their apathy, they do nothing to help you succeed and are waiting to see who the "winners" are before signing on. They need to be pressured in order to elicit their cooperation.

♦ *Communication goals*: During the initial phase in the position, you will communicate to your staff what needs to be accomplished. Do not ask what should be accomplished—that is up to you to establish—but do ask them for input on how they envision accomplishing goals you have outlined.

♦ *Establish expectations*: Be clear about what you expect from each of your staff members to reach the team's goals. Be passionate about your mission. As the staff begins to appreciate your commitment to the process and sees that you are fair and open to their issues and concerns, they will start respecting you and cooperating with you to meet goals.

♦ *Be aware that managers are watching you*: During your first 6 months, your managers and supervisors will be monitoring your performance. Make sure you look professional when you go to work (wear clothes at least one step up from your staff), take management courses, seek out advice from your managers, study facility policies and procedures, seek a mentor in your facility (or outside) to show you the ropes, and do everything in your power to prove that you deserved the promotion (Rozny, 2011).

DEALING WITH NOT GETTING A PROMOTION

As professionals, most of us are looking for challenges in our work. One of the most obvious ways to seek additional challenges is to earn a promotion at your current place of work. When a sought-after promotion does not materialize and another colleague is chosen or someone is hired from outside instead, it makes sense to self-assess to determine why you did not get the promotion. Reasons for not getting a promotion fall into three different types of situations: those that relate directly to you, those that are dependent on other issues or people, and those that should not be issues at all (cvtips.com, 2013).

Issues That Relate to You

- ◆ Performance
- ◆ Quality of work
- ◆ Experience
- ◆ Expertise

These are the variables that you can control. The quality of your work is an important indicator of your workplace behaviors. Are you professional and effective in your treatment interventions? Do you maintain your work area in a neat, professional manner and provide quality documentation? The way you work is an indicator of how you will perform when greater responsibilities are placed upon you.

Issues That Relate to Other Influences

- ◆ Workplace relationships
- ◆ Competition from other qualified staff
- ◆ Employer policies
- ◆ Equal opportunity requirements

As important as your work skills are, your workplace relationships are as important as an indicator of your suitability for a promotion. This includes relationships with supervisors, colleagues, peers, and subordinates. If you have a history of not getting along with people, it will hamper your promotion potential. Maintaining positive relationships with your coworkers creates an impression of you as someone who has strong social and emotional intelligence skills, which are indicators of your suitability to move into a managerial position.

Even with strong interpersonal skills, you may run into the challenge of competition for the position from equally qualified colleagues. For example, Beatricia has been working in a large acute care hospital for 3 years. She has performed well and is well liked by peers and managers. Based on her strong performance, she is hoping to be promoted to senior occupational therapist. Her friend and colleague, Selma, is also vying for the same promotion. When the opening occurs, Selma gets the promotion because she had been working at the facility for a longer time. They were both equally qualified, so the longevity factor weighed in Selma's favor. In another example of a situation that may be outside your control, Mary, a senior therapist, gave her notice and Irwin, knowing he was next in line, was hoping for the promotion. Due to cutbacks, the administration decided not to hire a replacement for the departing therapist and eliminated the senior position (which paid more than the staff position) to save costs. Irwin remained in the staff position.

Another variable is the need to comply with equal opportunity regulations. Diversity is a very big goal for larger organizations. There are times when a facility will prefer to promote an equally talented coworker who helps improve the facility's diversity statistics.

Issues That Should Not Affect Promotion

- ◆ Personal relationships
- ◆ Nepotism
- ◆ Poor employment policies
- ◆ Ignoring equal opportunity requirements

If any of these is a reason for not getting a promotion, you might want to reconsider your place of employment. Promotions should be based on merit, and if it is clear that a facility is promoting based on factors other than merit, it may be time to move on. Example: Dr. Alan Leven, the director of a large special education school, hired his daughter, Ava, a psychologist with little experience, to serve as the school's assistant director. In this role, she was in charge of all of the occupational therapists. During Ava's tenure in the position, she seemed overwhelmed and did not attend to the needs of the children or the staff. She neglected basic duties, such as ensuring Individualized Education Programs were on site for all students, scheduling required meetings, and ordering equipment. The entire staff knew that she was incompetent and her lack of skill was negatively impacting the school's operations. When one brave professional reported the problems to Dr. Leven, he responded angrily and denied there was a problem. This created great frustration for the staff and impacted outcomes for the children. Eventually, the problem was uncovered by the board of directors of the school, and both the father and daughter were terminated.

Dealing With Your Feelings After Being Passed Over

When you have been overlooked for a promotion, it is very difficult to carry on in your position without feeling disappointed and rejected. These feelings are intensified when you have to work on a daily basis with the person who was promoted, especially if he or she is a friend. Some tips for dealing with these feelings of rejection include the following:

- Remain professional and support the successful candidate. This demonstrates your maturity and willingness to be a team player. Lack of cooperation can damage your reputation and could negatively impact your options should another promotion opportunity appear.
- Stay calm and collect your thoughts before reacting to the news. Hold back the negativity or you may be sorry later.
- Ask your supervisor for some feedback as to why you were passed over for the promotion and what you can do going forward to improve your chances.
- Based on feedback and self-assessment, develop a plan to improve any identified areas of weakness so you will be primed when the next opportunity comes along. This might include taking courses, volunteering in areas where you would like to learn more, or mentoring.
- Think about looking elsewhere. Sometimes you realize that there may not be enough upward mobility in a position or it is not the place you want to be in the long run. This is a good time to reevaluate your career and determine where you want to be in 1, 5, and 10 years (Benjamin, 2013).

IS IT TIME FOR YOU TO LEAVE?

Everyone has a bad day at work when they feel like quitting. However, it is often just a passing phase based on frustration. Is it just a bad day, or is it time to move on? How do you know the difference between real dissatisfaction with a job vs a bad day? How do you know that it is time to leave and how do you execute your plan?

There are always pros and cons for both leaving and staying. Employers like longevity and become suspicious of someone who moves around a lot. If you have been in one place for 2 years, you need not worry about moving on. You have demonstrated that you were able to succeed in your workplace as you maintained your job over a long period. However, if you have a history of leaving a job after 1 year or less, you should probably put a lot of thought into a move until you have more time under your belt, proving that you can stick with a position.

Staying too long can be just as bad as leaving too soon. Often, you can get very comfortable in the same routine and find that you are no longer growing professionally. You may be sleepwalking through the job—doing an adequate job, but with little enthusiasm and motivation. Signals of being stuck include talking about quitting but never doing anything about it; lack of interest in any other job possibilities at your facility (nowhere to go); or consistent underperforming, either because of lack of interest in what you are doing or because you lack the resources and support to improve your performance. If you find yourself in this position, it is useful to reflect on your professional goals. Ask yourself whether what you are currently doing is meaningful and challenging? What else would you like to do? Does the current environment offer this? It may be that there are opportunities for growth that you are not recognizing or you might be in a stagnant environment. At that point, you should consider your options. It is time to leave your job if the following applies:

- You are no longer valued. Do you get recognition for a job well done? Have you been passed over for a promotion or been denied a merit raise? Do you understand why? Both instances indicate that something is wrong. It may be a function of your performance, indicative of a conflict with a superior, or reflective of the culture of the facility. You need to assess whether it is you or them, and then figure out what to do to repair the situation.
- The job is making you sick. Stress can bring on many physical symptoms, such as headaches, anxiety, depression, and frequent colds. If your health is suffering from the pressures or tensions of a job, it may be time to move on.
- You are no longer challenged.
- Your ethics are being challenged. With increased financial pressures on facilities, you may be asked to perform at a level that is not conducive to quality interventions. You may be asked to do things that are morally suspect. You need to assess the situation to determine if there is an ethical challenge, and then decide how best to handle the situation. Sometimes you have no choice but to move on.
- You have built a bad reputation that cannot be mended.
- Your life situation has changed and the position no longer works for your lifestyle.
- You keep threatening to look for a job but you never follow through. There is a reason why you are thinking about leaving. You need to analyze why you are not following through.
- There is no place for you to move up or the upward options do not interest you.
- You feel mistreated. You should not tolerate an environment where you feel you are not respected or are mistreated or belittled by your superiors.
- The facility is having financial or managerial difficulties. A facility that is constantly reorganizing, downsizing, or changing leaders may be experiencing internal difficulties. If you believe that the facility is on the brink of closing (sometimes it is obvious, sometimes it comes as a complete surprise), it is a good idea to look elsewhere before you find yourself out of work.
- You dread going to work every day. No one should be miserable at work. It creates stress and impairs job performance.
- A better opportunity has come along (Sixwise.com, 2006).

Burnout is a term coined in the 1970s to describe a "psychological syndrome of emotional exhaustion, depersonalization, and reduced accomplishment. It is especially common in health care because our jobs focus on sickness and suffering. Burnout can lead to reduced performance, high turnover, and poor patient care" (Waite, 2012, p. 12).

Classic signs of burnout include feeling depersonalized, emotional exhaustion, feeling as though you are not accomplishing anything at work, and a loss of motivation (Waite, 2012). Burnout can happen in even the best work environments, especially in today's health care environment where productivity pressures have become commonplace. Feeling as though you do not have the time to do what you think your patients need due to time constraints can lead to stress and burnout. To avoid burnout, it is important to have balance in your life. Take some time off if you have not had a vacation in a while. Everyone needs time away from their work. Make sure that you develop after-work activities that you enjoy, be it exercise, painting, or group sports. Burnout is a leading cause of staff turnover. A good employer will recognize that burnout is common in health care and will be alert for signs of it so that the right support can be provided to help the practitioner get through it.

If the burnout is chronic and unyielding, it may be time to think about moving on.

Before making the decision to leave your current job, make sure that you have looked at the risks of leaving. By quitting, you may damage existing relationships, lose income, or blemish your resumé. Only you know the specifics of your situation and you must carefully weigh the factors. In a *Harvard Business Review* article by Amy Gallo (2013), it is estimated that people usually get 10 chances to quit a job in their lifetime, which works out to an average of every 4 years. If you are changing things up more than that, facilities may look at you as a serial job changer. This can hurt your reputation and make people think twice about hiring you.

LOOKING FOR A NEW JOB

Once you have determined that it is time to leave your job, you must carefully think through your job search strategy. The strategy will be somewhat different from the one used when you were a new graduate because you now have a position to protect. You will probably want to keep your job search confidential as you will not want your current employer to know you are looking. The following recommendations should help you in your search for a new job:

- Do not let your boss know that you are looking. That silence should carry forward to everyone else in the organization. Once one person knows, he or she will talk about it with others and it may get back to the wrong person. Do not share the information that you are looking with anyone. (Note: Some facilities might fire you on the spot if it is known you are looking. This is not common, but it happens.)

- Do not use your work computer in your job search. Do not search for jobs, send your resumé, or store your resumé on your computer at work. Someone is bound to see your screen, and everything on your work computer is available to your employer.

- Do not give your work phone number or e-mail to potential employers. Try to perform all search-related calls during your breaks or lunch hour out of ear shot of others.

- Stay quiet about job interviews. Obviously, when people know you have interviews, they also know you are looking to leave. However, another variable to consider is that you do not want others to know about your possible job opportunity as they may seek to get in on it. **Example**: Lena, an occupational therapist, was looking for a per diem position. She accidentally overheard another occupational therapist at her job talking about a position she applied for at an outpatient facility through a placement agency. Lena decided to call the facility directly and got hired before her coworker ever made it for the interview.

- Make interview appointments before or after work, or use a vacation day. In a health care setting, it is pretty obvious that something is up when you leave in the middle of the day. In addition, you are usually dressed a little better than normal when you are going for an interview. (Tip: Change back into your normal clothes to avoid suspicion.) Avoid speculation and try to schedule the meeting when no one will notice.

- Identify references other than your current employer to provide to a possible new employer. Typically, a prospective employer will want to call references from your current employer. Of course, once that happens, the current employer will know you are looking elsewhere. Make sure you have references outside of your current position to avoid a sticky situation.

- Be aware that, frequently, someone at the interview site will be acquainted with someone at your current job. When this happens, the person at the new site will probably call his or her acquaintance at your current job to get the "low down" on you. Such unofficial references are very common and can hold a lot of weight since they are more candid. That is why you must be on good terms with everyone and never burn bridges. You never know who on the job might be informally asked about you as a coworker (Abott, 2011; Benjamin, 2013).

Finding Job Leads When You Are Working

Many of the techniques used in Chapters 2 and 3 can be utilized when looking for a new job as well. Placement agencies can be a good source of leads, along with online and print ads. One of the best sources of job leads is through professional networking. The best jobs often never make it past the word-of-mouth stage. If you are not networking, you may miss out on one of these opportunities. The best advice is to stay actively engaged in professional activities, such as attending courses, volunteering in local associations, keeping in touch with former colleagues and classmates, and joining supervision groups and any other activities where you come in contact with other professionals both in and out of your discipline.

Answering the Question, "Why Are You Leaving Your Job?"

This question will be inevitably asked when interviewing for a new position. Only you know the real reason you are leaving, but some reasons are better than others when trying to impress a potential employer. Here are some productive answers to the question:

- I was no longer feeling challenged in my work. It is really important to me to be happy at work and I did not want to let my discontent get in the way of how I was performing.
- There was not enough room for growth in my current facility. I'm looking for new challenges.
- I did not have access to the population I want to work with at my current job. I want to expand my repertoire.
- I would like to work in a larger department where I could learn from my colleagues.
- I was laid off from my position due to budget cuts.
- After several years in the same environment, I wanted a more team-oriented approach.
- I'm ready to take on more responsibility (e.g., supervision, administration, management, student education).
- I do not feel that my skills are being fully utilized in my current job (and be ready to explain why).
- My family situation has changed and I am looking for a position with more (or less) of a time commitment and responsibility.
- I left my former position to spend more time with my family. Circumstances have changed and I am ready to commit to a full-time position (Doyle, 2013).

HOW TO LEAVE YOUR JOB

As we discussed previously, there are many reasons why people voluntarily leave their jobs. They may not like the workload, the population, the commute, their colleagues, or the pay, or they may just be looking for another experience. The important thing to remember is that you want to leave on the best possible terms. As said before, the field of occupational therapy is very small. The networking process is very active and underground information about colleagues is often passed around. The people you have worked with before are likely to pass your sphere again. A former colleague might even be the one making a hiring decision on your behalf in the future. You will definitely want to secure a positive letter of reference from your current employer after you leave. Be sure to leave in a classy and professional manner.

Do Not Leave a Job in an Improper Fashion

- Do not leave impulsively when angry. Often, we work under less-than-favorable circumstances, and we fantasize about quitting in a big way. When you find yourself thinking about quitting suddenly and telling your supervisor what you think of him or her and the facility, stop and calm down. Think about the consequences and try to identify a more productive way of getting out of a bad situation.
- Do not tell people off. You may want to tell certain colleagues what you really think of them, but disregard this idea. You never know who may cross your path again one day.
- Do not walk out the door without proper notice; it is very unprofessional. Your colleagues and clients are counting on you, and a sudden departure does not allow your facility to make proper plans to cover your responsibilities.
- Do not leave without securing another job. It is human nature that people want to hire people who are employed—they just appear more valuable and desired. It is best to secure another job before leaving the old one. This also gives you more choice in what to accept because you are not desperate to secure work. The exception to this is if you want to take time off for yourself and do not need the income and benefits.
- Do not speak negatively to or about your coworkers or your supervisor as you are preparing to leave. You do not want to make enemies at this late stage. Hold your negative comments or share them with unrelated parties outside of the workplace.
- Do not damage or take property. This can be considered a criminal act that can jeopardize your professional career.
- Do not leave your workspace dirty or unkempt. Clean out your personal things, return all equipment and devices, and leave a clean workspace for the next hire.
- Do not leave without completing all of your progress notes and other projects that were assigned to you (Rosenberg McKay, 2013).

Proper Steps When Leaving a Job

- Give appropriate notice. When leaving your current position, it is typical to provide your supervisor with at least 2 weeks' notice (or whatever may be documented in your contract, if you have one) so that your department and coworkers can prepare for your departure. This gives them time to recruit another therapist and redistribute the workload.
- Provide an official letter of resignation. The letter should be typed and include the date you are writing it and your supervisor's name, title, department, and facility address. It should begin with a positive statement about your current position and lead into the fact that you are resigning from your position with the date of departure at least 2 weeks from the date of the letter. Be sure to express thanks to your supervisor for the working environment and the learning opportunities offered. The letter should be on your letterhead (which you can compose yourself) or personal stationary.

    How to write a termination letter:
    ◇ Type the letter and keep a copy for yourself.
    ◇ Deliver the letter in person.
    ◇ Remember to sign your name.

Sample Resignation Letter

Your Name
Your Address
Your Phone Number
Your Email
Date
Mr. Eric Kettle
Occupational Therapy Supervisor
Zigfield Hospital
380 Katekarf St.
Mattapan, MA 01876

Dear Mr. Kettle,

I am writing this letter to inform you of my resignation from my position as staff occupational therapist. My last day of employment will be Friday, March 16, 2013, which includes my required two weeks' notice.

Although I have enjoyed my time working here and have learned a lot, I have secured a new position with a different population that offers me the opportunity to grow in a new direction. I have gained valuable experiences under your supervision and appreciate all you have done to foster my growth as a professional.

Sincerely,
Your Name   (Adapted from best-job-interview.com, 2013.)

- Do not brag to colleagues about the new job. Although you are excited about your new opportunity and it is appropriate to share that excitement, be aware that your colleagues and patients may have mixed feelings about your leaving. Do not criticize your current facility to the staff or patients. They are all staying and may be not want to hear how antiquated, cramped, or poorly located the facility is.
- Remove any personal contacts and e-mails from your computer and pack up your personal belongings, leaving the space clean for the next therapist.
- Write a brief e-mail to the facility's staff and send it 1 or 2 days before you leave, letting them know how much you appreciate them and sharing the news of your new career move, for example:

Dear All,

I would like to let you know that I am leaving the facility as of Friday, May 13. Although I have loved my time here, I have accepted a new position with greater responsibility and the chance to work with patients with traumatic brain injuries.

It has been a pleasure to work here with you. The team here has been generous, caring, and supportive, helping me to grow as a clinician and a human being. I will miss my coworkers and patients but hope we will keep in touch. My new e-mail is eviloria@hotmail.com.

Thank you for the opportunity to work with all of you.

Sincerely,
Elissa Viloria
                                                       (Adapted from best-job-interview.com, 2013.)

- Be aware that the human resource director may ask for an exit interview. This is a meeting in which he or she will ask you in confidence to provide feedback about your experience working there. The director may probe you to determine if there are things your employer could have done to avoid your resignation or make things better for the future. This is where your employer may learn that the pay was too low, the workload too high, or your workspace was cramped and not conducive to improved productivity. Make sure your answers are diplomatic and offer solutions to problems you faced. This information assists the facility to improve its procedures and environment. This is not the time or place for negative attacks. Keep the interchange very professional and positive.

- Do not bad mouth your employer or any of your coworkers to your replacements at the old facility or your associates at your new position. This only makes you look bad and will make them suspicious that you will be talking about them behind their backs as well.

- Be sure to ask for a written reference. Although you may assume that you will always be able to get in touch with your former supervisor when you need him or her to provide a reference, that is not always the case. People move and things change. If your boss is willing, try to get a typewritten reference on facility letterhead before you leave. Include this letter in your portfolio for future use. Often, when a written reference is provided, potential employers will not even bother calling references. By securing a written reference, you are protected in the event that you lose touch with your reference.

INVOLUNTARY TERMINATIONS

This is the term that is used to refer to a situation where you lose your job against your will. Employers give many reasons for terminating an employee. Your termination could be labeled as a firing, layoff, downsizing, or redistribution of work. When someone hears any of these words spoken, they mean one thing—he or she is out of work. If this happens, it is important to react professionally. Remain calm and use the time to find out more information about why you are being let go.

If you are being fired for poor performance, your dismissal should not come as a shock. In most instances, employees are aware that they are heading down the firing line because they get reprimands and warnings from supervisors for unsatisfactory work or receive poor performance reviews. You can always ask to see your file and request a meeting with human resources to discuss the firing if you feel you were given no warning. Conduct of a criminal act, such as theft or abuse, is cause for immediate termination.

After delivering the news about the firing, most employers ask the employee to leave right away so other employees are not disrupted. Do not feel insulted if you are immediately asked for your keys and name badge and are given a few minutes to pack up your personal possessions. Be prepared for your computer access to be blocked. This is standard procedure. Many times, the employer will provide you with a small severance package, perhaps 2 weeks' pay or 1 additional month of health coverage. Typically your final paycheck is ready for you when you leave or will be mailed to you within the week.

If your position is being eliminated due to downsizing or budget issues, it is also best that you leave quietly and professionally. There is always a chance that you could be rehired if things change for the better. Being professional is the key here as you want your supervisor to recognize your value and consider you first for rehire.

Note: When you are terminated, you no longer have the opportunity to gather some of your professional work for inclusion in your portfolio. It is a good idea to keep your resume updated. Keep a copy of professional products you have created. For example, a documentation form you designed, a research project you created, a professional conference you created and produced, in-services you provided, program protocols you developed, etc. It is also a good idea to have sample progress notes and evaluations (with identifying information removed) in case a new employer would like to see a sample of your writing skills. Constantly fine-tune your portfolio so that it is always ready when you need it.

Benefits and Insurance Issues When Terminating a Position

Whether you leave a position voluntarily or involuntarily, it is important that you consider your health insurance needs, especially if you suffer from a chronic health condition. Often, when leaving a job and taking a new one, there is a waiting period before you are covered by health benefits, and your prior benefits will likely be terminated the day you leave. It is important to keep in mind that the federal government has established laws that allow you to self pay for your health and dental benefits after you leave your employment under Consolidated Omnibus Budget Reconciliation Act (COBRA). COBRA gives workers and their families who lose their health benefits the right to continue them for a proscribed period of time. Qualified individuals are required to pay the entire premium for coverage up to 102% of the cost to the plan.

Know your rights as an employee by asking the human resources department at your facility for information.

SUMMARY

At some point in one's career, most therapists will decide they want to move up in their organization or move on to another more challenging position. This desire is predicated by a variety of reasons, whether it be a desire to assume managerial or supervisory responsibilities, work with a different population, experience a different environment, achieve greater job growth potential, take on more responsibilities, or work in a better location with more convenient hours (and the list goes on and on).

This chapter serves as a guide to help occupational therapists identify what their next steps should be and how to implement their plans in the most professional way possible. Starting with the decision to move on or up, guidance is provided for securing a promotion at the current job, dealing with the emotional ramifications of not getting a sought-after promotion, searching for a new job while still employed, and giving notice in the most productive way possible. By following a professional path when making the change, one ensures that their reputation remains intact.

DISCUSSION QUESTIONS/ACTIVITIES

1. List five ways you can enhance work skills, exposure, and reputation so that it leads to a future promotion.
2. Choose a partner. One is the occupational therapist and the other the supervisor. Develop a strategy for asking for a raise. Role play the request. Afterward, discuss what went well and what did not. What would you have done differently?
3. Invite a local representative from the AOTA or your local or state occupational therapy organization to speak to the class about getting involved in local or national issues related to the profession.
4. Name five ways you could improve upon your networking efforts. List specific activities or people you would contact to spread the word that you are looking for a new position.
5. Invite three experienced occupational therapists or certified occupational therapy assistants to the class for a panel discussion on "moving on." Prior to the visit, the class should break

up into groups of four and identify questions to ask. For example, how did you know it was time to leave your job? Did you ever get fired? Did you ever get promoted? What was it like to manage your friends? Describe a difficult time you had at work that made you want to quit. Did you quit or did you resolve the situation? Identify your own questions.

REFERENCES

Abott, N. (2011). 3 tips: How to find a new job while still working. Retrieved from http://www.glassdoor.com/blog/3-tips-find-job-working/.

Benjamin, T. (2013). How to deal with not getting a job promotion. Retrieved from http://www.ehow.com/how_12007130_deal-not-getting-job-promotion.html.

best-job-interview.com. (2013). How to quit your job. Retrieved from http://www.best-job-interview.com/how-to-quit-your-job.html.

cvtips.com. (2013). Promotions: Dealing with not getting the promotion. Retrieved from http://www.cvtips.com/career-success/promotions-dealing-with-not-getting-the-promotion.html.

Doyle, A. (2013). Job interview question: Why are you leaving your job. Retrieved from http://jobsearch.about.com/od/interviewquestionsanswers/a/interviewleave.htm.

Gallo, A. (2013). Is it time to quit your job? *Harvard Business Review*. HBR Blog Network. Retrieved from http://blogs.hbr.org/hmu/2013/01/is-it-time-to-quit-your-job.html.

Halter, J. (2011). How to manage your ex peers after a promotion. Retrieved from http://www.streetsmart-leader.com/2011/03/06/how-to-manage-your-ex-peers-following-a-promotion.

Hansen, R. (2013). Moving up the ladder: 10 strategies for getting yourself promoted. Retrieved from http://www.quintcareers.com/getting promoted strategies.

Klaus, P. (2011, July 10). Don't fret. Just ask for what you need. *New York Times*, pp. SB-7

Reed, S. (2010). How to ask for a promotion or raise – a guide for you. Retrieved from http://ezinearticles.com/?How-to-Ask-for-a Promotion-or-Raise---A-Guide-for-You&id=4298021.

Rosenberg McKay, D. Five things not to do when you leave a job: How to move on with class. Retrieved from http://careerplanning.about.com/od/jobseparation/a/leave_mistakes.htm.

Rozny, N. (2011). Career advancement: how to deal with a promotion. Retrieved from http://www.myfoot-path.com/mypathfinder/career-advancemen-how-ro-deal-with 0a-promotion.html.

Stoval, Q. (2013). How to ask for a promotion in an email. Retrieved from http://www.eHow.com.how_6681278_ask-promotion-email.htm.

Sixwise.com. (2006). Twelve signs it is really time to leave your job. Retrieved from http://www.sixwise.com/newsletters/05/07/06/12-signs-it-is-really-time-to-leave-your-job.htm.

Waite, A. (2012). Battling workplace burnout: Practitioners discuss keys to job satisfaction and lower turnover. *OT Practice*, 28(18).

INDEX

abilities, definition of, 23
abuse, in health care, 115-116
academic course work, 210
accommodation, in conflict handling, 77
Accreditation Council for Occupational Therapy Education, 215
acronyms, defining, 102
adjustment period, in organizational socialization, 4
Advanced Practice program, 208
Age Discrimination in Employment Act, 110-111
age-related competencies, 201
agreeableness, 6-7
agreement, gender differences in, 96
American Occupational Therapy Foundation, 215
Americans with Disabilities Act of 1990, 110-111
anger, communication during, 43-44
anticipatory organizational socialization, 8, 10
AOTA (American Occupational Therapy Association)
    Advanced Practice program, 208
    "Continuing Competence Plan," 204
    local salary data of, 222
    mentoring resources of, 212
    "Model Continuing Competence Guidelines for Occupational Therapists and Occupational Therapy Assistants: A Resource for State Regulatory Boards," 209
    Occupational Therapy Code of Ethics and Ethical Standards, 120-121
    OT Practice, 207
    Professional Development Tool, 205, 209
    Specialty Certification program, 208
apologies, 44, 54, 83, 95
appearance. *See also* dress codes and dress recommendations
    in communication, 50
    professional, 24-25

application, employment, 157
arguments, gender differences in, 95
arrogance, 27
assertive approach, in conflict resolution, 80
autonomy, 120-121
avoidance, in conflict handling, 77-78

Baby Boomers (born 1945-1964), characteristics of, 96-102
background checks, 157
behavior
    at conferences, 214
    in empathy, 20
    ethical, 120-121
    gender issues in, 93-96
    generational differences in, 96-102
    of new employees, 7-8
    professional, 15-30
    uncivil, 190
beneficence, 120
benefits, 175-184, 233
billing, fraud and abuse in, 115-116
biologic variations, in different cultural groups, 91
bisexual community, 103-105
blame game, conflict from, 76
board certification, 215
body language, 41, 49
    controlling, 51
    in interview, 168
    in listening, 52
body orientation, gender differences in, 95
breathing, for self-regulation, 40
burnout, 227-228
business letters, 55-56